Praise for *Sports Nutrition for Endurance Athletes,* 2nd Edition

"Working with Monique has taken me to the winning edge in my sport. She has helped guide me to become an Olympian and World Champion in the sport of cycling. Whether you are going for the gold or have other ambitions, we are all up against highly trained and motivated athletes. To find that competitive edge, take the next step by adding the nutritional component to your daily training regime. Reading Monique's book is a great place to start."

—*Kristin Armstrong, 2006 World Time Trial Champion, Two-Time U.S. National Time Trial Champion, Former U.S. National Road Race Champion, Two-Time Pan American Games Medalist, 2005 World Time Trial Bronze Medalist*

"I have always believed that the top Ironman athletes train very similarly, and that winning or losing comes down to nutrition and mental toughness. I know I would not have won two Ironman World Championships without focusing on my nutrition every day. Monique does a fantastic job covering everything you need to know about daily and racing nutrition. *Sports Nutrition for Endurance Athletes* sets the standard for getting you fueled to the finish line."

—*Tim DeBoom, Two-Time Ironman World Champion*

"A must-read whatever your competitive goals may be. Monique's vast knowledge is evident, and this book will serve as a complete source for all your nutritional inquiries. From making optimal food and fluid choices, to meal planning and timing, to event-specific needs, this book has it all."

—*Alan Culpepper, Two-Time U.S. Olympic Runner, Three-Time U.S. Cross-Country Champion, Two-Time U.S. 10K Champion, Former U.S. 5K Champion*

"With all the 'science' behind sports nutrition, *Sports Nutrition for Endurance Athletes* offers an accurate and clear direction for today's competitive rowers. The information complements how I handled my diet as an athlete, and the direction I offer both light- and heavyweight rowers today."

—*John Riley, Two-Time U.S. Olympic Rower, Eleven-Time U.S. National Champion, Former U.S. National Team Coach*

"*Sports Nutrition for Endurance Athletes* is a comprehensive nutritional guide to help athletes maintain their energy levels and maximize their ability to perform in endurance events. The cycling chapter offers race-day specific advice for cyclists in all events—road, off-road, and cyclo-cross."

—*Dede Demet Barry*, *2004 Olympic Time Trial Silver Medalist, Former U.S. National Criterium and Road Race Champion, Two-Time World Championship Team Time Trial Medalist, Six-Time U.S. National Championship Medalist*

"[To] race nonstop for days on end, tackling challenging disciplines like mountain biking, trekking, kayaking, rappelling, and mountaineering in some of the most extreme environments found on earth . . . the paramount importance of nutrition cannot be overstated. Proper nutrition often separates those who win from those who go home before the race is over.

This comprehensive yet accessible manual makes sports nutrition easy to understand and carry out. I highly recommend *Sports Nutrition for Endurance Athletes* to both the beginner athletes I coach and the professionals I race with."

—*Travis Macy*, *Professional Adventure Racer and Coach*

"Monique's chapter on rowing provides rowers of all levels with an excellent introduction to the physiological demands of the sport and the appropriate nutrition to meet those demands. Together, this chapter and the rest of the book give a solid nutritional framework for all endurance athletes."

—*Julie McCleery*, *World Championship Bronze Medalist, Former U.S. National Rowing Team Member*

SPORTS NUTRITION FOR ENDURANCE ATHLETES

SECOND EDITION

Monique Ryan, MS, RD, LDN

BOULDER, COLORADO

Acknowledgments

For over two decades endurance sports have contributed a great amount of enjoyment to both my sports nutrition career and my own sports participation. The second edition of this book is dedicated to endurance sport athletes and to my love of endurance sports and competition. A special thank you to all the athletes, clients, and coaches, who have allowed me to be part of their endurance sport experiences and invited me to share my sports nutrition knowledge with them.

Of course producing this book would not have been possible without the hard work and support of everyone at VeloPress. From the moment a second edition of the book was proposed, it was clear that a dedicated and enthusiastic team was behind this project. I give many thanks to Renee Jardine, Dave Trendler, Jade Hays, Iris Llewellyn, Jen Soulé, and Liza Campbell for all of their invaluable contributions.

SPORTS NUTRITION FOR ENDURANCE ATHLETES, SECOND EDITION
Copyright © 2007 by Monique Ryan

Ironman® is a registered trademark of the World Triathlon Corporation.
XTERRA® is a registered trademark of TEAM Unlimited.

VeloPress
1830 North 55th Street
Boulder, Colorado 80301-2700 USA
303/440-0601 · Fax 303/444-6788 · E-mail velopress@insideinc.com

Cover design by Anita Koury
Cover photo by Chris Milliman
Interior design by Erin Johnson Design
Part-opener art by iStockphoto Images

Distributed in the United States and Canada by Publishers Group West

Cataloging-in-publication data for this book is available from the Library of Congress

For information on purchasing VeloPress books, please call 800/234-8356 or visit www.velopress.com.

07 08 09 / 10 9 8 7 6 5 4 3 2

Contents

Introduction

WHEN THE FIRST EDITION OF *Sports Nutrition for Endurance Athletes* was published in 2002, triathletes, cyclists, runners, swimmers, and adventure racers devoured the wealth of practical, sport-specific nutritional advice found within its covers. Over the years, it has been rewarding and gratifying to hear from readers, clients, and coaches across North America that the book has been an indispensable tool and resource for their training and race programs. With the ever-increasing participation in endurance sports, it seemed only logical to write the second edition that you are now holding in your hands. As a dedicated endurance athlete, you take your nutrition plans very seriously, and whether this book has found you at the start, peak, or post-event phase of your training season, you deserve to have the latest and best cutting-edge nutrition strategies.

While endurance athletes were digesting and absorbing the sports nutrition guidelines in the first edition, research in the practical application of sports nutrition and performance continued to expand and flourish. The second edition of *Sports Nutrition for Endurance Athletes* provides updated guidelines that are scientifically sound and practical for athletes participating in endurance and ultraendurance sports.

This book is ultimately about improving the quality of your training and performance in events and competition, but endurance athletes know that good health also means lasting participation in their chosen sport. Part I is filled with updated information on the links among your daily food choices, optimal health, and disease prevention, with a perspective that supports your daily hours of dedicated training and longevity in your endurance career.

Part II contains the greatest amount of updated material, with the well-researched principles that truly distinguish your diet as an endurance athlete. From your perspective, nutritional timing and portioning are everything. The section on immediate post-training nutritional recovery has been expanded, the information about hydration and electrolyte strategies for training and competition has been fine-tuned, and the nutritional guidelines for muscle building have been updated. Most important, Part II outlines how to adjust and periodize your nutritional intake for the various training cycles so that your daily training diet can be tailored more specifically to each training block and to each exercise session within these blocks. Current recommendations on the proper use of the ever-expanding offering of sports nutrition and dietary supplements and ergogenic aids will help you use these products wisely and safely.

Part III explains how to apply sports nutrition principles to training and competition in each highlighted endurance sport. Each chapter contains detailed practical guidelines for various racing distances and disciplines. The race nutritional strategies of an Ironman® competitor differ from those of a short-course triathlete, and fueling strategies for a mountain bike race differ from those of a cycling road race. This part of the book specifies how to adapt the general principles to your specific sport. A new chapter on applied nutrition for rowers has been added so participants in this demanding endurance sport now have a detailed nutrition resource.

As before, this book addresses nutritional strategies relevant to recreational athletes, serious age-groupers, and elite endurance athletes. Whatever your goals and level of participation, an optimal sports nutrition plan is ultimately about making your participation in your sport more effective, more rewarding, and just plain fun.

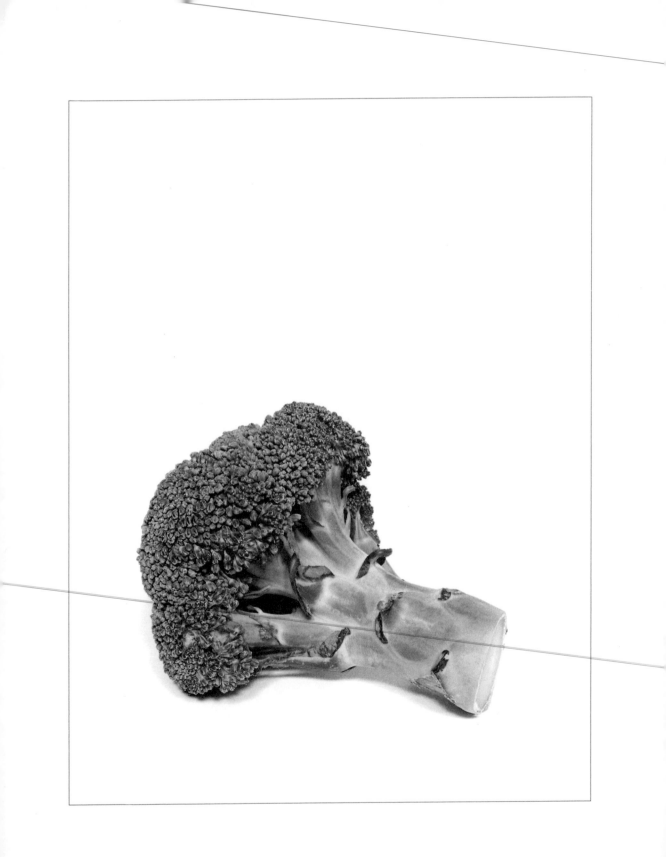

PART I

YOUR DAILY PERFORMANCE DIET

Optimal Food and Fluid Choices for Endurance Training and Health

P roper nutrition is essential for any athlete, but it plays a particularly important role for endurance athletes because of the special demands and stresses of their sport. Whether you are an enthusiastic recreational participant or a serious endurance sport competitor, the subject of nutrition—part art and part science—is one that is well worth mastering. It involves choosing the proper foods, but knowing how much to eat—and when to eat it—is just as important as knowing what to eat. Eating right for your training regimen and competition schedule allows you to replace the fuel you burn during training and supplies the ingredients required to build strength and muscle. As you begin to focus on optimal nutritional recovery from day to day, and from workout to workout, your efforts will be rewarded. You will derive the maximum benefit from your exercise program, and when you arrive at the start of an event or race, you will be in top nutritional shape. The bottom line is that when your diet meets the nutritional demands placed upon your body, you will perform at your best.

Bodies trained and primed for endurance sports require premium fuel for staying healthy throughout the season. If you suffer from lackluster training days, injuries, and more than a fair share of colds and bouts of flu, you may not be making the highest-quality fuel choices. When it comes to daily diet, endurance sport athletes need to obtain each of more than forty-five different nutrients required for optimal functioning of the human body.

Part I of *Sports Nutrition for Endurance Athletes* provides guidelines for building a training diet that will promote optimal health and a strong immune system. This section also identifies the most nutritious sources of carbohydrates, proteins, and fats; how to balance them for optimal training and health; and how to meet the fluid, vitamin, and mineral intakes necessary to build the foundation of a cutting-edge sports diet and good health.

Like any good diet, an endurance training diet simply emphasizes high-quality foods, variety, and balance among the food groups. But this wide-angle view of the endurance training diet is not enough—one needs to take a closer look to truly learn how to use nutrition to enhance performance. Many categories of foods are complex and provide several nutrients that work in tandem to keep an athlete's body well nourished and healthy. Which foods complement each other, and how can one best approach meals and snacktimes throughout the day? How can an athlete make sure there is enough variety in his or her diet? Within each food group are nutrient-packed choices that are minimally processed, fresh, and wholesome. It is best for your lasting good health that you avoid the highly processed foods so prevalent in the North American diet. But how can this best be achieved? Chapters 1 to 3 focus on the details of applying solid nutritional principles to sports nutrition for the endurance athlete.

Quality eating for training and good health takes knowledge and planning, and having a working knowledge of food groups is a key first step. Foods can be categorized in different ways. We often think of basic outlines, such as the government food pyramid, or even systems used by a variety of commercial diet programs. But these food group systems simply do not work for the endurance athlete. Foods are more often grouped according to carbohydrate, protein, and fat content, as the proper balance of these nutrients is required for optimal training and recovery in endurance sports. However you look at it, there is an optimal combination of food groups that come together to produce a cutting-edge diet for each endurance sport and for every individual athlete. Some individuals may find that placing a strong emphasis on fruit and vegetable intake enhances their training and performance, especially because of the excellent immune system boost these foods provide. These athletes will likely focus on plant protein sources and may obtain most of their fat intake from nuts and seeds rather than oils, or may or may not prefer to have a significant amount of dairy products in their diet.

While grouping and categorizing foods can be useful in planning a healthy endurance sports diet, it can also lead to oversimplification. The next step in planning a healthy training diet is to look at some of the choices available within each of the main food groups to see what nutrients they provide. For example, some oils can be highly processed and are a very poor nutritional choice, while others are relatively healthy and can be beneficial. Animal proteins can contain varying levels of fat, and some meats are much too high in fat to be a regular part of any serious athlete's diet. Skim milk and yogurt, in contrast, contribute carbohydrates in addition to high-quality protein. Grains can be wholesome, high in fiber, and even provide small amounts of protein, or they can be highly processed and nutritionally very poor.

Ultimately, the goal is to come to appreciate which choices are the most nutritious and to design a diet plan that works for you. How you portion and time these healthy foods is what distinguishes your endurance training diet from an everyday diet geared toward good health.

TABLE **I.1**	NUTRIENTS FOR THE ENDURANCE DIET

NUTRIENT	FUNCTIONS	FOOD SOURCES
Carbohydrates	Primary high-energy fuel source during exercise Replenish body stores of glycogen Provide dietary fiber	Grains, breads, cereals, rice, pasta Fruit and fruit juices Vegetables Dairy and soy milk, yogurt
Fat	Provides essential fatty acids Provides fat-soluble vitamins Adds flavor to foods Used as a fuel source Protects and insulates body organs Component of cell structures	Liquid oils Margarine and butter Nuts and seeds Avocado Fish
Minerals	Involved in energy production Play role in building body tissue Play role in muscle contraction Involved in oxygen transport Maintain acid-base balance of blood	Fruits and vegetables Lean protein foods Whole grains Oils, nuts, and seeds
Protein	Provides essential amino acids Required for maintaining and developing muscle and other body tissue Essential component of enzymes, hormones, and antibodies Needed for the formation of hemoglobin	Meat, poultry, fish, cheese, eggs Soy, dried beans, lentils Dairy and soy milk, yogurt
Vitamins	Enhance energy production Involved in tissue repair and protein synthesis Play role in red-blood-cell formation Act as antioxidants	Fruits and vegetables Lean protein foods Whole grains Oil, nuts, and seeds
Water	Carries oxygen and nutrients to cells Plays a role in digestion Cools the body through sweat production Has important role in many cellular processes Significant component of muscle tissue	Tap water Bottled water Fruit juices, dairy milk, soy milk Solid foods that contain water, such as fruits, vegetables, yogurt

Table I.1 outlines the functions and food sources of many of these important nutrients. More information on how to determine food portions and how to time meals and snacks to complement your training program is provided in Part II.

1

DAILY HYDRATION
ESSENTIALS

Drinking It In

WATER IS ONE OF THE MOST ESSENTIAL nutrients for the endurance athlete. Some two-thirds of your total body weight is water, and this remarkable substance plays an important role in every major organ and system keeping you alive. We've all seen the need for hydration in a sweat-logged athlete. But for the athlete, the distraction of competition can make it easy to forget to keep drinking water. Many athletes also have not taken the time to learn valuable hydration strategies. While much research and emphasis has been placed upon an endurance athlete's fluid intake directly before, during, and after training or racing, emptying your bottles of fluid during a swim, bike ride, rowing session, or run is only one of many hydration strategies essential for top performance. Paying attention to daily fluid intake on nonactive days is also important. Nevertheless, daily water and fluid intake is often a secondary nutritional consideration, and many athletes frequently fall short on the everyday consumption of this life-sustaining nutrient.

Years of hydration research indicate that athletes should try to prevent even mild levels of dehydration. Although an athlete may not always be aware of how much he or she is sweating, even relatively small fluid losses during training and competition can be significant enough to hinder performance. And sweating doesn't take place only during hot weather; it takes place in cool weather and during winter sports as well. Studies demonstrate that even in thirst-inspiring hot weather, athletes usually fail to replace all the fluid that is lost through sweat during training and competition. To prevent any adverse performance effects, every athlete should arrive for training sessions optimally hydrated, and to do so means staying on top of your daily fluid intake.

WATER: THE FIRST NUTRIENT

Much marketing fuss has been made about the optimal ingredients for the fluids that athletes require. But before the plethora of sports-related drinks and designer fluids flooded the market, there was simply water. Water is basic and unpretentious and flows naturally into an active sport life with no packaging or gimmicks attached. Don't take basic H_2O for granted. Carbohydrates may be the premium fuel for your energy tank, but when you are about to train or compete in your sport, your fluid stores should be topped off as well.

Water plays an integral role in the optimal functioning of your body both during training and during rest and recovery. Well-hydrated muscles are high in fluid content—in fact, water makes up to 70 to 75 percent of an athlete's muscle tissue. Fat tissue is relatively low in water content, at about 10 percent. Consequently, muscular athletes will have high water content when adequately hydrated. Water is stored in many body compartments, and it moves freely among these various spaces. About two-thirds of your body's water is stored inside your cells, giving them their shape and form. The rest of the water in your body surrounds these cells and flows within your blood vessels. Even bones, though seemingly solid, are about 32 percent water. Water plays a role in cooling the body and also provides structure to body parts, protecting important tissues such as your brain and spinal cord and lubricating your joints. When fluids become depleted through sweating, both your cells and blood decrease in water content and volume.

Athletes should appreciate that water is also the main component of their blood. Blood performs the important function of carrying oxygen, hormones, and nutrients such as glucose to your cells. The protein content of blood, muscle, and other tissues also holds water in those tissues. Muscle glycogen holds a considerable amount of water, and water removes lactic acid from exercising muscles, which can be an advantage to athletes who are well hydrated. Water aids digestion through saliva and stomach secretions, and it eliminates waste products through urine and sweat. Water is also essential for the proper functioning of all your senses, particularly hearing and sight.

Clearly the role water plays in maintaining your overall health is extremely important. That's why you can't live without water for more than a few days. But the role that water plays in your performance is equally vital. Being even slightly underhydrated dramatically impedes top athletic performance. As the primary component of sweat, water plays a major role in body temperature regulation. It is water that enables you to maintain a constant body temperature under various environmental conditions because it allows you to continually make adjustments to either gain or lose heat.

Your fluid balance is simply the result of your intake of fluids versus your output of fluids. Intake is the net result of the water and other hydrating fluids we consume, the water in some of the foods we eat, and the metabolic water produced by your body. When you are not training, urine output represents your greatest fluid loss, or output, but sweating during exercise can result in significant fluid losses, even in cold weather and during intense workouts in the gym. Fluid is also lost in feces and in the air you exhale; through exposure to warm or humid weather, living in a dry climate, or living and training at altitude all increase fluid losses; and when traveling, especially by plane.

Most people have heard the oft-quoted recommendation to consume eight 8-ounce cups of fluid (a gallon, or about 1.9 L) daily, mainly in the form of water. In 2004, when much public attention was focused on dietary water requirements, the Food and Nutrition Board of the Institute of Medicine released Dietary Reference Intakes (DRI) for water and various electrolytes. Because of the large variations in water needs among individuals, the IOM panel established Adequate Intake (AI) levels of 130 ounces, or 16 cups (3.8 L), daily for men and 95 ounces, or 12 cups (2.9 L), for women.

But of course daily fluid losses can vary greatly depending on your level of training, whether you are male or female, and your own individual sweat rate. The daily fluid needs of active males can increase to 4.75 quarts (4.5 L), but requirements for male endurance athletes can often be in excess of 10.5 quarts (10 L) daily. There is less data on women, but they likely need about one-half to one quart less fluid daily than men. Estimating fluid requirements beyond the basic AI recommendations is really about replacing fluid at a rate close or equal to your own individual sweat rate and total sweat losses for a particular day of training. Further guidelines for replacing sweat losses are provided in Chapter 5.

At rest, the fluids your body needs can be slowly replenished throughout the day as you make a conscious effort to drink enough water every one to two hours to replace these fluid losses. You should be aware, however, that climate, clothing, and other factors can affect daily water requirements. While thirst is often thought of as the primary human drive that pushes us to drink, it is important for athletes not to rely on thirst alone but to develop regular drinking habits and behaviors to maintain a good level of daily hydration. By the time someone becomes thirsty, his or her body has already sensed a decrease in the level of fluids or an increase in sodium concentration. So in reality, you get thirsty only when you have already experienced significant fluid losses or alterations in your sodium status, both of which are affected by the prolonged periods of sweating that endurance athletes regularly experience. By then, an athlete's performance level would already have decreased. So for an endurance athlete in training, one of the most important concepts to learn is that it is unwise to rely on thirst for daily hydration needs. Doing so may result in falling short of both optimal fluid intake and optimal performance or recovery. And relying on thirst is especially unwise for seasoned masters athletes, because as we get older our thirst mechanism becomes an even poorer sensor of our body's fluid needs.

TABLE **1.1**	CAFFEINE CONTENT OF FOODS AND FLUIDS

PRODUCT	SERVING SIZE	CAFFEINE CONTENT
Coffee		
Coffee, grande, Starbucks	16 oz. (480 ml)	550 mg
Coffee, tall, Starbucks	8 oz. (240 ml)	250 mg
Coffee, brewed, drip	8 oz. (240 ml)	185 mg (95–290 mg)
Coffee, brewed, percolated	8 oz. (240 ml)	130 mg (65–270 mg)
Coffee, instant	8 oz. (240 ml)	105 mg (50–190 mg)
Espresso, double, Starbucks	2 oz. (60 ml)	70 mg
Espresso, Starbucks	1 oz. (30 ml)	40 mg (30–50 mg)
Coffee, decaffeinated	8 oz. (240 ml)	5 mg (3–8 mg)
Espresso, decaffeinated, Starbucks	1 oz. (30 ml)	5 mg
Tea		
Tea, black, loose leaf	8 oz. (240 ml)	25–110 mg
Tea, oolong, loose leaf	8 oz. (240 ml)	12–55 mg
Tea, green, loose leaf	8 oz. (240 ml)	30 mg
Iced tea	12 oz. (360 ml)	70 mg
Soda		
Mountain Dew	12 oz. (360 ml)	54 mg
Coca Cola	12 oz. (360 ml)	46 mg
Diet Coke	12 oz. (360 ml)	46 mg
Dr. Pepper	12 oz. (360 ml)	46 mg
Pepsi Cola	12 oz. (360 ml)	38 mg
Other		
Hot cocoa	12 oz. (360 ml)	8–12 mg
Milk, chocolate	8 oz. (240 ml)	5–8 mg

CAFFEINE

In North America, about 90 percent of adults regularly consume caffeine, mainly in liquid form, whether from cola, tea, coffee, or other caffeine-laced beverages. Caffeine is also present in cocoa and chocolate. Given this statistic, it is safe to assume that most endurance athletes ingest caffeine on a daily basis and perhaps even during training and competition. While proper use of caffeine can enhance physical performance (see Chapter 7), it has long been labeled as a diuretic, or a substance that actually increases fluid losses by increasing urine production. Athletes have often been cautioned to limit daily caffeine and not to count caffeine-containing beverages toward total daily fluid intake.

But in recent years scientists have challenged this assumption about caffeine. Reassessments of existing data and new studies on the effects of caffeine on the hydration status of athletes show that, while caffeine often does act as a mild diuretic, stimulating urine production from the kidneys, it does not produce a greater increase in urine volume when compared with the same volume of water or caffeine-free fluid consumption. One study compared the effects of caffein-ated and noncaffeinated beverages (both caloric and calorie-free) on the daily hydration status of healthy males. Over a twenty-four-hour period, there were no significant hydration differences among the various beverages. Another study had athletes rehydrate with a caffeinated beverage between exercise periods. The researchers found little evidence to support that caffeine can slow down an athlete's efforts to rehydrate.

Endurance athletes can rest assured that a moderate daily intake of caffeine of about 1.4 to 2.7 milligrams per pound (3–6 mg/kg) of body weight daily should not compromise their daily hy-dration status when consumed within the context of a well-balanced diet. Caffeine intakes safely falling into this range would be 230 to 460 milligrams of caffeine for a 170-pound (77 kg) man, or 190 to 380 milligrams for a 140-pound (64 kg) woman. A can of soda contains about 40 to 45 milligrams of caffeine, but the amount of caffeine in a cup of coffee varies widely depending on how the coffee is brewed (for the caffeine content of some foods and beverages, see Table 1.1). Avoid excessive doses of caffeine, however, as high amounts are associated with side effects such as nervousness, gastrointestinal upset, irritability, and insomnia. Higher doses can also nega-tively affect your hydration status and do not result in performance improvements much beyond the moderate doses.

ALCOHOL: THE NONNUTRITIVE NUTRIENT

One would hope that endurance athletes would be among those inclined not to drink alcohol, given their greater awareness of health issues and their desire to perform well in training and competition. Still, many who do drink may not be aware of how it can affect their athletic perfor-mance. It is important for an athlete to use alcohol sensibly, as it does not play any role in physi-cal recovery and could have mild or even serious detrimental effects upon your performance.

Abuse of alcohol can impair health by contributing to cirrhosis of the liver and other diseases, and drunk driving is always dangerous and irresponsible. Alcohol is a widely abused drug, with a significant number of problem drinkers or abusers, and can lead to many kinds of health and social problems. Of course, alcohol should never be consumed during pregnancy. But let's take a look at the implications of alcohol specifically for endurance sports enthusiasts.

Although alcohol is considered a drug, it provides calories just as foods do but at fairly high levels. As far as your body is concerned, alcohol is merely an onslaught of empty calories. These calories are not used for energy in the same way as carbohydrates, proteins, and fats. Beer and wine contain only small amounts of carbohydrates and only trace amounts of protein, vitamins, and minerals. In fact, alcohol can interfere with how your body uses vitamins and minerals. Half an ounce of pure ethanol is the equivalent of one drink—that is, 12 ounces (360 ml) of beer (150 calories), 4 ounces (120 ml) of wine (100 calories), or 1.25 ounces (38 ml) of liquor (100 calories). Despite originating from fermented carbohydrates, alcohol is metabolized in your body as fat. Alcohol by-products are converted into fatty acids, which are stored in your liver and sent to your bloodstream. For this reason, alcohol is not the best nutrient choice if your goal is to be a lean athlete. Consuming four or more drinks daily raises your odds of developing obesity by 46 percent.

In the media much has been made of alcohol's protective effects against heart disease. Like fruit and vegetables, red wine and dark beer contain antioxidants called *polyphenols,* which are believed to protect against cancer. But while moderate amounts may raise the desirable and protective high-density lipoprotein cholesterol (HDL), too much alcohol may actually increase your risk of heart disease. Three or more alcoholic drinks daily can raise your blood pressure as well as the level of harmful blood fats in your body called *triglycerides,* which, when combined with a low amount of the good cholesterol, HDL, makes for a health profile associated with an increased risk of heart disease. Consumed in excess over a long period, alcohol may not only elevate blood pressure but also increase the risk of stroke and, of course, liver damage. Excessive intake of alcohol also increases risk of mouth, esophageal, stomach, liver, breast, and colon cancer. Even one drink a day can slightly raise breast cancer risk in women. Chronic alcohol abuse also increases the risk of developing osteoporosis and can accelerate aging of the brain.

Consuming too much alcohol too soon after training or racing can impede recovery. Alcohol is a diuretic that causes your body to lose more fluid than it takes in. That's why you need to replace losses even after drinking moderate amounts of alcohol. Alcohol may also interfere with glycogen synthesis. Athletes with soft tissue damage or bruising may also want to consider that alcohol is a blood vessel dilator. Consuming alcohol after exercise may aggravate swelling or bleeding and impair healing. These types of injuries are usually treated with ice, which is designed to constrict blood flow to the injured parts.

Excessive alcohol consumed shortly before training, or even the night before, can impair fine motor ability and coordination, increase risk of dehydration, and weaken fuel stores. Alcohol adversely affects your brain's ability to process information and therefore delays your reaction times. Know your limits, and be aware of how they change with your training and fitness level. Keep in mind that people metabolize alcohol at different rates depending on their body size. Average-sized men metabolize slightly less than one drink per hour, whereas smaller men and women take longer to metabolize this same amount.

Underage drinking is also a problem. High school and college athletes participating in endurance sports should be aware of alcohol's harmful effects. Parents of any teenager should emphasize that alcohol consumption can result in long-term health risks. But young athletes also need to understand that alcohol and hangovers affect performance. Alcohol can disrupt fluid balance and temperature regulation, impair fine motor skills, and cause subpar practices and competitive performance.

Adult athletes can have an occasional drink, but they must drink in sensible amounts. If you do choose to indulge once in a while, have a large glass of water with each alcoholic drink. Consider that when you are resting from your sport, your top priority as an athlete is recovery. Too much alcohol can compromise how effectively you recover.

DAILY HYDRATION ESSENTIALS

It is essential that you stay on top of your fluid needs by drinking a minimum of 11 to 16 cups (2.7–3.8 L) of fluid daily for basic hydration requirements when not training. Try to drink on a schedule of 8 ounces (240 ml) every hour. Water should make up about half of your daily fluid intake, but you can also receive hydration benefits from other fluids. Juice, dairy milk, soy milk, soup, and various sports nutrition supplements can be good choices. Some foods—especially fruits and vegetables—contain a high percentage of water and can also contribute fluid to your daily diet. Endurance athletes with very high energy requirements can consume high-calorie drinks such as juices and smoothies to assist them in meeting their fluid, carbohydrate, and energy needs. Caffeinated beverages can be incorporated into your diet in reasonable amounts, but they should not be your first choice prior to and after training. Overdoing your caffeine intake can also interfere with your sleep patterns and make you nervous and jittery.

You can monitor your hydration status by checking the color and quantity of your urine. Clear or lemonade-colored urine reflects adequate fluid intake, while darker or apple juice–colored urine, or a smaller volume of urine, indicates that you need to step up your fluid intake. Urine tends to be more concentrated when you first wake up, but it should become clearer throughout the day. You should urinate at least four full bladders every day. Certain vitamin supplements can

DAILY HYDRATION STRATEGIES

- Start your day with hydration in mind. Consume liquids such as juice, dairy milk, or soy milk at breakfast. Liquid hot cereals and juicy fruits, such as melons, also contribute to your fluid intake. A moderate dose of a caffeinated beverage is fine in the morning.
- Don't rely mainly or solely on caffeinated beverages for your hydration needs, however. After a moderate intake of caffeine, you can have decaffeinated coffee, decaffeinated tea, herbal tea, and other caffeine-free beverages.
- Carry water with you at all times—when you drive or commute, while you are at work or school, and just about everywhere else as well.
- Incorporate real fruit juices, soy or cow's milk, yogurt, and water into meals or snacks.
- Spruce up your water with lemon, lime, or a small amount of juice for flavor.
- Consume 24 ounces (720 ml) of fluid 2 hours before exercising, and another 8 to 16 ounces (240–480 ml) 30 minutes before exercising to ensure that you start training well hydrated.

darken urine, so volume rather than color may be a better indicator of hydration status if you take them. Regular monitoring of your weight during heavy training periods can also be helpful in judging fluid balance. If you notice significant weight losses at morning weigh-ins, this may be an indicator of chronic dehydration.

It is definitely worthwhile to focus on your daily fluid intake and make the effort to improve in this area. Athletes who have developed techniques for increasing their fluid intake have consistently found that improved hydration results in enhanced recovery and higher energy levels. Improving your hydration levels is really very simple. Just plan ahead and make sure that water and other hydrating fluids are available for consumption throughout the day. This will ensure that you begin your training sessions with a well-hydrated body.

FILTERED, BOTTLED, OR TAP?

With the advent of the burgeoning bottled water market, you may have wondered whether it may be in your best interest to buy your water on a regular basis, or even to filter your water at home. For healthy adults, tap water in the United States is a very safe option, but that doesn't mean that you shouldn't make your water safer, and many American consumers are considering new water options. Over the past several years, purchases of home filtration systems have increased. Americans consumed more than 7.5 billion gallons of bottled water in 2005 alone. The Environmental Protection Agency (EPA) estimates that 90 percent of drinking water is safe.

Tap water does contain substances other than water. Depending on where you live, it can provide varying levels of minerals such as calcium, sodium, magnesium, iron, zinc, lead, and mercury. Keep in mind that tap water is also fluoridated in the majority of the country. While calcium may be beneficial, lead and mercury are not. As a health-minded athlete and consumer, you may also be concerned about microbial contamination and pesticide residues in water.

Tap water is regulated under the strict standards of the EPA, but there are some contaminants that the EPA does not regulate. Your local water municipality is required to supply you with an annual "Right to Know Report" every July. This report lists contaminants detected in your drinking water and notes any violations that have occurred in the past year. Your water provider is also required to test for microbes several times daily. You can contact your local water municipality to obtain the names and numbers of certified testing labs to have the water from your own tap checked. Levels of lead and copper in your water may be higher than official reports because of deterioration of household plumbing and faucets.

If you discover that your water is not of the best quality, filtered water may be a viable option. Many filters attach right to the tap and can filter out lead and other contaminants. Another convenient filtering method is a pour-through filter that can be placed in a special pitcher and kept in your refrigerator to be used as needed. More expensive filters include an under-the-sink model that requires a permanent connection to your water pipe. Reverse osmosis filters are considered the best of this type and can filter out lead, mercury, minerals, some pesticides, and microorganisms. Whole-house filters are the most expensive and are installed where the water meets the main water pipe. The benefit is that this type covers all the water used in the house.

CONTINUES

FILTERED, BOTTLED, OR TAP?   continued

You may also determine that bottled water is a convenient option for reaching your recommended daily water intake, though there is no guarantee that it is microbe-free or safer than tap water. About one-quarter of all bottled water comes from municipal water supplies. Bottled water can also be spring water, mineral water, well water, or distilled water. Unlike tap water, which is regulated by the EPA, bottled water is regulated by the Food and Drug Administration (FDA). It is not tested for the parasites cryptosporidium or giardia, and it is tested only once weekly for microbes. It is convenient, however, and many consumers like the taste of certain brands.

An independent organization called NSF International sets standards for and certifies water filtration systems. Its Web site, at www.nsf.org, lists filters and the contaminants that each is certified to reduce in your water. Look for a filter with a pore size of less than 1 micron in diameter. Be sure to follow the manufacturer's directions for replacement of the filter cartridge.

It is also a good idea to look for brands of bottled water that maintain the NSF International certification. To do so, water bottlers must send daily samples for microbial testing to an independent lab and maintain records of filter changes and other quality checks. You can also determine if your brand of water is NSF certified by visiting the NSF's Web site.

New varieties of bottled water include fortified waters, fitness waters, waters supplemented with vitamins and herbs, and oxygen-enriched water. Some of these waters simply provide flavor for individuals who do not want to drink plain water, and for this reason they do encourage good fluid intake. Some contain only a small number of calories, while others may provide more calories per bottle than consumers realize. Check labels to determine the number of calories per serving and the number of servings per bottle. Some of the new designer waters may contain artificial sweeteners. Herbal and vitamin-enhanced waters may not provide significant amounts of these nutrients per serving; however, if you drink them frequently you could potentially consume enough to take in too much of some of these substances. Currently there is no scientific backing for the idea that consuming oxygen-enriched water can boost energy by increasing the oxygen content of red blood cells, as the advertisements for these products claim.

2

ENERGY NUTRIENTS FOR OPTIMAL
HEALTH AND PERFORMANCE

Building a Solid Nutrition Base

BEING AN ENDURANCE ATHLETE COMES WITH a number of perks: You get to spend many hours outdoors doing a sport that you love, you enjoy the health benefits of being in top physical shape, and, not least, you can consume generous portions of a variety of delicious and healthy foods. The endurance athlete's diet is definitely not one of restriction and self-sacrifice. Because these athletes regularly participate in vigorous physical activity year-round, they have many days and training cycles that demand a high energy intake. The training hours they put in on a weekly basis require them to take in adequate amounts of carbohydrates, proteins, and fats. Consuming enough of these nutrients allows them to replace fuel stores used in training, make the most of recovery time between training sessions, and ultimately, arrive for competition in the best form possible with fuel to burn.

But this doesn't mean that endurance athletes can eat just anything they feel like eating. Training bodies rely on premium, high-quality fuel for staying healthy. This chapter focuses on the foods that should provide the foundation of your daily training diet and discusses how your food choices impact your health, immune system, and well-being. Popular diets often promote a specific balance of carbohydrates, proteins, and fats, but some of these, such as the low-carbohydrate diets so prominent in the media over the past few years, raise serious concerns for endurance athletes, especially because of their recommendation to eliminate many of the healthy grains and fruits that are so important for good nutrition. Well-designed clinical studies have repeatedly demonstrated that as the duration and intensity of an endurance athlete's training increase, so does his or her need for carbohydrates. Just how much of this fuel an athlete requires for various training days is outlined in Chapter 4. This chapter focuses on the best food choices for endurance athletes rather than on portion sizes, total calories, and gram counts. If you are an endurance athlete, the first step you must take is to forget everything you've heard about the pitfalls of consuming a high-carbohydrate diet—that is, everything but one idea: The restrictive diets that launched the carbohydrate-phobia craze did provide dietitians with an opportunity to highlight the importance of consuming nutritious carbohydrates rather than sugar-loaded sweets and empty calories.

CARBOHYDRATES: THE ATHLETE'S FUEL

CLASSIFYING CARBOHYDRATES: FROM SIMPLE TO COMPLEX TO INDEXING

Endurance athletes should appreciate that carbohydrates are a major source of fuel. While nutrition plans should always be personalized to an athlete's training program, medical history, and genetics, if your carbohydrate intake does not provide a sufficient amount of fuel for your training and recovery, you will not perform at your best. Of course, your carbohydrate choices should be of the highest quality possible.

Many athletes are familiar with the traditional classification of carbohydrates. Simple carbohydrates, which are often called "sugars," consist of one or two molecules. One-molecule carbohydrates, or monosaccharides, include glucose, fructose (found in fruit), and galactose and are the easiest to digest. Two-molecule carbohydrates, or disaccharides, include sucrose, lactose (found in milk), and maltose and are also relatively easy to digest. Carbohydrates that contain three to twenty molecules are oligosaccharides. This category includes many manufactured carbohydrates, such as maltodextrins (found in some sports drinks), as well as corn syrup and high-fructose corn syrup. Oligosaccharides also include healthy carbohydrates such as rafinnose and stachyose, which are found in legumes. Other complex carbohydrates, or polysaccharides, are composed of more than twenty and sometimes up to thousands of carbohydrate molecules joined together. This group includes amylose and amylopectin. The vast majority of carbohydrates in the plant world, such as those found in cereals, rice, corn, potatoes, and wheat, are polysaccharides. Complex carbohydrates should be a main source of carbohydrate energy for an athlete. Glucose polymers, a string of glucose molecules, are also complex carbohydrates and can be found in sports drinks and carbohydrate gels. Complex carbohydrates provide indigestible fiber, such as cellulose, hemicellulose, gums, and pectins, and are very important for gastrointestinal health and disease prevention.

All of this may sound overly complex at first. Is it really necessary to know how to classify carbohydrates and to understand the scientific terminology in order to simply frame a healthy training diet? The short answer is yes. The reason is that it is important for endurance athletes to appreciate that they may incorporate different types of carbohydrates into their diet at different times. For example, a wide variety of sports drinks, gels, and recovery drinks now contain various types of simple or manufactured complex carbohydrates. Are these products healthy or useful, and if so, at what points in your training day or cycle? When choosing among them, what should you look for? You can use them wisely and keep them in perspective if you have a basic knowledge of the science of carbohydrates. Some of these manufactured carbohydrates may be marketed as "complex" because they are made of chains of molecules that are seemingly superior to the simple sugars found in similar products. They are designed to quickly deliver energy to your working muscles during exercise because they are easily tolerated in the gut and easily digested. These carbohydrates are not necessarily more nutritious than others or superior in terms of providing health benefits or boosting athletic performance, however. There is no particular reason to consume them when you are not in the midst of vigorous physical exercise. They can, however, do the job they were designed to do—fuel your body during exercise. If you like the taste and your digestive system tolerates them well, they may be worthwhile and right for you.

Keeping up-to-date on the science of carbohydrates also allows the endurance athlete to distinguish fact from fiction when it comes to dietary advice. For years nutrition experts said that simple carbohydrates such as fructose and other sugars caused a rapid rise and subsequent fall in blood sugar levels that resulted in fatigue, and that these sugars were therefore less nutritious. Conversely, it was maintained that complex carbohydrates resulted in a more gentle blood glucose rise and occurred in more nutritious foods. In the world of black-and-white thinking, simple carbohydrates were considered "bad" and complex carbohydrates "good." Although this classification might seem logical, scientific data from the past decade indicate that the advice is outdated. What endurance sport athletes should be concerned about is the quality of the carbohydrates they are consuming on a daily basis, emphasizing nutritious and wholesome sources while decreasing nutrient-poor, refined sources. Wholesome carbohydrates provide vitamins, minerals, and fiber, while refined carbohydrates mainly come from processed foods that provide little other than calories.

In reality, wholesome carbohydrates are not always of the complex variety, and refined carbohydrates are not always simple sugars. Fruit contains simple carbohydrates but is packed with nutrients, whereas products made from white flour, such as white bread, contain complex carbs but often have a much lower vitamin and mineral content. Grain sources are much more nutritious in their natural state. For optimal training and good health, choose wholesome carbohydrates. They are a very important component of your diet because they are higher in nutritional value.

In addition to being wholesome or refined, carbohydrates can be categorized according to how they affect blood sugar (or blood glucose) levels. The belief that simple carbohydrates cause a rapid rise in blood glucose and that complex carbohydrates cause a slower rise is outdated.

TABLE **2.1**	GLYCEMIC INDEX AND GLYCEMIC LOAD OF FOODS

FOOD, PORTION	GRAMS CARBOHYDRATE PER PORTION	GLYCEMIC LOAD PER PORTION	GLYCEMIC INDEX FOR 50 GRAMS
High-Glycemic Foods (GI > 70)			
Potato, baked, 6½ oz. (200 g)	29	27.3	94
Rice, instant, 5 oz. (200 g)	42	36.5	87
Corn Flakes, 1 oz. (30 g)	25	21.5	86
Rice Krispies, 1 oz. (30 g)	29	24	82
Total cereal, 1 oz. (30 g)	25	19	76
Waffle, 2 oz. (60 g)	25	19.3	76
Cheerios, 1 oz. (30 g)	25	18.5	74
Watermelon, 8 oz. (240 g)	12	8.6	72
Bagel, white, 2¼ oz. (70 g)	35.5	25.5	72
Millet, 5 oz. (150 g)	34.8	24.7	71
Bread, white, 2 oz. (60 g)	26.8	18.8	70
Moderate-Glycemic Foods (GI 55–70)			
Shredded Wheat, 1 oz. (30 g)	21.7	14.6	67
Pineapple, 4 oz. (120 g)	9.6	6.3	66
Oat kernel bread, 2 oz. (60 g)	25.6	16.6	65
Raisins, 2 oz. (60 g)	42.7	27.3	64
Muffin 2 oz. (57 g)	27.7	17.2	62
Couscous, 5 oz. (150 g)	14.3	8.7	61
Spaghetti, white, durum wheat, 6 oz. (180 g)	44.3	25.6	58
Muesli, 2 oz. (60 g)	32	17.9	56
Oat Bran, raw, 2 oz. (60 g)	30	16.5	55

CONTINUES

Research has demonstrated that each carbohydrate food produces its own unique blood glucose profile, which does not correlate with the simple-versus-complex classification.

The ranking system that describes the blood glucose profile of a food is referred to as the *glycemic index,* which represents the effect a particular food has on the rate and amount of increase in blood glucose. In this system, a blood glucose profile of 50 grams of pure glucose is given a glycemic index of 100. Other carbohydrates are tested in 50-gram doses and compared with glucose. High-glycemic foods are generally considered to have a glycemic index of greater than 70.

TABLE **2.1**	GLYCEMIC INDEX AND GLYCEMIC LOAD OF FOODS continued		
FOOD, PORTION	**GRAMS CARBOHYDRATE PER PORTION**	**GLYCEMIC LOAD PER PORTION**	**GLYCEMIC INDEX FOR 50 GRAMS**
Low-Glycemic Foods (GI < 55)			
Buckwheat, 5 oz. (150 g)	28.8	14.6	51
Bread, whole-grain, 2 oz. (30 g)	23.0	12.0	51
Banana, ripe, 4 oz. (120 g)	23.9	12.1	50
All-Bran, 2 oz. (60 g)	36.8	18.4	50
Rice, brown, 5 oz. (150 g)	47.7	23.9	49
Porridge oatmeal, 8 oz. (250 g)	20.3	9.9	48
Sweet potato, 5 oz. (150 g)	26	12.5	48
Grapefruit juice, 8 oz. (260 g)	15.7	7.5	41
Pear, Bartlett, 4 oz. (120 g)	11.3	4.6	40
Apple, 4 oz. (120 g)	14.6	5.9	33
Yogurt, fruited, 6½ oz. (200 g)	33	10.9	32
Milk, skim, 8 oz. (259 g)	13	4.1	32
Spaghetti, whole-meal, 4 oz. (120 g)	30	9.6	28
Peach, 8 oz. (240 g)	15	4.2	28
Lentils, 5 oz. (150 g)	14.9	4.1	28
Kidney beans, 5 oz. (150 g)	24	5.5	23

SOURCE: WWW.GLYCEMICINDEX.COM.

Moderate foods are in the 55 to 70 range, and foods with a score of less than 55 are considered low on the glycemic scale.

Table 2.1 provides an abbreviated list of the glycemic index ranking of high-carbohydrate foods, while a more extensive listing is provided in Appendix A. Interestingly, fruits generally have a low glycemic index, despite containing simple carbohydrates, whereas white potatoes, which contain complex carbohydrates, have a high glycemic index. Many factors influence the glycemic index of a food, including the type of fiber in the food, how the glucose molecules in the food are connected, and the way the food is prepared.

Individuals with specific health concerns such as diabetes who need to control blood glucose and elevated blood lipids can manipulate their carbohydrate intake according to their benefit based on the glycemic index of the foods. The glycemic index can also play a role in treating

CONSIDER THE GLYCEMIC LOAD

The glycemic index (GI) is a ranking of carbohydrates based on their immediate blood glucose effects. The glycemic load (GL) builds on the GI of a food to provide a more meaningful measure of how your body responds to the carbohydrates you consume. That's because the GL takes portion sizes into consideration. Not all carbohydrate food portions supply the 50-gram dose used in glycemic index testing; often an actual person may consume a much smaller amount.

Glycemic load is the glycemic index of a food multiplied by the total grams of carbohydrates in the portion used, which is then divided by 100. One GL unit is approximately equal to the glycemic effect of 1 gram of glucose. To make practical use of this information, one can add up the total GL of all carbohydrate foods eaten throughout the day and determine whether one is eating high or low on the GI/GL scale. The total GL for the day in the typical American diet ranges from 60 to 180. On a low-GL day the GL units will add up to less than 80, whereas on a high-GL day the total will be greater than 120. The general equation is:

GL = GI x grams of carbohydrates per serving ÷ 100

Let's compare the GL of carrots with corn, for example. Carrots have a GI of 92, which is high, whereas corn has a more moderate glycemic index of 60. We'll assume that our hypothetical diner eats one-half cup of each, and that both are cooked. The math for carrots works out as follows:

92 x 6 = 552, and 552 ÷ 100 = 5.52

Carrots have a GI of 92. One-half cup of cooked carrots has 6 grams of carbohydrates. The carrots have a GL of 5.52. The math for corn works out as follows:

60 x 20 = 1,200, and 1,200 ÷ 100 = 12

Corn has a GI of 60. One-half cup of cooked corn has 20 grams of carbohydrates. The corn has a GL of 12.

Although carrots have a higher glycemic index than corn, the GL of carrots is lower than that of a similar portion of corn. Many moderate- to high-GI foods may not be consumed in the 50-gram portion test dose and could have a low GL. Alternately, a typical portion of a food that seems to rank low on the GI scale may actually have a high GL ranking. A low GL for a carbohydrate serving is 10 or less, a moderate GL may range from 11 to 19, and a GL of 20 or more is high.

individuals diagnosed with a condition called metabolic syndrome that is characterized by insulin resistance, or problems with the ability to use insulin appropriately. Ongoing research utilizes the glycemic index to help fine-tune dietary recommendations for individuals with these health concerns. But athletes may also be able to use the glycemic index to their performance advantage by developing specific recommendations for manipulating carbohydrate intake before, during, and after training and competition. These sports nutrition applications of the glycemic index is reviewed in Chapters 4 and 5. For their daily diet, endurance athletes should experiment with various unprocessed, nutrient-dense, whole-grain carbohydrate foods to determine what works best for them, taking their individual food preferences and schedules into account.

GO FOR THE GRAINS—THE WHOLESOME ONES

With the advent of carbohydrate-restricted diets, the group of carbohydrates most often eliminated and heavily restricted is grains. This is unfortunate because wholesome grains are good sources of carbohydrates, fiber, and B vitamins. Because they are so concentrated in carbohydrates, they are excellent choices for replenishing your body's carbohydrate stores—namely, muscle and liver glycogen, which becomes depleted from intense and demanding training sessions. Grains are easily obtained in the North American diet, but unfortunately many of the most accessible ones are refined grains rather than whole grains. Just as there are "good fats" and "bad fats" (a topic explored later in this chapter), in the typical North American diet there are good carbohydrates and bad carbohydrates.

For both optimal health and top performance (especially during the winter months), choose whole grains whenever possible. Whole grains literally come from the entire grain, which includes the endosperm, germ, and bran portion of the grain, thereby retaining all the desirable nutrients. In contrast, when refined grains are produced, the bran and germ are separated from the starchy endosperm. The endosperm is then ground into flour.

Whole grains are packed with vitamins, minerals, and phytochemicals, which have powerful antioxidant and disease-fighting properties that cannot be obtained from white bread, processed cereals, white rice, and even many "enriched" multigrain breads. Some of the phytochemicals found in whole grains include oligosaccharides, flavinoids, lignans, phytates, and saponins, many of which have powerful antioxidant properties. Whole grains also provide vitamin E and selenium. Studies have shown that regular consumption of whole grains can help to prevent heart disease, diabetes, and certain cancers, yet surveys indicate that most Americans consume less than one serving of whole grains daily. Consuming grains such as whole oats, barley, and bran can reduce the glycemic load of your diet. High-fiber, whole-grain breads that contain whole seeds have an even lower glycemic index.

Include a variety of whole grains in your diet. Even making simple changes, such as using brown rice instead of white rice and whole-wheat pasta instead of semolina pasta, will be beneficial. Buy 100 percent whole-grain breads and look for "whole grain" on the package, which indicates that more than half of the weight of the product comes from whole grains.

Athletes who are tired of the same wheat- and rice-based grain choices also have a few more adventuresome options to choose from. There are many whole-grain alternatives, including amaranth, kasha (buckwheat), quinoa, spelt, and teff (see Table 2.2). They may take a bit more cooking time than pasta, rice, and potatoes, but they are nutritious and add variety to the diet. You can experiment with various seasonings to flavor these wholesome grains.

Whole grains should be an important part of your diet because of the nutrients and carbohydrates that they provide. But you should also place a strong emphasis on fruits and vegetables, not only for their carbohydrate content but also because of the great health benefits that they

TABLE **2.2**	**WHOLE-GRAIN ALTERNATIVES**	
GRAIN	**DESCRIPTION**	**PREPARATION**
Amaranth	High in protein and fiber Good source of vitamin E	Boil and eat as a cereal. Cook 1 c. grain in 3 c. water for 30 min.
Barley	High in soluble fiber	Cook 1 c. grain in 3 c. water for 45 min.
Bulgur	High in fiber, folate, magnesium, and iron	Cook 1 c. grain in water or broth for 10–12 min.
Kasha (buckwheat groats)	Excellent source of magnesium High in fiber	Serve as a cereal, as pilaf, or in pancakes. Cook 1 part groats in 2 parts water for 15 min.
Millet	A staple in Africa High in minerals	Serve with meat or cook as a cereal. Cook 1 c. grain in 2¼ c. water for 25–30 min.
Oats	Source of cholesterol-lowering fiber High in protein	Avoid instant varieties; steel-cut are more nutritious. Cook 1 c. oats in 4 c. liquid for 20 min.
Quinoa	Excellent source of B vitamins, copper, iron, and magnesium	Oatmeal-like cereal. Rinse before cooking to remove bitter coating. Cook 1 c. grain in 2 c. water for 20 min.
Spelt	A distant cousin to wheat High in fiber and B vitamins	Used to make breads and pastas. Can be used in pilafs. Cook 1 c. grain in 4 c. water for 30–40 min.
Teff	Rich in protein Good source of iron and calcium	Cook 1 c. grain in 3 c. liquid for 15–20 min.

GETTING IN THE GRAINS

The U.S. Department of Agriculture (USDA) 2005 Dietary Guidelines recommend that adults eat at least three servings of whole grains every day. One slice or 1 ounce (30 g) of bread or 1 ounce (30 g) of cereal equals one serving.

Find whole-grain cereals that you enjoy and make them a regular part of your breakfast every day. Good choices include oatmeal, Fiber One, Go Lean, Heart to Heart, All-Bran, Raisin Bran, Original Shredded Wheat, and Grape Nuts. Read labels to make sure one of the first ingredients is wheat bran, whole wheat, whole-grain wheat, cornmeal, or whole oat flour. You should choose cereal primarily for its fiber content. Aim for at least 5 grams per serving, but 8 grams per serving is even better. Remember that added sugars listed on the label, such as cane sugar, evaporated cane juice, and high-fructose corn syrup, have no real nutritive value and simply add empty calories. Also look out for hydrogenated oils (see section entitled "Fat: Facts and Figures" later in this chapter).

Choose whole-grain breads as well, and don't rely on the color, texture, or even fiber content of the bread to judge its true whole-grain content. Bread that is 100 percent "whole grain" is best, and "enriched" wheat flour is not whole-grain. The terms "multi-grain" and "7-grain" do not guarantee a whole-grain product, nor does "made from whole grain." Try to choose a whole-grain bread with a short ingredients list, and look out for breads that contain high-fructose corn syrup. Some breads labeled as "soft," "light," or "double fiber" may have added fiber or improved texture, but they do not necessarily contain the healthy phytonutrients found in true whole-grain products. For a lighter texture, try bread made from "white whole wheat," though many of these breads are not 100 percent whole-grain.

Start by making whole substitutions for the grains you eat the most, such as rice and pasta. Just using brown rice instead of white rice will add fiber to your diet. One-quarter cup of dry brown rice contains 2 grams of fiber. Whole-grain pasta can provide up to 6 grams of fiber per serving (2 oz. dry pasta).

Look for the whole-grain stamp of approval developed by the Whole Grains Council. This stamp depicts shafts of wheat and the words "whole grain" followed by one of three terms: "100%" if all grain ingredients are whole-grain, "Excellent Source" for at least 16 grams of whole-grain ingredients per serving, and "Good Source" for 8 grams or more of whole-grain ingredients per serving.

offer. In fact, some health organizations and health researchers believe that fruits and vegetables should constitute the majority of our carbohydrate intake. Studies have shown that eating more fruits and vegetables can reduce your risk of heart disease, stroke, and some types of cancer. How you put together your sport diet will ultimately depend on your food preferences, need for convenience, personal health considerations, and carbohydrate training requirements. But chances are that boosting fruit and vegetable intake would be a step in the right direction for any athlete interested in optimal performance when cycling, rowing, running, or swimming.

FRUITS AND VEGETABLES: THE HARVEST OF CHAMPIONS

Fruits and vegetables are especially distinguished by the thousands of substances that they provide which protect our bodies from disease. These phytonutrients act as antioxidants and counteract the cellular damage that we encounter every day. Fruits and vegetables are also great sources of the immune-boosting vitamin A and the antioxidant beta-carotene, as well as other health-enhancing carotenoids. They also supply ample amounts of vitamin C, another important antioxidant and vitamin that performs many essential functions in your body, and the mineral potassium. In this section we will review not only some nutrient-packed fruit and vegetable choices for your training diet but also excellent sources of specific vitamins, minerals, and antioxidants.

Filling Up on Fruit

Because fruits and vegetables are so packed with disease-fighting nutrients, the American Heart Association and the American Cancer Society both recommend five or more servings daily. Fresh fruits, dried fruit, and fruit juice can also provide the endurance athlete with a significant and concentrated source of carbohydrates that provide energy for training and fuel for recovery.

All fruits are nutritious, but some choices are extremely nutritious. Tropical fruits such as papaya, mango, kiwifruit, and guava have wonderfully high levels of vitamin C and carotenoids, which are potent antioxidants. Carotenoids are also found in significant amounts in deep yellow or orange-colored fruits such as apricots, cantaloupe, and nectarines. Citrus fruits such as oranges and grapefruits are known for being great sources of vitamin C. Also found in fruits are phytonutrients such as catechins, flavonols, stilbenes, allicin, quercetin, ellagic acid, anthocyanins, limonin, zeaxanthin, and lutein, which appear to be increasingly important to maintaining good health.

The best way to obtain a variety of phytonutrients is to consume a variety of fruits. Dried fruits and real fruit juices will provide the most concentrated sources of carbohydrates for athletes with higher energy needs. Dried fruit, however, will not be as great a source of vitamin C, though it may provide more minerals and fiber than fresh fruit because it is so concentrated. Try to avoid dried fruits prepared with sulfites if you are sulfite-sensitive. (Sulfites are preservatives that trigger allergic reactions in some individuals.) Fresh fruits are also great sources of fiber and the highest in nutrients.

While the warm summer months are associated with a wide variety of fresh fruits, fresh produce is often not as abundant or reasonable in cost during the winter months. Choose fresh and eat fresh whenever possible, but don't disregard frozen and canned choices to keep a healthy supply of fruit in your diet year-round. The nutritional value of fresh fruits is too high to ignore, but any source of fruit is better than none. Flash freezing and other new technologies trap vitamins, minerals, and phytochemicals in fruit immediately after they are harvested, when produce is at its peak. When you peruse the supermarket aisles, purchase enough fresh fruits and vegetables to last three to four days, the amount of time it takes fresh fruit to lose its nutritive value when sitting in your refrigerator. If you shop twice weekly, pick up another fresh fruit stash later in the week. If you shop once a week (and it can be challenging to keep up a healthy sport diet if you shop any less frequently), buy a variety of frozen or canned fruit.

Choose your frozen and canned fruits carefully. Avoid frozen brands that add extra sugar or syrup and canned varieties that are packed in heavy syrup, as this preparation adds nonnutritive calories. Opt for fruit canned and packed in light juice and frozen fruit where the fruit is the sole ingredient on the package label. If you miss those delicious summer raspberries and blueberries at certain times of the year, don't forget the frozen version. Check for organic fruit in the frozen food aisle as well; it is increasingly becoming available in mainstream stores. Frozen fruits should move about freely in the package; when they have fused into a solid block of ice, some nutrient loss has already occurred. Also avoid packages that are sweating or stained with the color of the fruit that is inside; this appearance indicates that the package was partially thawed and refrozen before reaching the supermarket. Once-thawed frozen fruit can be a bit more waterlogged than its fresh counterparts. Frozen fruits work well on top of hot cereals, pancakes, and waffles, and they are perfect for smoothies, which are great recovery drinks for endurance athletes.

Finding Veggie Heaven

Like fruits, vegetables provide a wide variety of vitamins, minerals, phytonutrients, and fiber to enhance your health. While a wide variety of vegetables are available in the spring and summer months at supermarkets and farmers' markets, great winter vegetable choices include broccoli, bok choy, Brussels sprouts, potatoes, sweet potatoes, and of course winter squash.

All vegetables are good, healthy choices, but some stand out, nutritionally speaking, and are even more concentrated in nutrients than fruit. Color is often a good indicator of a higher nutrient content in vegetables. Some stellar options include carrots, sweet potatoes, and red peppers, which are high in carotenoids. Spinach and romaine lettuce are good leafy choices for their vitamin C, folate, and phytonutrient content. Another group of vegetables that contain not only beta-carotene and vitamin C but also the cancer-fighting phytonutrients called "indoles" are broccoli, cauliflower, bok choy, collards, Brussels sprouts, and kale.

Each day try to consume a variety of colorful vegetables that are yellow, orange, red, and deep green. Choose large servings of vegetables when you eat at home, as it can be challenging to obtain quality vegetable choices when eating out. Buy fresh vegetables when you know you will consume them within a few days, and store them in the refrigerator crisper drawer. When buying fresh, remember that carrots tend to retain their nutritive value a bit longer, whereas kale, broccoli, and green beans lose nutrients a bit more quickly. If your crisper drawers have humidity settings, set the level to high humidity for leafy green vegetables to extend freshness. Most other vegetables do best at a lower humidity setting, and some, such as tomatoes and onions, are best left out at room temperature.

Frozen vegetables are a good second choice. Frozen produce may even provide more beta-carotene because it is protected from light by packaging. Fresh tomatoes contain lycopene, a powerful antioxidant; canned and jarred tomatoes and tomato sauces contain even higher levels of

TABLE **2.3**	TOP FRUIT AND VEGETABLE CHOICES

GOOD SOURCES OF VITAMIN C	GOOD SOURCES OF CAROTENOIDS AND VITAMIN A	GOOD SOURCES OF PHYTONUTRIENTS
Artichokes	Apricots	100% real fruit juices
Blackberries	Broccoli	Apples
Broccoli	Cantaloupe	Asparagus
Brussels sprouts	Carrots	Beets
Cauliflower	Guava	Blackberries
Kiwifruit	Kale	Blueberries
Mangoes	Mangoes	Cabbage
Okra	Nectarines	Cherries
Oranges	Peaches	Cirtus fruits
Papayas	Romaine lettuce	Cruciferous vegetables
Peas	Spinach	Grapes
Pineapples	Sweet peppers	Kale
Potatoes	Sweet potatoes	Onions
Strawberries	Swiss chard	Tomatoes
Tangerines	Winter squash	Watermelons
Tomatoes		

available lycopene. Frozen and canned vegetables are preferable to fresh choices that have been sitting in your crisper too long, and they are a good winter alternative to your delicious summer farmers' market produce. Frozen vegetables, like frozen fruits, should also move freely about in the package, indicating they have retained the full force of their nutritional value.

Avoid overcooking your vegetables in order to preserve all the wonderful nutrients they contain. Steaming above water level is the best choice for preserving nutrients in cooked vegetables, whereas boiling or allowing any contact with water during the cooking process results in the highest nutrient losses. When microwaving vegetables, use as little water as possible to preserve nutrient content, and check for doneness frequently to avoid overcooking them.

FITTING IN FIBER—EVERY DAY

Besides their many other benefits, wholesome and unprocessed foods provide the fiber that is such an important component of your diet. Despite the wide selection of high-fiber food choices at the supermarket, Americans obtain only about 14 grams of fiber daily, less than half of the recommended intake of 25 to 38 grams. This typical amount is not enough to obtain all of the known health benefits of fiber. Diets high in fiber can help prevent heart disease, diabetes, stroke, high blood pressure, cancer, diverticulitis, and constipation. Fiber is also available in supplement form, but it is best to obtain most of your fiber from food so that it can work its wonders in conjunction with other nutrients.

Fiber is made up of a group of indigestible carbohydrates found in plant foods. It is calorie-free, as it is not absorbed by the body. Fiber in food products may be natural dietary fiber or manufactured functional fiber, with the total sum of these two fibers being the fiber amount listed on food labels. For decades, fiber has been divided into two main categories, water-soluble and water-insoluble fiber. Both types are found in every fiber-rich food, though one usually predominates, and it is important to obtain fiber from a variety of sources. Insoluble fiber is the most familiar form and is found in wheat bran, whole-grain cereals, dried beans and peas, vegetables, and nuts. This type of fiber aids digestion, moves potentially cancerous substances through the colon, and keeps colon function regular. Water-soluble fiber acts more like a sponge and can help control blood glucose and blood cholesterol levels. Good sources of water-soluble fiber include whole oats, oat bran, some fruits, and dried beans. Fiber can also increase your feeling of fullness after consuming a meal, a useful tool for individuals trying to reduce their caloric intake and lose weight.

If you need more fiber in your diet, increase your intake slowly and drink plenty of water. Most fruits and vegetables average 2 to 3 grams of fiber per serving. Dried peas and beans are loaded with fiber, providing 6 to 8 grams per one-half cup. Whole grains can provide 2 to 3 grams of fiber per serving. Check labels to make the best choices. Nuts and seeds are also great sources.

SIFTING THROUGH THE SUGARS

For many of us, sugar is contained in foods that we view as treats or even comfort foods. Perhaps as an active athlete you feel that there is some room for sugar in your diet. There is no denying that sugar is a significant part of our diet, with Americans estimated to consume, on average, over 60 pounds (27 kg) yearly.

"Sugar" commonly refers to simple carbohydrates composed of single and double carbo-hydrate molecules. Glucose, fructose, and galactose are the monosaccharides, or single molecule carbohydrates, that serve as the carbohydrate building blocks of our diet. Disaccharides are composed of two molecules and include sucrose (table sugar) and lactose (milk sugar).

Depending on the food choices you make, the sugar in your diet is either added sugar, which is simply sugar added to food, or naturally occurring sugar, which is a natural component of foods and therefore not added in processing, preparation, or at the table. The key to smart sugar consumption is choosing the healthy natural sugars and downplaying the nonnutritive added sugars. Naturally occurring sugars include the fructose found in fruits and the lactose found in milk and yogurt. The health benefits of these foods are reviewed in other sections of this book. The food sources of these sugars are highly nutritious and contain a wide range of vitamins and minerals.

Added sugars are quite the opposite and are often found in foods low in nutritional value. Sucrose, commonly referred to as table sugar, is found mainly in dessert and snack foods with very limited nutritional value. Particularly prevalent is high-fructose corn syrup (HFCS), an added sugar produced by chemically altering cornstarch that is cheaper and sweeter than sucrose. HFCS is made up of about 55 percent fructose and 45 percent glucose. Some HFCS has higher fructose levels, at 90 percent, for an even sweeter flavor. HFCS is added to a variety of food products, including baked goods, breads, cereals, ketchup, soft drinks, and many other items, so read labels carefully. One-third of all the sugar consumed in the United States is the HFCS in soft drinks.

Recently there have been concerns regarding HFCS. Some experts contend that increased intake of HFCS is directly linked to the growing rate of obesity and type 2 diabetes in the United States. Other experts counter that it is simply the empty calories consumed from HFCS-containing products that contribute to obesity, and that weight gain is not inherent to the sweetener itself. Of course, all experts agree that this sugar is found in foods with very little nutritional value that are high in refined carbohydrates.

CONTINUES

SIFTING THROUGH THE SUGARS   continued

In many cases fruit juice is an excellent example of a natural sugar product gone bad. Any fruit juice you consume should be 100 percent juice, and not a juice drink or blend that provides some HFCS. But even real fruit juice is higher in simple sugar than whole fruit counterparts. Fruit juice also provides no fiber. Look for "100 percent fruit juice" on labels and try to avoid the cheap fillers of apple juice and white grape juice. Read the ingredient list carefully. The juices that appear at the beginning of the list are present in the greatest quantity. Juices with color tend to have more antioxidants and phytonutrients, so purple grape juice, for example, is better than white grape juice.

Sugars can make foods more palatable and need not be completely eliminated from your diet. But how much added sugar is too much? Nutritional surveys and logic indicate that as added sugar intake increases, intake of several vitamins and minerals decreases. Processed sugar calories should not replace appropriate servings of fruits, vegetables, whole grains, and low-fat dairy products, or the quality of your diet will suffer. The World Health Organization recommends limiting free sugars—that is, added sugars and the sugar occurring naturally in fruit juice—to no more than 10 percent of daily calories, a proportion significantly lower than the National Academy of Science guideline of no more than 25 percent of daily calories. One recent study estimates that 20 percent of our carbohydrate intake and 10 percent of our total calorie intake come from corn syrup alone.

Although you should try to minimize sugar in your diet, you do not have to eliminate it completely. The occasional dessert or piece of candy after a meal is fine as part of a well-balanced diet. If your active lifestyle demands an intake of 2,400 calories daily, your sugar intake should not exceed 240 calories. This leaves room for some treats in a daily diet filled with wholesome choices. You can also aim for an intake of no more than 10 teaspoons of sugar daily. One teaspoon of sugar equals 4 grams.

Nutrition labels do not distinguish between added sugars and natural sugars in a food, however. Only the "total sugars" are listed, and this total can include both types. You can determine if added sugars are a major ingredient by referring to the ingredient list. Some added sugars to look for on the label include beet juice, brown rice syrup, cane syrup, corn syrup, corn sweetener, crystalline fructose, dextrose, evaporated cane juice, fructose, high-fructose corn syrup, invert sugar, malt syrup, maltodextrin, and sucrose. The closer the terms are to the beginning of the ingredient list, the greater the amount of added sugar in the product.

High-fiber foods should be part of your daily diet but may not be the best choices immediately before training and close to competition, as they may cause intestinal discomfort with exercise. For the athlete who benefits from a comfortable stomach and intestinal system during exercise, fiber intake is not only about health but also about consuming the correct amounts at the safest times.

PROTEIN POWER

While wholesome carbohydrates are a staple in an athlete's diet, endurance athletes interested in maximizing power and strength as well as building endurance also need adequate amounts of protein foods for top performance. Power athletes especially gravitate toward high protein intakes, but endurance athletes need high amounts of protein as well. This is because you burn some level of protein during training, you have a higher level of muscle mass than your sedentary counterpart, and you need to recover from the muscle damage that can occur during training.

Protein plays an important role in the growth, repair, and maintenance of muscles and other tissues in your body, such as tendons, ligaments, skin, hair, and nails. It is also required to form hormones, enzymes, and neurotransmitters, all of which perform essential functions in your body, and it is the key component of your immune system. Protein is needed for the formation of hemoglobin, the substance that carries oxygen to the exercising muscles, and can even serve as a fuel source during endurance exercise if your body's carbohydrate stores run low. Protein is also crucial to controlling fluid volume in the body and maintaining water balance.

Proteins are composed of amino acids, which are the building units that create protein-based tissues. We obtain amino acids from the protein-containing foods we consume and from the breakdown of our muscle tissue. Amino acids that can be manufactured by our body are considered nonessential to our diet, as it is not required that we consume them from food. Conversely, amino acids that we cannot manufacture in our body are considered essential to our diet and must be obtained in adequate amounts for good health and optimal performance. Both essential and nonessential proteins perform all the important functions required of proteins. The terms can be misleading: In reality, "nonessential" amino acids are just as essential as "essential" ones to the proper functioning of the human body—we just do not need to obtain them from the foods we eat.

Proteins that we consume are digested into smaller protein molecules called polypeptides and eventually into the individual amino acids, which then go to the amino acid pool in your body. These amino acids can be drawn upon to synthesize protein-based tissues or can be used as energy if carbohydrate stores run low. The best way to ensure that your body can manufacture all the needed proteins is to consume a wide array of amino acids from a variety of foods and consume an adequate number of calories. With these ingredients, your body can synthesize proteins as needed.

The dietary protein intake of an endurance athlete can easily make up 15 to 20 percent of his or her daily energy consumption, though amounts of 12 to 15 percent may be more than adequate on many training days. Higher amounts are needed when there has been greater muscle damage from hard training. More protein is burned for fuel when your body's stores of carbohydrates or glycogen run low. Burning protein for energy creates some metabolic waste, however, and it is not the most efficient or cleanest way for an endurance athlete to burn fuel. This use of protein for training fuel is best prevented by eating a diet adequate in carbohydrates and by consuming carbohydrates during training.

For many athletes, daily protein intake actually exceeds protein requirements. Our culture encourages large protein portions, so generally our athletes get plenty of protein to meet their body's needs. Some athletes, however, may restrict certain foods in an attempt to limit or avoid fat intake, possibly placing themselves at risk. Consuming inadequate protein can interfere with regulation of metabolism in the formation of hormones and enzymes. Insufficient protein can also hinder muscle recovery in the hours after training because of protein's essential role in the building and repair of muscle tissue. Your protein requirements can change depending on your current training cycle and day-to-day variations in your training program, but on even the most demanding training days it should not be difficult to obtain adequate amounts of protein in your diet. If you consume too much protein, your body can either store the excess as fat or burn it for energy—which, again, is to be avoided.

Animal foods such as lean meats, poultry, fish, and eggs are the foods most concentrated in protein. Many of these animal proteins are also good sources of iron and zinc. High-quality plant sources of protein include soy products such as tofu and tempeh, dried peas and beans, and lentils. Low-fat dairy products are also an excellent source of protein as well as of the mineral calcium. What is important for optimal health is to choose lean protein sources, as this will reduce your intake of saturated fat. Too high an intake of saturated fat is a risk factor for developing heart disease. Table 2.4 lists the protein content of certain foods per specified portion. Try to emphasize leaner choices of beef, lamb, and pork to limit your intake of saturated fat. Cheese is also high in saturated fat. Plant foods can also contribute to your total daily protein intake, although they do not provide the same quality or amount of protein as animal sources do. More discussion of protein choices and protein requirements for specific types of training is provided in Part II.

FAT: FACTS AND FIGURES

Fat is an important part of anyone's diet, but the role it plays for an endurance athlete is somewhat different from the role it plays for the typical sedentary person. Although fat is well-known

TABLE **2.4**	**PROTEIN CONTENT OF FOODS**

FOOD	PORTION	PROTEIN (g)
Animal foods		
Chicken, white	3 oz. (100 g)	25
Pork, lean	3 oz. (100 g)	23
Beef, lean	3 oz. (100 g)	21
Fish, white	3 oz. (100 g)	20
Eggs	2 whole	13
Legumes and soy products		
Tofu, firm	4 oz. (120 g)	20
Lentils, cooked	1 c. (240 ml)	18
Kidney beans, cooked	1 c. (240 ml)	17
Tempeh	½ c. (120 ml)	16
Black beans, cooked	1 c. (240 ml)	15
Soy milk	1 c. (240 ml)	10
Dairy products		
Milk	8 oz. (240 ml)	8
Yogurt	6 oz. (180 ml)	8
Cheese	1 oz. (30 g)	7
Nuts and seeds		
Peanut butter	2 tbsp. (40 ml)	8
Sunflower seeds	1 oz. (30 g)	6.5
Almonds	1 oz. (30 g)	6
Cashews	1 oz. (30 g)	4.5
Vegetables		
Potato	5 oz. (150 g)	5
Broccoli	1 c. (240 ml)	5
Carrots	1 c. (240 ml)	2

as a concentrated source of calories, and often shunned for that very reason, it does play several key roles in keeping you healthy. Most important, fat is a source of nutrients known as *essential fatty acids.* Just as you need to obtain vitamins and minerals in your daily diet, the two essential fatty acids, linoleic acid and alpha-linolenic acid, must also come from the foods you eat.

BEING A VEGETARIAN ATHLETE

In recent years, many nutritionally aware athletes have decreased their intake of specific proteins, such as meats high in saturated fats. Some have gone a step further and replaced animal proteins with plant proteins. Vegetarians are individuals who have consciously made the choice to completely exclude animal foods from their diet, or to include only specific animal foods, such as dairy products, eggs, or fish, and obtain a significant portion or all of their protein from plant foods. Whether these dietary modifications are for health, environmental, ideological, or taste-related reasons, vegetarians need to pay close attention to their nutrition program to ensure adequate protein consumption and sufficient intake of specific vitamins and minerals. Vegetarian athletes must design a well-balanced diet suited to their training program.

"Vegetarianism" is a term that actually incorporates a range of dietary exclusions. A plant-based vegetarian diet may refer to one of the following descriptions:

Semi- or Near-Vegetarians: Eat small amounts of fish, poultry, eggs, and dairy products and avoid red meat.
Pesco-Vegetarians: Eat fish, dairy products, and eggs.
Lacto-Ovo Vegetarians: Eat dairy products and eggs.
Ovo-Vegetarians: Eat eggs.
Vegans: Eat no animal foods whatsoever.

If you are a vegetarian, you need to carefully choose foods that provide specific nutrients in your diet. These nutrients include protein, of course, but also iron and zinc, and—particularly if you exclude dairy products—vitamin B12, calcium, and vitamin D.

CONTINUES

Essential fatty acids help maintain the integrity of cell membranes and play a role in the growth, reproduction, and maintenance of skin tissue as well as general body functioning. Another important function of fat is its role in the transport and absorption of the fat-soluble vitamins A, D, E, and K as well as the carotenoids. Of course, fat can also add a wonderful flavor to our meals and make them more filling and satisfying.

Much has been made of the quantity of fat consumed in the North American diet. A high fat content often characterizes convenience foods, restaurant meals, and especially fast foods. Fats are a concentrated source of calories, and excess fat beyond your requirement does not provide optimal fuel for your body and can even crowd out valuable complex carbohydrates and proteins.

Throughout this book, the unique considerations of vegetarian athletes will be addressed in regard to specific nutrients. Of course, any athlete can choose to include more plant sources of specific nutrients—including high-quality plant proteins—in his or her diet. Plant foods are filled with health-promoting minerals and other nutrients. Vegetarians appear to have a lower risk of developing hypertension, certain cancers, heart disease, and diabetes. A plant-based diet also supplies plenty of carbohydrates for replenishing body-fuel stores after training. Filling up on whole grains, fruits, and vegetables benefits any endurance sport athlete. Milk and yogurt, though sources of high-quality protein, add nice amounts of carbohydrate to your diet as well.

Like a diet containing meat and other animal protein, a vegetarian diet can be well planned and support your training efforts, or it can be overly restrictive, poorly planned, and counterproductive.

Generally, endurance athletes may need anywhere from 20 to 25 percent of their dietary calories to be derived from fat. Consuming excess fat, or "fat loading," does not appear to improve performance. But it is important that endurance athletes consume adequate fat to replace the fat stored in the muscle for fuel, especially on days that include four or more hours of training. It is fairly easy to consume plenty of fat in the typical North American diet, and lowering your fat intake to the right balance for optimal training takes planning and knowledge. Another important consideration is that many North Americans don't consume the best types of fat and may need to increase their intake of specific essential fatty acids. Oils, butter, and margarine are all fats, also referred to as *lipids*, but they differ in some of their characteristics. Lipids that are solid at room temperature are called "fats," while lipids that are liquid at room temperature are called "oils."

Fat comes in several chemical forms, some of which are healthier than others. Depending on their composition, fats are categorized as *saturated* or *unsaturated*. Unsaturated fats include both polyunsaturated and monounsaturated fats. Currently the American Heart Association sets the recommended range of fat intake as from 15 to 30 percent of total calories. Exceeding this range may increase the risk of heart disease, while going below it could result in essential fatty acid insufficiency in some individuals. The most important general rule is to limit the amount of saturated and hydrogenated fats, or *trans fats*, that you consume to 10 percent or less of your total caloric intake in order to prevent heart disease. Saturated fats and the trans fat produced from hydrogenation of liquid oils raise the harmful low-density lipoprotein (LDL) cholesterol, and trans fat can also lower the beneficial high-density lipoprotein (HDL) cholesterol. Undesirable saturated fat is found mainly in fatty animal foods such as cheese and whole-milk products, fatty cuts of meat, highly processed lunchmeats, butter, lard, and shortening. Palm, palm kernel, and coconut oil are three highly saturated plant oils sometimes found in processed foods and commercial baked goods.

Trans-fatty acids are created from liquid oils that are "partially hydrogenated." Hydrogenation turns liquid corn oil into margarine sticks and increases the shelf life of commercial products that contain the altered oils. Some common sources of trans fat are cookies, crackers, and snack chips. Check labels to limit hydrogenated oils as much as possible, particularly if they are listed as one of the first several ingredients. If you consume margarine, choose products that list "liquid oil" as the first ingredient and that are marked as being "trans-fat free" per serving. Labels now list the trans fat content of a serving and can be marked as containing zero grams of trans fat if they have less than 0.5 gram of trans fat per serving.

Unsaturated fats can help lower LDL cholesterol when they replace saturated fats in your diet. Corn oil, safflower oil, sunflower oil, and walnut oil are all polyunsaturated. These oils should make up no more than one-third of your total fat intake and should be consumed in liquid form. Most health-care professionals advocate that monounsaturated fats constitute the majority of your fat intake. Many cultures that consume ample amounts of olive oil seem to have a decreased risk of heart disease, and monounsaturated fat seems to be the fat of choice for other health concerns as well. Good monounsaturated oils include olive oil, canola oil, avocado oil, almond oil, and hazelnut oil. Table 2.5 outlines the types of fats contained in various oils.

Unfortunately, what has gotten lost in some of this heart-healthy advice about monounsaturated oils is that some polyunsaturated fats should also be included in your diet. Linoleic and alpha-linolenic essential fatty acids are both polyunsaturated fats, but they differ greatly in how they affect health. Linoleic acid is from a family of fats known as "omega-6" fats; alpha-linolenic acid is from the "omega-3" family of fats. Two other omega-3 fats, and two of the most potent, are docosahexaenoic acid (DHA) and eicosapentaenoic acid (EPA), both of which are abundant in fish such as salmon and tuna. The body can convert alpha-linolenic acid in plant foods to the more potent EPA, though only about 10 percent of the alpha-linolenic acid consumed is converted in this way.

DHA and EPA are of great interest to health experts. Consuming these fats, as well as alpha-linolenic acid, is necessary to produce hormone-like compounds that can reduce unnecessary blood clotting, boost immune function, and reduce inflammation. High intakes of DHA and EPA may help to prevent heart disease and stroke and may improve conditions such as rheumatoid arthritis and depression. Conversely, excess linoleic acid can produce hormones that lead to inflammation, promote blood clotting, and constrict arteries. Linoleic competes with alpha-linolenic

TABLE **2.5**	PERCENTAGES OF FAT IN VARIOUS OILS		

OIL	% SATURATED	% POLYUNSATURATED	% MONOUNSATURATED
Canola	6	32	62
Hazelnut	7	11	82
Flaxseed	7	75	18
Safflower	7	79	14
Almond	8	19	73
Walnut	9	67	24
Grapeseed	10	73	17
Sunflower	11	69	20
Corn	13	62	25
Olive	14	9	77
Pumpkin seed	15	53	15
Soybean	15	61	24
Sesame	15	44	41
Margarine (tub)*	17	34	24
Wheat germ	17	61	22
Peanut	18	34	48
Rice bran	26	28	46
Cottonseed	27	54	19
Lard	41	12	47
Palm kernel	85	2	11
Coconut	92	2	6

*ALSO CONTAINS SOME TRANS-FATTY ACIDS. DIFFERENT BRANDS OF MARGARINE CONTAIN VARYING LEVELS OF HYDROGENATED OILS. SOME LABELED AS TRANS-FAT FREE ARE AVAILABLE.

acid, DHA, and EPA for use by the body; it is best not to consume an excess of linoleic acid and to make sure that you consume enough of the healthy omega-3 fatty acids.

Keep in mind that all of these essential fats are good for you. But what is desirable is to obtain the proper balance of essential fatty acids in your diet. Most North Americans consume an excess of linoleic fat (omega-6) and need to increase their intake of alpha-linolenic acid, EPA, and DHA (omega-3). Table 2.6 will guide you in choosing food sources of these fats. Try to emphasize fatty fish, and use soy and canola oils. Although olive oil is an excellent source of the healthy monounsaturated fat, it supplies very little of the essential fatty acids. Other good plant

TABLE **2.6**	FOOD SOURCES OF ESSENTIAL FATTY ACIDS

FOODS RICH IN ALPHA-LINOLENIC OMEGA-3 FATTY ACIDS

Food	Portion	Alpha-Linolenic Acid Content (g)
Flax oil	1 tbsp. (20 ml)	6.6
Canola oil	1 tbsp. (20 ml)	1.6
Soybean oil	1 tbsp. (20 ml)	1.0
Walnut oil	1 tbsp. (20 ml)	1.4
Flaxseed, ground	1 tbsp. (20 ml)	1.8
Soy nuts, roasted	½ c. (120 ml)	1.8
Tofu, firm	½ c. (120 ml)	0.7
Soy milk	1 c. (240 ml)	0.4
Legumes	½ c. (120 ml)	0.05
Oat germ	2 tbsp. (40 ml)	0.2
Wheat germ	2 tbsp. (40 ml)	0.1
Sardines	2 oz. (60 g)	0.28
Spinach, cooked	1 c. (240 ml)	0.15
Kale, cooked	1 c. (240 ml)	0.13
Almond butter	2 tbsp. (40 ml)	0.12

FOODS RICH IN EPA AND DHA OMEGA-3 FATTY ACIDS

Food	Portion	EPA + DHA Content (g)
Farmed Atlantic salmon	3 oz. (90 g), cooked	1.8
Herring, cooked	3 oz. (90 g), cooked	1.7
Wild Atlantic salmon	3 oz. (90 g), cooked	1.6
Blue fin tuna	3 oz. (90 g), cooked	1.3
Sockeye salmon, canned	3 oz. (90 g), cooked	1.3
Atlantic mackerel	3 oz. (90 g), cooked	1.0
Farmed rainbow trout	3 oz. (90 g), cooked	1.0
Wild rainbow trout	3 oz. (90 g), cooked	0.8
Sardines, canned	3 oz. (90 g), cooked	0.8
Swordfish	3 oz. (90 g), cooked	0.7
Mussels	3 oz. (90 g), cooked	0.7
Sole	3 oz. (90 g), cooked	0.4
Tuna, white meat, canned	3 oz. (90 g), cooked	0.2
Wild catfish	3 oz. (90 g), cooked	0.2
Farmed catfish	3 oz. (90 g), cooked	0.1
Atlantic cod	3 oz. (90 g), cooked	0.1

CONTINUES

TABLE **2.6**	FOOD SOURCES OF ESSENTIAL FATTY ACIDS continued

FOODS RICH IN LINOLEIC AND OMEGA-6 FATTY ACIDS

Food	Portion	Linoleic Acid Content (g)
Safflower oil	1 tbsp. (20 ml)	10.1
Sunflower oil	1 tbsp. (20 ml)	9.2
Corn oil	1 tbsp. (20 ml)	7.8
Soybean oil	1 tbsp. (20 ml)	6.9
Walnuts	1 oz. (30 g)	11
Soy nuts, roasted	½ c. (120 ml)	9.0
Brazil nuts	1 oz. (30 g)	7.0
Pecans	1 oz. (30 g)	6.0
Tofu, firm	4 oz. (120 g)	5.4
Peanuts	1 oz. (30 g)	4.5
Peanut butter	2 tbsp. (40 ml)	4.4
Almonds	1 oz. (30 g)	3.0
Almond butter	2 tbsp. (40 ml)	3.8
Wheat germ	2 tbsp. (40 ml)	0.8
Flaxseed, ground	1 tbsp. (20 ml)	0.5

SOURCES: USDA NUTRIENT DATABASE, RELEASE 14, 2001; USDA NUTRIENT DATABASE, RELEASE 15, 2002.

sources of alpha-linolenic acid are leafy green vegetables, walnuts, and flaxseed. Several foods are listed under both essential fatty acid headings, as they are rich in both. Though scientists are still formulating specific recommendations, aim for a minimum of 2 grams of omega-3 fatty acids daily.

To emphasize the best fat choices, you can balance your intake in the following way:

- Consume fish such as salmon, light tuna, sole, and tilapia twice or more weekly.
- Emphasize soy and canola oils and related products, and use olive oil as well.
- Have green leafy vegetables, walnuts, and ground flaxseeds in your diet.
- Choose the leanest cuts of red meat possible.
- Limit fatty cheeses.
- Emphasize poultry, beans, lentils, and soy protein in your diet.
- Control margarine intake and choose products with liquid oil as the first ingredient.
- Avoid processed foods that contain partially hydrogenated oils and trans fats.

CONSUMING FISH OILS SAFELY

Fish is good for you because it is a great source of omega-3 fatty acids, which can reduce disease risk and enhance health. But when you consume fish, it would be appropriate to take into consideration choices that will minimize your mercury intake. Mercury is present in our air and water and when converted to methyl-mercury can accumulate in fish and humans. Methyl-mercury is a known toxin to developing fetuses, small babies, and children and is now considered a potential threat to adults as well. Mercury can damage the brain and nervous system and cause symptoms such as fatigue and hair loss.

The health benefits of eating fish do outweigh these risks, if you make good choices regarding the type and amount of fish consumed. Currently the American Heart Association recommends eating fish twice weekly. Generally you can keep your total fish portions to about 12 ounces weekly, though mercury's effects are somewhat dose related based on body weight.

Next, try to choose types of fish that tend to be low in mercury. Those highest in mercury are shark, swordfish, king mackerel, and tilefish. Other high-mercury fish are fresh tuna, red snapper, orange roughy, and marlin. Some types of fish and shellfish that tend to be lower in mercury are shrimp, salmon, pollack, catfish, tilapia, sardines, and sole. Canned white albacore tuna contains more mercury than canned light tuna and should be limited. Other fish fairly low in mercury are haddock, herring, and whitefish.

Many salmon lovers are also concerned about the cancer-causing polychlorinated biphenyls (PCBs) in fish. Testing indicates that both farmed and wild salmon are contaminated with PCBs, with the farmed varieties containing much higher amounts. Farmed varieties from both the United States and Canada contain lower amounts of PCBs than those from European countries, but the levels present in all farmed salmon are much higher than in wild varieties. When it is in season, choose wild Alaska salmon, which is lowest in PCBs. Canned salmon, which comes almost exclusively from the wild Alaskan variety, is also a good choice. Since September 2004, all seafood has been labeled as farmed or wild. The country of origin is also now marked. This labeling requirement should be a great help to consumers who wish to include fish in their diet on a regular basis without including harmful toxins.

Fish oil supplements are another option for obtaining DHA and EPA omega-3 fatty acids in your diet. In fact, it may be safer to take fish oil supplements than to eat the amount of fish needed

CONTINUES

CONSUMING FISH OILS SAFELY   continued

to obtain the same level of these beneficial substances. Lab analysis has shown supplements to be free of mercury, PCBs, and dioxins. Mercury accumulates in the muscle tissue of fish, not the fat tissue that is the source of most fish oil. One exception is cod liver oil, which comes from fish liver, where toxins do accumulate. Fish oils are also processed to remove any toxins. Look for brands that have been "distilled" or "deodorized."

If this option appeals to you, discuss taking fish oil supplements with your physician. Some people with heart disease may be placed on therapeutic doses ranging from 1 to 3 grams daily, but the higher doses require medical monitoring. Large doses can sometimes cause nausea or burping. People who take blood-thinning medications, who have a history of a bleeding stroke, or who are scheduled for surgery should not take EPA and DHA supplements. If you take a fish oil supplement, choose a brand that contains both DHA and EPA in the highest level that you can tolerate in one pill. Supplements are better absorbed when taken with meals.

3

VITAMINS, MINERALS, AND
ELECTROLYTES

The Nuts, Bolts, and Spark Plugs of Your Diet

AS AN ENDURANCE ATHLETE, you no doubt have more than a passing interest in getting the vitamins and minerals you need in your diet. These nutrients are important for everyone, but for an endurance athlete they are crucially important. Because of your training and the stress it imposes on your body, you may need higher amounts of vitamins and minerals than your sedentary counterparts. And, as an athlete, you have a highly vested interest in keeping your immune system healthy so that illness does not put a halt to training, especially during the peak of race season. Athletes have long been advised by sports dietitians to consume high-quality foods for an optimal nutrient intake, but many advertisers touting their products suggest that athletes require megadoses of specific nutrients. Some endurance athletes rely on high-dose supplementation, and vitamins and minerals are now added to many sports nutrition products such as energy bars and recovery drinks. Are the claims of these advertisers correct? Vitamins and minerals are indeed essential to good health and maximum performance, but how much of these essential ingredients do you need?

Of course, choosing foods that provide you with adequate amounts of vitamins and minerals is necessary for optimal performance. Vitamins and minerals are essential for metabolizing energy, building body tissue, maintaining fluid balance, and carrying oxygen in the body. Vitamins and minerals also play a role in reducing the oxidative stress that is brought on by endurance training. Correcting any dietary inadequacies could even improve your performance. Depending on your health status, typical dietary intake, and specific nutrient needs, you may need to supplement your diet in an educated fashion. Certain groups of athletes may benefit from nutrient supplementation beyond the basic assurance of a daily multivitamin and mineral supplement. However, research has not conclusively proven that taking "extra" amounts of vitamins and minerals when no deficiency is present will enable an athlete to train harder or longer. In fact, in some cases taking too many supplements can be harmful—large doses of the fat-soluble vitamins A, D, E, and K, for example, can be toxic, and megadoses of even some of the water-soluble vitamins can cause problems.

Although all vitamins and minerals—in the correct amounts—are important components of anyone's diet, endurance athletes should be aware of the nutrients that are especially suitable for meeting their unique health and training needs. A well-balanced diet that includes a wide variety of nutritious foods can provide ample amounts of vitamins, minerals, and phytochemicals. And as an endurance athlete, you have higher energy needs than the average sedentary person because of the time you spend training, which means that you can eat more of the nutrient-rich foods your body requires. You should also keep in mind that nutrients exist together in foods in the proper balance, which is not the case with capsules, pills, and specially formulated powders or drinks. This chapter discusses your vitamin and mineral requirements for exercise, the functions of these nutrients in your body, optimal food sources of these nutrients, and appropriate reasons and guidelines for supplementation.

VITAMINS

Vitamins, any of thirteen organic compounds found in small amounts in foods, play important roles in many physiological processes. During prolonged or vigorous exercise, extra demands are placed on your body that intensify these processes—in other words, your body has to work extra hard to train, to perform in competition, and to heal during the recovery phase, and this work draws upon your body's vitamin and mineral reserves. To ensure that these body processes function optimally, you should try to maintain high levels of these nutrient reserves. Although inadequate intake of vitamins is known to result in deficiencies, whether it will adversely impact your performance depends on the extent of the deficiency. Extreme deficiencies are not very commonplace in North America, and many dietary inadequacies can be corrected by making the proper food choices.

Athletes most likely to have problems with an inadequate vitamin intake are those following a restricted-calorie diet for weight loss, those who have adopted an extreme or fad diet, and sometimes, those on a restrictive vegetarian diet. Overall, however, athletes training and competing in endurance sports can greatly minimize their risk of vitamin deficiency by consuming a wide variety of nutrient-dense foods and adequate calories to match their training needs.

Vitamins play a major role in catalyzing energy-production reactions from body-fuel stores. For instance, a number of B vitamins are essential to converting carbohydrates into energy for

OPTIMAL HEALTH AND DIETARY REFERENCE INTAKES

The Dietary Reference Intake (DRI) system, developed by the Food and Nutrition Board of the National Academy of Sciences in the 1990s, is designed to reflect the health goals of the twenty-first century. It is hoped that rather than merely preventing nutrient deficiencies, these latest guidelines for nutrient intakes will optimize health by reducing the risk of chronic diseases such as heart disease, cancer, and osteoporosis.

The DRI system includes four classifications:

Recommended Daily Allowance (RDA): The RDA is the amount of a nutrient that should decrease the risk of chronic disease for most healthy individuals in a specified age group and gender. It is based on estimating the average requirement plus an increase to account for individual variation. The RDA may serve as a goal for individuals who desire to ensure adequate daily nutrition. You may also see the term "% Daily Value" or "%DV" on food labels. The Daily Value is a reference number based on the RDA and developed to help consumers determine whether a food contains a little or a lot of a specific nutrient. On the Nutrition Facts label, %DVs are based on a 2,000-calorie diet. If a food contains over 20 percent of the Daily Value in one serving, it is considered to be a good source of that nutrient.

The RDA is a good starting point for athletes who wish to determine the nutritional adequacy of their diet. Athletes of all ages are likely to have energy requirements higher than the average person, and some vitamins and minerals are required to process this energy. Endurance athletes may also have a higher nutrient intake than the average person, however, simply because of their high energy needs and quality food choices.

Adequate Intake (AI): The AI is used when there is not enough scientific evidence to set an RDA. It is a recommended daily intake based on observed or experimentally determined approximations of nutrient intake by a group of healthy people. The AI can be used as a goal for individual intake when an RDA does not exist.

Estimated Average Requirement (EAR): The EAR is the nutrient value estimated to meet the requirements of half of the healthy individuals in a given group. The EAR represents the average nutrient intake required to maintain a specific body function. For example, the EAR for vitamin C is set at a level that prevents scurvy, a deficiency disease. The EAR is used to develop the RDA, assess adequacy of intakes, and plan diets for population groups.

CONTINUES

Tolerable Upper Intake Level (UL): The UL is the highest daily intake level of a nutrient, from both food and supplement sources, thought to be within safe limits. If it is exceeded, individuals may experience adverse or toxic health effects. This is not a recommended amount, but rather an upper limit. For most nutrients, the UL refers to the total amount obtained from food intake, fortified foods, and supplements. This number can provide guidance to athletes who consume numerous such fortified foods, take various vitamin and mineral supplements, and frequently use sports nutrition products that are supplemented with nutrients.

muscular contraction. Vitamins themselves do not directly provide energy, which must be obtained from consuming carbohydrates, protein, and fat. The vitamins B12, B6, and folic acid play an important role in the development of red blood cells, which deliver oxygen to your exercising muscles. Vitamins are also involved in tissue repair and protein synthesis. Several vitamins, such as E and C, are antioxidants that protect cells from potentially toxic free radicals. Free radicals are unstable molecules produced by oxygen-related reactions in the body and have been implicated in contributing to a number of diseases. Each vitamin is unique in the functions it performs in the body and in how it interacts with other dietary nutrients.

Vitamins are separated into two classifications: fat-soluble and water-soluble. Your body may contain large stores of the fat-soluble variety—A, D, E, and K. Deficiencies of these nutrients are rare, though excessive intakes may have toxic effects. The water-soluble variety—which includes vitamin C and the eight B vitamins, thiamin (B1), riboflavin (B2), pyridoxine (B6), niacin, B12, folacin, biotin, and pantothenic acid—are not stored in your body in significant amounts. Harmful effects of excessive intakes of these water-soluble vitamins are not as likely, though there are exceptions. Appendix B provides a list of vitamins, their functions, Dietary Reference Intakes (DRIs), and food sources.

B VITAMINS

Because of their role in processing energy from the metabolism of carbohydrates, B vitamins have received much attention from athletes. However, several of these vitamins are easily obtained from a variety of carbohydrate-rich foods, such as breads, cereals, brown rice, wheat germ, and vegetables, and certain B vitamins are also found in protein-rich foods that are found in relatively high amounts in the high-energy athlete's diet, such as dairy milk and yogurt, pork, fish, and poultry. Often the intake of the B vitamins easily exceeds the RDAs when an endurance athlete consumes the calories required for training and competing from a healthy diet.

THIAMIN AND RIBOFLAVIN

Thiamin, or vitamin B1, is present in a wide variety of food sources besides whole grains, including nuts, dried peas and beans, and pork. It plays an important role in deriving energy from carbohydrates. A thiamin deficiency is unlikely to occur in athletes. Many athletes with high energy needs likely consume thiamin well above the current RDA of 1.2 milligrams daily.

Riboflavin is also involved in energy production from carbohydrates, proteins, and fats. Vegetarians should pay attention to their riboflavin intake, as milk, meat, and eggs are good sources. Some plant sources include brewer's yeast, wheat germ, soybeans, avocados, green leafy vegetables, and enriched bread and cereals. Training for your sport may slightly increase your riboflavin requirements, but the higher amounts are easily met in a well-balanced diet.

PYRIDOXINE AND NIACIN

Pyridoxine, or vitamin B6, is found mainly in whole-grain cereals, brown rice, wheat germ, bananas, legumes, fish, and poultry. This vitamin is closely linked to protein metabolism, the manufacture of muscle and hemoglobin, and the breakdown of muscle glycogen. Athletes who consume adequate calories should get plenty of vitamin B6 in their diets. Though most water-soluble vitamins are easily excreted, excess supplementation of B6 can present a problem. Doses of more than 1 gram daily over several months may cause numbness and even paralysis. Symptoms have also been experienced with chronic doses as low as 200 milligrams daily.

Niacin is involved not only in carbohydrate, protein, and fat metabolism but also in glycogen synthesis and cellular metabolism. Good food sources of niacin are meat, whole or enriched grains, nuts, seeds, and dried beans. Because niacin occurs in such a wide variety of foods, it is relatively easy to obtain enough of it in your diet. In fact, excess niacin from oversupplementation can block the release of free fatty acids, resulting in greater use of muscle glycogen and thereby depleting a limited energy source for exercise. Large doses may actually reduce performance.

VITAMIN B12

Vitamin B12 plays a major role in red blood cell development, folic acid metabolism, and DNA development, among other important functions. Your vitamin B12 needs are easily met by consuming animal foods, but vegetarian athletes, especially strict vegans, should pay close attention to their B12 intake. If you consume eggs and dairy foods, your intake levels should be fine. The only plant foods that can be counted on for their B12 content are those that have been fortified with this vitamin, such as soy milk, soy burgers, and some breakfast cereals. Plant proteins such as tempeh and miso may not contain the active form of vitamin B12, however. The human intestinal tract does make some vitamin B12, but this form is generally not well absorbed.

Although the Recommended Daily Allowance (RDA) for this vitamin is relatively low, a deficiency can have serious implications and even lead to irreversible nerve damage. Vegans who do not regularly consume fortified foods should take a vitamin B12 supplement providing 100 percent of the Daily Value (DV), and consume foods fortified with B12.

Megadoses of this vitamin are not needed or recommended. However, endurance athletes have routinely taken high doses of this vitamin for years, often injecting the nutrient during periods of heavy training. There is no evidence to suggest that this improves performance.

FOLACIN

Folacin is a B vitamin that has deservedly received much increased attention from health professionals over the past several years. *Folacin* is the collective term for folate, folic acid, and other forms of the vitamin. Folate is the form found naturally in foods, and folic acid is the form of the vitamin found most often in your body and added to foods and supplements. Folic acid is actually absorbed twice as well as the folate that occurs naturally in foods.

Since January 1998, manufacturers have been required to add folic acid to all enriched products, including flour, bread, rolls, grits, cornmeal, rice, pasta, and noodles. There is good reason for this fortification. Obtaining enough folic acid in the early weeks of pregnancy can significantly reduce the risk of neural tube defects such as spina bifida in newborns. Prior to fortification, most Americans consumed only about 200 micrograms of folic acid daily, falling short of the recommended 400 micrograms. Fortification will prevent a significant number of neural tube defects.

But this fortification may not only benefit pregnant women and newborns. Evidence is building that folic acid may reduce the risk of heart disease, stroke, and certain cancers. Folic acid helps reduce blood levels of the amino acid homocysteine. Researchers are still trying to determine if high levels of homocysteine are a strong predictor for heart disease and stroke. Keeping homocysteine low also requires adequate intake of the vitamins B6 and B12. Thirty percent of all older Americans don't produce enough stomach acid to absorb the B12 found in foods. Synthetic B12, however, doesn't have this stomach acid dependency. Connections between folic acid and the prevention of cervical cancer and colorectal cancer, through prevention of damage to DNA, have also been suggested.

Many researchers suggest that individuals over the age of fifty take a supplement providing the RDA of folic acid, B12, and B6 (high doses are not advised). Older individuals are also more likely to take medications that interfere with folic acid absorption.

TABLE **3.1**	FOLATE-RICH FOODS	
FOOD	**PORTION**	**FOLATE CONTENT (mg)**
Lentils, cooked	1 c. (240 ml)	358
Yeast, brewer's	1 tbsp. (20 ml)	312
Liver, beef	3 oz. (90 g)	285
Garbanzo beans, cooked	1 c. (240 ml)	282
Kidney beans, cooked	1 c. (240 ml)	229
Turnip greens, cooked	1 c. (240 ml)	171
Asparagus, boiled	6 spears	131
Beans, white, baked	1 c. (240 ml)	122
Orange juice	1 c. (240 ml)	110
Spinach, raw, chopped	1 c. (240 ml)	108
Mustard greens, cooked	1 c. (240 ml)	103
Broccoli, cooked	1 c. (240 ml)	78
Romaine lettuce	1 c. (240 ml)	76
Endive	1 c. (240 ml)	72
Wheat germ, raw	¼ c. (60 ml)	70

Of course, every athlete should increase the intake of folate-rich foods because of folate's relationship to maintaining red blood cells. Folate deficiencies can lead to alterations in protein synthesis and a type of anemia called *megaloblastic anemia*. Try to obtain folate from fresh foods, since it is easily destroyed by long storage times and common cooking techniques. Romaine lettuce is a great source; for other examples, see Table 3.1.

BIOTIN AND PANTOTHENIC ACID

Biotin plays a role in glucose production, in carbohydrate metabolism, and in the synthesis of glycogen and proteins. It is found in egg yolks, peanuts, walnuts, pecans, and yeast. Because biotin can also be synthesized by bacteria in the intestines, a biotin deficiency is rare. Pantothenic acid is part of a compound, coenzyme A, that plays an important role in carbohydrate, protein, and fat metabolism. Pantothenic acid is found in a wide variety of foods, with meat, whole grains, beans, and peas being the best sources.

TABLE **3.2**	FOOD SOURCES OF VITAMINS C AND E	

FOOD	PORTION	VITAMIN C (mg)
Pepper, green	1 large	130
Orange juice	1 c. (240 ml)	124
Cranberry juice	1 c. (240 ml)	108
Grapefruit juice	1 c. (240 ml)	94
Broccoli, cooked	½ c. (200 ml)	90
Brussels sprouts, cooked	7	85
Strawberries, raw	1 c. (240 ml)	85
Orange, navel	1	80
Kiwi	1 medium	75
Cantaloupe pieces	1 c. (240 ml)	70
Cauliflower, cooked	1 c. (240 ml)	65
FOOD	**PORTION**	**VITAMIN E (IU)**
Wheat germ oil	1 tbsp. (20 ml)	25
Sunflower seeds	1 oz. (30 g)	21
Almonds	1 oz. (30 g)	11
Sunflower oil	1 tbsp. (20 ml)	10
Wheat germ	1 oz. (30 g)	5
Margarine, soft	1 tbsp. (20 ml)	3
Mayonnaise	1 tbsp. (20 ml)	3
Brown rice	1 c. (240 ml)	3
Mango	1 medium	3
Asparagus	4 spears	2

VITAMIN C

Another water-soluble vitamin of interest to and heavily marketed to athletes is vitamin C. Several important functions of this vitamin impact athletes. It is necessary for the formation of connective tissue, cartilage, bone, skin, and tendons and is involved in the healing of wounds, fractures, and bruises. It also plays a role in the production of certain hormones and neurotransmitters that are secreted during exercise, in iron absorption, and in the formation of red blood cells. This vitamin is also strongly promoted because of its role as a powerful antioxidant. Symptoms of vitamin C deficiency could impair athletic performance.

Despite being a water-soluble vitamin that is easily excreted, the human body actually has a pool of vitamin C stores ranging from 1.5 to 3 grams. Serious vitamin C deficiencies are rare because fresh or frozen fruits and vegetables are so abundant in our food supply. Though vitamin C is readily available from food, athletes often consume vitamin C supplements. Correcting a deficiency clearly improves performance, but research does not demonstrate that vitamin C supplements enhance performance when a vitamin C deficiency is not present.

Nevertheless, because exercise places stress on the body, moderate amounts of vitamin C above the RDA of 75 to 90 milligrams may be appropriate for athletes. Some scientists have recommended 200 to 300 milligrams daily, which can be obtained from a diet abundant in fruits and vegetables. Research indicates that 200 milligrams daily of vitamin C leads to full saturation of this nutrient in the plasma and white blood cells, which supports optimal immune function. Vitamin C supplements may reduce the symptoms and duration of upper respiratory tract infections, which may be more likely to occur following strenuous physical efforts. Vitamin C also plays an important part in the healing process when there is injury or muscle soreness. However, contrary to popular belief, most studies have not found that vitamin C supplementation helps to prevent the common cold.

A diet rich in fruits and vegetables provides ample amounts of vitamin C as well as other healthful substances found in those foods (see Tables 3.2 and 3.3). Avoid excessive intake of vitamin C supplements reaching 1,000 to 3,000 milligrams daily, which can cause side effects such as diarrhea and kidney stones. The safe upper limit is 2,000 milligrams daily.

VITAMIN E

Vitamin E receives much attention from athletes because of its role as a potent antioxidant. It prevents the oxidation of unsaturated fatty acids in cell membranes and protects the cell from damage. Vitamin E is widely distributed in foods and stored in the body, so vitamin E deficiencies are rare. The current DRI is 15 International Units (IU). Polyunsaturated oils such as soybean, corn, and safflower are the most common sources of vitamin E. Other good sources are fortified grain products and wheat germ (see Table 3.2).

Experiments on vitamin E supplementation at altitude have produced some interesting results, but more research is required, especially to determine whether any real performance benefits are possible. Because of its antioxidant effects, vitamin E may also be beneficial to athletes training in high-pollution areas. Endurance athletes should supplement with vitamin E carefully, however. One study assessed oxidative function in triathletes who supplemented with 800 IU of vitamin E in the weeks leading up to an Ironman triathlon. This level of vitamin E supplementation was actually found to increase oxidation rather than decrease it.

TABLE **3.3**	SUPER SOURCES OF CAROTENOIDS*

FOOD	PORTION
Apricot, dried	6 halves/pieces
Broccoli, cooked	½ c. (120 ml)
Cantaloupe	1 c., chunks (240 ml)
Carrot, raw	1 medium
Collard greens, cooked	½ c. (120 ml)
Grapefruit	½ medium
Kale, cooked	½ c. (120 ml)
Mango	1 medium
Mustard greens, cooked	½ c. (120 ml)
Orange	1 medium
Papaya	½ medium
Pepper, red, raw	½ medium
Pumpkin, cooked or canned	½ c. (120 ml)
Spinach, raw	½ c. (120 ml)
Sweet potato, mashed	½ c. (120 ml)
Tangerine	1 medium
Tomato sauce	½ c. (120 ml)

*INCLUDES ALPHA-CAROTENE, BETA-CAROTENE, B-CRYPTO-XANTHIN, LUTEIN/ZEANTHIN, AND LYCOPENE.

Though no performance benefits have been firmly established, vitamin E supplements may also be recommended for possible prevention of chronic diseases, especially heart disease. Some researchers currently feel that a daily supplement dose of 100 to 200 IU is safe and appropriate, though more research on the highest safety dose is required. People with a bleeding disorder or who are taking an anticoagulant medication or statin medication (designed to lower elevated blood lipids) should be cautious and first check with their physician before taking vitamin E. If you do take a vitamin E supplement, choose one that provides the natural source of the vitamin.

CAROTENOIDS AND VITAMIN A

Beta-carotene is one of 600 carotenoid pigments that give fruits and vegetables their yellow, orange, and red colors. Carotenoids are also abundant in green vegetables. While carotenoids are not vitamins, many act as antioxidants and also protect cells from free radicals.

The carotenoids most commonly found in blood and tissues are alpha-carotene, beta-carotene, lycopene, beta-cryptoxanthin, lutein, and zeaxanthin. Only alpha-carotene, beta-carotene, and beta-cryptoxanthin can be converted to vitamin A in the body. Research is just beginning to determine how specific carotenoids can boost immunity and protect the heart and eyes from chronic disease.

To obtain a variety of carotenoids in your diet, aim for at least five servings combined of fruits and vegetables daily, focusing mainly on yellow-orange, red, and dark green choices. You can easily obtain ample amounts in your diet.

Taking a supplement with carotenoids requires some caution, particularly in the case of beta-carotene supplements, which were found to increase cancer in smokers. If you do supplement, stay under 3 milligrams daily. You should also keep in mind that carotenoids interact with one another. Supplementing with one carotenoid may impair the absorption of others. Carotenoids are converted to vitamin A as the body requires. But vitamin A supplements can be highly toxic at greater than the daily RDA of 5,000 IU. Besides, foods high in carotenoids may provide health-promoting substances not found in supplements. It's quite possible that these protective nutrients work best when they are packaged together.

VITAMINS D AND K

Because of vitamin D's important role in bone building, it is covered below in the section on calcium, although it also plays other important roles in maintaining good health. Vitamin K is also essential to bone health and is needed for the formation of prothrombin, which is required for blood to clot properly.

MINERALS

Like vitamins, minerals are involved in energy metabolism and also play important roles in building body tissue, in maintaining and strengthening the skeleton, in enabling the muscles to contract properly, in transporting oxygen as needed throughout the body via the red blood cells, in maintaining the acid-base, or pH, balance of the blood, and in regulating normal heart rhythm—all important for top athletic performance. Weak bones can contribute to the development of stress fractures, and an acid-base imbalance can affect endurance and energy metabolism so that fuel is not utilized as efficiently as possible during training. Minerals are involved in the metabolism of carbohydrates, proteins, and fats and in obtaining energy from an important fuel source, phosphocreatine.

There are two classes of minerals, both important to optimal body functioning. The macro-minerals are present in relatively large amounts in the body and include calcium, phosphorus, and magnesium. Trace or microminerals include iron, zinc, chromium, copper, and selenium. Several minerals also function as electrolytes and play important roles in fluid balance. Sodium, chloride, and potassium are of special interest to the endurance athlete because they are three of the electrolytes lost in sweat. Magnesium and calcium also function as electrolytes and are lost in sweat in smaller amounts. Many of the recommendations for sodium that are made to the general public may not apply adequately to endurance athletes, who lose large amounts of sweat on a daily basis.

Altogether there are twenty-five essential minerals, each with its own unique functions. Minerals are obtained in our diet from the water we drink and from both plant and animal foods. Training-induced mineral losses can occur not only through sweat but through urine and gastro-intestinal losses as well.

Two minerals very important to the athlete are calcium, because of its essential role in maintaining healthy bone structure, and iron, which plays a crucial role in oxygen transport. Sodium is also important because of the potential sweat losses of this mineral and the negative performance effects that can result from excess loss.

CALCIUM

Calcium is the most abundant mineral in the body. Ninety-eight percent of calcium is found in bone, a dynamic tissue that is constantly being broken down and rebuilt. The remaining 2 percent of calcium is circulating in your bloodstream and contained in your teeth.

Calcium circulating in your blood has a significant effect on metabolism and physiological functions. It is involved in all types of muscle contraction, including contractions of the heart muscle, skeletal muscle, and smooth muscle found in blood vessels. By activating a number of

TABLE **3.4**	CALCIUM AND VITAMIN D REQUIREMENTS	
AGE	**CALCIUM (mg)**	**VITAMIN D (IU)**
19–50 years	1,000 (men and women)	200
51–70 years	1,200 (men or women on hormone replacement therapy—HRT) 1,500 (not on HRT)	400
> 70 years	1,200 (men or women on HRT) 1,500 (not on HRT)	600

TABLE **3.5**	FOOD SOURCES OF CALCIUM

GREAT SOURCES (300 mg per portion)	**PORTION**
1% milk	8 oz. (240 ml)
Skim milk	8 oz. (240 ml)
Orange juice, calcium fortified	8 oz. (240 ml)
Collard greens, cooked	1 c. (240 ml)
Rhubarb, cooked	1 c. (240 ml)
Yogurt	6–8 oz. (200–240 ml)
Mackerel, canned	3 oz. (90 g)
Sardines, canned, w/ bones	3 oz. (90 g)
Salmon, canned, w/ bones	3 oz. (90 g)
Swiss cheese	1 oz. (30 g)
Blackstrap molasses	2 tbsp. (40 ml)
GOOD SOURCES (200 mg per portion)	**PORTION**
Bok choy, fresh	1 c. (240 ml)
Broccoli, cooked	1 c. (240 ml)
Kale, cooked	1 c. (240 ml)
Mustard greens, cooked	1 c. (240 ml)
Soybeans, cooked	1 c. (240 ml)
Turnip greens, cooked	1 c. (240 ml)
Brick cheese	1 oz. (30 g)
Cheddar cheese	1 oz. (30 g)
Colby cheese	1 oz. (30 g)
Edam cheese	1 oz. (30 g)
Mozzarella cheese	1 oz. (30 g)
Instant breakfast	1 packet
Sesame seeds	2 tbsp. (40 ml)

CONTINUES

enzymes, calcium also plays a role in both the synthesis and breakdown of muscle and liver glycogen. It is involved in nerve impulse transmission, blood clotting, and secretion of hormones. These physiological functions of calcium take precedence over formation of bone tissue. If the diet is low in calcium, it can be pulled from the bone to meet these more urgent needs.

Calcium deficiency can develop from inadequate intake or from increased calcium excretion. Strenuous exercise increases sweat loss of calcium. One of the major health concerns associated

TABLE **3.5**	**FOOD SOURCES OF CALCIUM** continued

FAIR SOURCES (100 mg per portion)	PORTION
Cottage cheese, 1%	1 c. (240 ml)
Navy beans, cooked	1 c. (240 ml)
Pinto beans	1 c. (240 ml)
Swiss chard, cooked	1 c. (240 ml)
Tempeh, cooked	1 c. (240 ml)
Shrimp, cooked	6 oz. (200 g)
Lobster, cooked	6 oz. (200 g)
Frozen yogurt	½ c. (120 ml)
Pudding	½ c. (120 ml)
Tofu	½ c. (120 ml)
Parmesan, grated	1½ tbsp. (30 ml)
Skim milk, dry	1 tbsp. (20 ml)
Figs, dried or fresh	5 medium
Orange	1 large

with inadequate intake of calcium is osteoporosis, a disorder in which bone mass decreases and susceptibility to fracture increases. Optimal bone building takes place until age twenty-five, but you can continue to build some bone until thirty-five years of age. After this age, your efforts should focus on maintaining your current level of bone mass.

Hormonal status, more specifically estrogen loss, also contributes significantly to the development of osteoporosis, making women more susceptible to this disease after menopause occurs, though men can also develop osteoporosis. Hormonal status in younger female athletes plays an important role in bone health. Extra calcium is recommended for female athletes with absent or irregular menstruation and for post-menopausal athletes. Weight-bearing exercise such as running and weight training enhances calcium skeletal absorption, increases bone mass, and can help prevent bone loss at any age. Calcium recommendations for various ages are provided in Table 3.4.

Dairy products are very concentrated sources of calcium and for most individuals provide about three-fourths of their total calcium intake. Athletes who do not have a high intake of dairy products and vegan athletes need to focus on alternative plant sources of calcium intake and increase their intake of calcium-fortified foods. Try to choose low-fat options as much as possible. Some good plant sources of calcium are dark leafy greens, broccoli, bok choy, dried beans, and dried figs. Food sources of calcium are listed in Table 3.5. Some good fortified sources (check labels) are soy and rice milk, orange juice, cereals, tofu processed with calcium sulfate, and some types of energy bars. Look for products marked as "high" or "rich" in calcium or as an "excellent source" of calcium, as they contain more than 200 milligrams per serving.

Individuals who are lactose-intolerant can buy specially formulated lactose-free milk or take lactase supplement enzymes before consuming milk products. Yogurt and cheese have lower lactose levels than milk and may be well tolerated. You may also be able to tolerate small amounts of lactose-containing foods.

A well-balanced training diet should provide many of the essential nutrients needed to build and maintain healthy bones; however, a calcium supplement may also be indicated if your food intake is not adequate. If you do take a calcium supplement, find one that provides no more than 500 milligrams per pill, and take one pill at a time. Amounts greater than 500 to 600 milligrams will not be fully absorbed. Calcium carbonate should be taken with meals to increase absorption, while the calcium citrate form can be taken at any time. Avoid calcium made from oyster shells, bonemeal, or dolomite as these sources may contain lead.

Vitamin D recommendations are also provided in Table 3.4 because this vitamin is essential for adequate calcium absorption, which is crucial to bone health. When there is inadequate vitamin D, we absorb only 10 to 15 percent of the calcium that we consume, compared with the typical 30 percent. Calcium and vitamin D also work together to prevent colon cancer in some high-risk individuals. Vitamin D may deserve its own separate billing as an important nutrient, as it may help prevent prostate cancer, autoimmune diseases such as type 1 diabetes, rheumatoid arthritis, and multiple sclerosis.

As we age, our bodies become less efficient at converting sunlight to vitamin D, one of the best sources of vitamin D. Good food sources of vitamin D are relatively limited. They include fatty fish, such as cod, mackerel, salmon, and sardines, and egg yolks. Fortified food sources of vitamin D include milk, soy milk, butter, margarine, and many cereals. If you spend a considerable amount of time in direct sunlight when participating in your endurance training, you could make adequate vitamin D from sunlight. Sunscreen does block vitamin D production, however, and safe sun exposure without sunscreen is estimated to be only ten minutes. Moreover, sun exposure of any length may not be adequate from October to April in the northern part of the United States and Canada. If you tan when outdoors, you should be making sufficient amounts of vitamin D in your skin. But because our ability to make vitamin D from sunlight also decreases as we age, older athletes and individuals with limited sun exposure living in northern climates, as well as vegetarians, may want to consider taking a vitamin D supplement. Vitamin D is often conveniently combined with calcium in supplement form and can also be obtained from a multivitamin.

Other nutrients besides vitamin D that are also an important part of building healthy bones are:

VITAMIN C: Plays a role in collagen production that helps hold bone together. A diet with plenty of fresh fruits and vegetables provides ample amounts.

VITAMIN K: Activates osteocalcin, which is needed for optimal bone strength. Good sources are dark, leafy green vegetables.

MAGNESIUM: Another important mineral for bone formation. Good sources are almonds, bananas, avocados, dried beans, lentils, nuts, tofu, wheat germ, and whole grains.

In contrast, some dietary factors are actually harmful to calcium absorption. Excess sodium, protein, and caffeine, for example, increase calcium excretion. Alcohol can also be damaging to bone cells. Try not to consume excessive sources of caffeine. Intakes of phosphorus—namely, from carbonated beverages—should also be limited, because too much of this mineral can upset the calcium balance in the body. Keep your protein intake at an appropriate level for training, but do not consume excessive and unneeded amounts from supplements.

Obtaining adequate calcium in your diet takes planning. Here are some tips for maximizing your calcium intake:

- Have a breakfast every day that includes high-calcium milk, yogurt, or a calcium-fortified soy product.
- Include a high-calcium food with three meals or snacks daily.
- Prepare or order low-fat milk or soy milk smoothies whenever possible.
- Make some great stir-fried vegetables for dinner that include one of the following: bok choy, kale, broccoli, and leafy greens.
- Add reduced-fat cheeses to sandwiches.
- Drink a glass of calcium-fortified orange juice on a regular basis.
- Buy tofu high in calcium for stir-fries and other recipes.

IRON

Many athletes are aware of the important role that iron plays in exercise metabolism. Hemoglobin transports oxygen in the blood, and myoglobin transports oxygen in the muscle. Both of these oxygen-carrying molecules require iron for optimal formation. Many muscle enzymes involved in metabolism require iron. Other iron compounds facilitate oxygen use at the cellular level. It makes sense, then, that poor iron status could impair these functions and exercise performance.

The body storage form of iron, ferritin, is used as an indicator of iron stores, as are transferrin and hemoglobin. About 70 percent of the iron in your body is involved in oxygen transport, while the other 30 percent is stored in the body. Iron deficiency that is not corrected can progress to anemia, and anemia causes fatigue and intolerance to exercise.

Iron deficiency is the most common nutrient deficiency in the United States. It is estimated that 22 to 25 percent of female athletes are iron-deficient, with 6 percent having full-blown anemia. When iron stores are low, total hemoglobin drops and the muscles do not receive as much oxygen. Normal hemoglobin levels for males are 14 to 16 grams per deciliter, with anemia classified as less than 13. The normal range for women is 12 to 14 grams per deciliter, with anemia diagnosed at less than 12 grams per deciliter. Blood work can be interpreted to determine whether you have early iron deficiency or full iron-deficiency anemia. However, remember that endurance training can affect your blood measurements of iron. Training produces an increased blood volume, which dilutes hemoglobin, making it appear low in some athletes when iron stores are adequate. This increased blood volume often occurs at the start of a training program and has no harmful effect on performance. In fact, this increased blood volume means that your heart can pump more blood to your working muscles, enhancing oxygen delivery.

Data clearly indicate that true iron-deficiency anemia will impair exercise performance. Although we have less information regarding the performance effects of a low ferritin level, athletes may experience symptoms of fatigue and poor recovery with this condition. Of course, it makes sense to treat low ferritin levels so that full-blown iron-deficiency anemia does not develop and to improve any recurring symptoms. Your blood work should be monitored by a physician, and any required treatment should be carried out under a physician's supervision.

Inadequate dietary intake of iron is the most common cause of iron deficiency and anemia. Women with heavy menstrual blood loss may also experience iron deficiency. Strenuous exercise can increase iron sweat loss, precipitate gastrointestinal bleeding, and decrease iron absorption. In addition, heavy training may accelerate red blood cell destruction from mechanical trauma such as runners experience when pounding their heels on pavement. Training at altitude can place an athlete at risk for developing iron deficiency as well. Development of iron deficiency is also associated with low-calorie diets, vegetarian diets, very high-carbohydrate diets containing only small amounts of animal protein, and various fad and unbalanced diets.

Iron is obtained from food in two forms. Heme iron is found in animal foods—good sources are lean meat and dark poultry (see Table 3.6). About 10 to 30 percent of heme iron is absorbed from the intestines. Nonheme iron is found in plant foods—dried peas and beans, whole-grain

TABLE **3.6**	IRON CONTENT OF SELECTED FOODS	

SOURCES OF HEME IRON	PORTION	IRON (mg)
Liver, beef, cooked	3 oz. (90 g)	6
Beef, cooked	3 oz. (90 g)	3.5
Pork, cooked	3 oz. (90 g)	3.4
Shrimp, cooked	3 oz. (90 g)	2.6
Turkey, dark, cooked	3 oz. (90 g)	2
Chicken, breast, cooked	3 oz. (90 g)	1
Tuna, light	3 oz. (90 g)	1
Flounder, sole, salmon	3 oz. (90 g)	1
SOURCES OF PLANT IRON	**PORTION**	**IRON (mg)**
Cereal, iron-fortified	1 oz. (30 g)	2–18
Cream of wheat	¾ c. (200 ml)	9
Lentils	1 c. (240 ml)	6
Instant breakfast	1 packet	4.5
Kidney beans, canned	1 c. (240 ml)	3.2
Baked potato, with skin	1 medium	3
Prune juice	8 oz. (240 ml)	3
Wheat germ	¼ c. (60 ml)	2.6
Apricots, dried	10 halves	1.7
Spaghetti, enriched, cooked	½ c. (120 ml)	1.4
Bread, enriched	1 slice	1

products, apricots, and raisins are good sources. About 2 to 10 percent of nonheme iron is absorbed. Nonheme iron absorption is compromised by the phytates, phosphorus-containing compounds, found in many vegetables and whole grains.

Consuming meats and plant iron sources together can enhance iron absorption from plant foods. Small amounts of red meat in bean chili, spinach with chicken, and turkey with lentil soup combine heme and nonheme iron. Vitamin C–containing foods also enhance plant iron absorption. Try having orange juice or strawberries with fortified cereal, for example.

To boost iron intake, try these recommendations:

- Incorporate lean meat regularly into your diet. Have small amounts several times weekly.
- Try adding small amounts of red meats to your favorite recipes, such as stir-fries, soups, pasta sauces, and casseroles.
- Mix heme-iron foods with nonheme choices, such as bean chili with dark turkey meat.
- Incorporate iron-fortified cereals into your diet. Avoid cereals with a high bran content, as they contain phytic acid, which binds with iron and decreases absorption.
- Consider increasing fish and shellfish in your diet for their iron content.
- Increase your intake of plant iron such as whole-grain cereals, legumes, and green leafy vegetables. Have them with a vitamin C–containing food to improve iron absorption.
- Prepare green leafy vegetables by blanching them for 5 to 10 seconds to remove the oxalate they contain, which decreases calcium absorption.
- Athletes training at altitude, female athletes, and vegetarians may want to consider a supplement that provides 100 percent of the Daily Values for iron and other trace minerals, such as zinc and copper, to ensure that they obtain adequate amounts of these nutrients. Many multivitamins contain this amount of iron, so check labels.

As an endurance athlete, you should also have your hemoglobin, hematocrit, and ferritin stores monitored regularly—whether you take iron supplements or not. Taking excess iron from supplements does carry some risk, especially if you take a supplement containing greater than 100 percent of the RDA for iron. Higher doses of iron—even a daily dose of 25 milligrams—can inhibit absorption of zinc and copper. It is important that you do not self-diagnose or attempt to treat your own low iron stores; rather, have your blood work evaluated by a physician and follow his or her advice.

Excess iron supplementation may also adversely affect individuals who have a genetic predisposition to iron overload. Iron overload, a condition known as hemochromatosis, is a genetic disorder that affects 1 in every 200 people. This condition can result in excess iron deposits in the heart, liver, joints, and various body tissues, with the potential for damaging these tissues. High levels of iron supplements can also lead to gastrointestinal intolerance and constipation.

ZINC

Zinc is another important mineral for athletes who train hard. An adequate amount of zinc keeps your immune system strong and promotes healing of wounds and injuries. Zinc is also a component of several enzymes involved in energy metabolism and is involved in protein synthesis. Like iron, though, excess zinc can be too much of a good thing: Oversupplementing with zinc can interfere with absorption of other minerals.

MULTIVITAMIN AND MINERAL SUPPLEMENTS

Athletes training in endurance sports have the distinct advantage of being able to eat more than their sedentary counterparts. With a focus on quality food choices, this generally means a diet filled with variety and nutrients. While a multivitamin and mineral supplement does guarantee that you will obtain all the Daily Values (DVs) for vitamins and minerals, it is not the same as eating food. Nutrients from foods tend to be optimally absorbed and will provide you with all the phytochemicals, undiscovered or otherwise, that are not in your supplement.

However, a supplement containing reasonable amounts of a broad range of vitamins and minerals may provide just that little extra insurance that endurance athletes who care about their health often seek. Athletes who consume fewer than 1,500 calories daily, or who have food allergies that restrict a significant number of choices from one food group, might want to seriously consider taking a vitamin and mineral supplement. Other athletes may have a unique situation that makes it difficult for them to obtain all the nutrients they need from the foods they eat: They may travel frequently, for example, or have disordered eating and erratic diets for some other reason. These athletes should also consider supplementation. Vegans and other vegetarians may need additional vitamin D, zinc, iron, B12, and riboflavin. Each athlete should make this decision based on his or her own situation and medical history. Picky eaters who restrict many foods, athletes at risk for osteoporosis, and women who are pregnant or planning a pregnancy may want to consider this option.

If you decide to take a multivitamin and mineral supplement, try to stick to the following guidelines:

- Choose a broad-range, balanced supplement of vitamins and minerals that provides 100 percent of the DV. These doses are known to be safe.
- Avoid supplements that contain an excess of minerals or any one mineral, as these nutrients compete with one another for absorption.
- Choose a supplement with the United States Pharmacopeia (USP) stamp of approval on the label to guarantee that it dissolves properly in your body.
- Choose a supplement in which the majority of vitamin A is actually beta-carotene, the precursor to vitamin A. Actual vitamin A, or retinol, should not exceed 3,000 IU daily.
- A blend of natural and synthetic supplements is fine. Look for a mix of vitamin E from tocopherols and tocotrienols. Don't pay more for "time-release" or "chelated" products.

CONTINUES

- Calcium and magnesium may need to be purchased separately as they are too bulky to be provided in high amounts in a regular multivitamin pill.
- If you take antioxidant supplements, keep doses to 100 to 200 IU vitamin E and 250 milligrams vitamin C.
- Choose a multiple in which the vitamin D source is D3, or cholecalciferol, the type that is best absorbed.
- Take your multivitamin with a meal or snack and plenty of water.
- Don't double up on the daily dose of vitamins. You may get too much of certain nutrients.
- Avoid megadoses, and be sure to account for any vitamins and minerals you may be taking from sports nutrition supplements.
- Individuals over fifty years of age can opt for iron-free formulas and should look for B6 and B12 content in the higher range.

It is also important to keep the use of antioxidant supplements in perspective, as they are strongly marketed to athletes. It is actually diets abundant in foods that contain antioxidant nutrients that have been shown to prevent cancer and other diseases. So don't discount the importance of increasing food sources of these nutrients. If you are concerned about the negative effects of free radicals, don't assume that supplementation is the key to solving the problem: The jury is still out on this issue. It is impossible to directly measure free radical production in humans. Although free radical by-products do increase with exercise, trained athletes may dispose of them more effectively as they make advances in their training—that is, their bodies may learn to cope with the negative by-products over time.

Moderate doses of vitamin C, beta-carotene, and other carotenoids are easily obtained with educated food choices. However, one nutrient that may be difficult to obtain at antioxidant levels on a diet that limits fat intake to the recommended 30 percent level is vitamin E. Good sources of this vitamin are high in fat, and one would have to consume large amounts of them to reach even the low antioxidant dose of 100 IU. Researchers still need to determine the optimal doses of antioxidant supplements required for preventing heart disease and cancer.

If you do supplement, do so wisely. A multivitamin and mineral supplement providing 100 percent of the DV should be safe and does not have to be expensive. But keep in mind that the hazards of vitamin and mineral overdosing are real and can be subtle. If you take a supplement, understand the good reasons for taking it and consume appropriate doses.

Good sources of zinc include red meat, turkey, milk, yogurt, and seafood—especially oysters. The zinc from animal foods is better absorbed than that found in plant foods. Plant sources of zinc include garbanzo beans, lentils, lima beans, brown rice, and wheat germ.

ELECTROLYTES

Several minerals exist as electrolytes, or small particles that carry electrical charges. Sodium is a major electrolyte in the body, as are potassium, chloride, magnesium, and calcium. Electrolytes can function in a number of ways to control metabolic activities in the cells. Because electrolytes are lost in sweat, they are of particular interest to endurance athletes. When you lose large amounts of sweat during periods of heavy training, you can also lose large amounts of electrolytes. Sodium plays key roles in fluid balance, nerve function, muscle contraction, and acid-base balance.

We know that sodium concentration in sweat varies widely among athletes and that some athletes are more prone to large sodium sweat losses than others. Heat-related problems during training and competition, such as hyponatremia (low blood sodium levels) and muscle cramping, have been linked to sodium losses in sweat as well as other factors. However, sodium does have other health implications not related to your training and racing program. The 2004 DRI recommendations are for North Americans to restrict their sodium intake to 1,500 milligrams daily, with the Tolerable Upper Intake Level (UL) at 2,300 milligrams of sodium per day. Scientific evidence indicates that cutting back on sodium can decrease the risk of developing high blood pressure, and that we develop a greater sensitivity to sodium as we get older. The typical American diet contains at least 4,000 milligrams of sodium per day.

Nevertheless, endurance athletes lose considerably more salt in their sweat than the average American. This is particularly true of athletes who are "salty sweaters," as indicated by the salt markings left on their clothes during long training sessions. Sodium is present in small amounts in most natural foods, but the majority of the sodium in the typical American diet comes from sodium added to processed foods and foods prepared away from home. About one-fourth of an average American's sodium intake comes from added salt. It is possible that endurance athletes who faithfully follow a diet based on natural foods could have a fairly low sodium intake.

Daily sodium needs vary widely among endurance athletes. Most endurance athletes should be encouraged to salt their food, and they should consume sodium-containing foods during periods of heavy training in warm weather conditions. For example, even an acclimatized female endurance athlete with a relatively low sweat rate can lose more than 2,000 milligrams of sodium through sweat loss during a two-hour training session; sodium losses during long weekend training sessions would be even higher. In contrast, a fitness enthusiast exercising for an hour may lose less than 1,000 milligrams of sodium during a typical exercise session; at this level, there is no risk of sodium depletion even if the individual has a low-sodium diet. The sodium needs of endurance athletes can drop off when sweat losses decrease during the shorter and less intense workouts during a recovery training cycle. One way endurance athletes can replace their lost sodium during a training session is by having sports drinks handy. They should be careful, however, not to overdo it and get too much sodium. Individual athletes should discuss the risks of too high a sodium intake with their physician, since family history of heart disease and other factors in each athlete's medical history should be taken into account.

Chloride is also a mineral and an electrolyte, and intake of chloride is often paired with sodium, as table salt is sodium chloride. Chloride losses can also occur during heavy sweating, but a diet with adequate amounts of sodium should also be adequate in chloride.

Potassium, magnesium, and calcium are also contained in sweat, though lost in smaller amounts. For some individuals, sweat losses of these nutrients could add up owing to high sweat volumes. Some sports drinks contain small amounts of these electrolytes to assist in replacing sweat losses during exercise.

Obtaining plenty of these three minerals in your daily diet is also important. Information on calcium in relation to bone health is provided earlier in this chapter, and food sources are listed in Table 3.5. Women and other individuals at risk for osteoporosis should take extra care with their calcium intake in view of possible sweat losses.

Magnesium is also an electrolyte and plays important roles in muscle contraction and glucose metabolism. Some endurance athletes training in hot and humid conditions for extended periods of time could lose fairly high amounts of magnesium in sweat. Consuming ample amounts of magnesium from good food sources such as milk products, nuts, whole grains, and green leafy vegetables is advised to ensure that the recommended intakes are consumed.

Ample amounts of the electrolyte potassium can be obtained in the diet by consuming plenty of fresh fruits and vegetables, low-fat dairy foods, and animal proteins. High intakes of potassium may also help in preventing the development of high blood pressure. A balanced diet can easily provide several thousand milligrams of potassium daily, and the DRI is 4,700 milligrams. Your body stores of potassium are actually quite large, and while being an athlete increases your daily requirement, your sweat losses are truly only a small percentage of your total body stores. More information on replacing electrolyte losses is provided in Chapter 5.

PHYTOCHEMICALS

Unlike vitamins and minerals, phytochemicals are not nutrients. Most phytochemicals—that is, plant chemicals thought to have health benefits—are found in carbohydrate-containing foods such as fruits, vegetables, and grains. Some phytochemicals you may have heard about are the allylic sulfides found in garlic, the flavonoids found in citrus fruits, the genistein found in soybeans, the indoles in broccoli and cauliflower, and the phytoestrogens in soy products, to name a few. To take advantage of these phytochemicals, eat plenty of fruits and vegetables, dried peas and beans, and soy products. Brightly colored fruits and vegetables produce anti-inflammatory and antioxidant pigments, and the deeper the color, the more phytonutrients a given food contains. Some of the best choices are green leafy vegetables, cruciferous vegetables such as broccoli and Brussels sprouts, citrus fruits, and deep red and orange fruits. Whole grains, though not colorful foods, are also high in phytonutrients. In the future, probably even more phytochemicals will be discovered.

YOUR TRAINING DIET

Fine-Tuning Your Diet for Top Performance

An endurance athlete's diet should begin with essential nutrition practices, as outlined in Part I. But how can a basic well-balanced diet be transformed into a scientifically sound, cutting-edge sports nutrition plan designed to support your endurance training program? Part II looks at the details of sports nutrition with an endurance athlete's specific needs in mind.

Chapter 4 describes the fundamentals of an endurance athlete's daily training diet. To assist you in understanding the nutritional demands of your diet, it reviews the fuel demands of the body's energy systems. The chapter will enable you to understand the role that your current training cycle plays in determining your daily training diet and to see how your nutritional requirements shift as your training program builds in preparation for an event or competition. Tables outlining your nutritional needs, food lists, and sample menus are provided.

Because the timing of specific food and fluid portions is also an essential component of a high-performance diet, Chapter 5 provides very specific guidelines for pre-exercise and immediate post-exercise nutrient intake. Guidelines for fuel, fluid, and electrolyte intake during training are also reviewed, as are pre-competition meals and nutritional strategies for an event or race training taper.

Chapters 4 and 5 explain sound methods of:

- Consuming enough energy, or balance of calories, for recovery from training during any training cycle, for tissue building in masters athletes, and for growth in younger athletes.
- Consuming enough grams of carbohydrates to match that day's training and to be adequately fueled for the next training session.

- Timing your intake of carbohydrates to expedite the process of muscle glycogen resynthesis.
- Consuming optimal amounts of protein for recovery, muscle tissue repair, and the maintenance of a strong immune system.
- Consuming healthy fats and good sources of essential fatty acids to balance out the diet and replenish muscle fat levels.
- Consuming adequate amounts of fluid and electrolytes, particularly sodium, after training to rehydrate and replenish body fluid levels.
- Timing your post-exercise meals and snacks to maximize recovery until the next training session, with special consideration for immediate post-exercise nutrition recovery guidelines.
- Practicing recovery nutrition at regular intervals to replenish fuel, fluid, and electrolyte stores.

Body composition is also an important consideration for endurance athletes, and Chapter 6 outlines healthy nutritional strategies essential to muscle building and healthy and appropriate weight loss. Because nutritional supplements surrounded by claims of performance improvements are so heavily marketed to athletes, Chapter 7 is devoted entirely to a review of the science, effectiveness, and safety surrounding these "ergogenic aids."

4

THE DAILY
TRAINING DIET

Eating for Optimal Recovery

AS AN ENDURANCE ATHLETE YOU MUST consume the right amount of energy, or calories, to meet the nutritional demands of your training program. During periods of moderate to heavy training, endurance work can be tough and tiring, and eating enough food is essential to completing longer exercise bouts at the intensities outlined in your program. The intensity and duration of your training also control the types of fuel your body demands and the type it will best utilize for energy on a daily basis. Because of their integral role in fueling endurance exercise and the limitations of your body's fuel stores, carbohydrates are the stars of your training diet, with protein and fat playing important supporting roles. Nutritional recovery is simply the process of eating properly, which provides you with the fuel to go from one training session to the next with the energy required. This recovery process may need to take place in 24 hours, or perhaps even 12, 8, or 4 hours, depending on your training schedule. Begin by choosing quality foods for your sports diet as covered in Part I. A review of the body's energy systems, also called its power systems, will help you to appreciate the integral role of proper fueling.

THE POWER SYSTEMS

Each endurance sport training plan has its own unique mix of body-fuel requirements. That is, during the various components of an exercise program, such as focused training cycles and events and competition, the body uses energy in different ways. Appreciating how your body uses fuel for exercise, how your specific training sessions affect energy use and fuel depletion, and how you can best refuel your body to replenish these energy stores is essential to your full nutritional recovery from one training session to the next. Because the way your body uses energy during training directly impacts the nutritional requirements of your sport, runners, cyclists, swimmers, rowers, triathletes, and adventure racers can benefit from a basic review and understanding of energy production and the fuel demands placed on the muscles. Specific nutritional strategies can enhance your body's energy systems and muscle-building efforts and thus affect your athletic performance.

Each energy systems uses different metabolic pathways to produce energy. How significantly each system will contribute to the energy required for exercise depends on the type of activity performed, which is determined by your sport and training program, by the intensity or speed at which you train, and by how long you train. Obviously, your training sessions can vary in intensity and makeup depending on whether you are building your aerobic system, endurance, or speed and whether you are swimming, rowing, running, or riding your bike. Some training sessions require quick bursts of activity, some require steady activity with some periods of faster movement or specific interval training, and others require that your muscles work slowly and continuously. Your nutritional needs during focused long-distance training differ from specific speed sessions.

Each of these types of training uses a different type of energy system. The energy to power intense activity is referred to as *anaerobic,* whereas the energy that powers moderate and steady activity and the recovery process is mainly *aerobic.* Anaerobic energy systems are not dependent on the availability of oxygen to produce energy, while the aerobic system requires the availability of oxygen to produce energy during exercise. In addition to a mix of aerobic and anaerobic training sessions, many endurance sport athletes use weight training or resistance training (a form of anaerobic exercise) to build muscle and strength specific to optimal performance in their sport, and need to follow specific nutritional guidelines for muscle building. While there are some very important and essential nutritional principles related to training, performance, and recovery for all endurance sport athletes covered in this part of the book, there are also nutritional strategies specific to each endurance sport in Part III.

Because the anaerobic system has two major subcategories, your muscles actually have three energy systems from which to obtain energy or fuel:

- The phosphagen (creatine-phosphate) system
- The anaerobic glycolysis (lactic acid) system
- The aerobic system

A high-speed activity such as sprinting demands the all-out effort of the anaerobic phosphagen system, which may provide energy for up to 10 seconds. This fuel is quickly depleted. Muscles can also use stored carbohydrates—primarily glycogen—for fuel through the anaerobic glycolysis system. This system is called upon when working at high intensities for longer than 10 seconds but also utilizes fuel supplied by the phosphagen system. There are still limits to this fuel supply, which lasts about 90 seconds or slightly longer, and your muscles will still tap into the aerobic system for energy. Anyone who works out in a sport that increases respiration for longer than a few minutes is familiar with the aerobic system—this is what gives a dance class at the gym the name "aerobics." But the true meaning of the term encompasses much more—joggers, brisk walkers, and people out for a bike ride on a Saturday afternoon are all using the aerobic system, which can fuel extended exercise efforts. Obviously, it comes into play when following your endurance training program—for example, when you bike for several hours or go for a long run during marathon training. Long workouts rely on the aerobic system for fuel because this system burns oxygen to provide energy for much longer periods of time than can be supplied by the anaerobic system. The aerobic system only predominates as a fuel source, however, when you are working at low to moderate intensities. Once the pace picks up and your muscles start working harder, oxygen cannot be supplied quickly enough, and it is back to predominately the anaerobic system. Eventually the anaerobic system runs low on fuel and you become fatigued. Fuel can also become depleted from the use of the lower-intensity aerobic system, but a well-fed athlete should be able to train at low to moderate levels for several hours.

Well-trained athletes are able to provide plenty of oxygen to their muscles when needed and limit their reliance on the anaerobic system, delaying fatigue. All of these systems, whether aerobic or anaerobic, work best when they have the right fuels available. Some of these fuels are easier to supply than others. Body-fat stores are in abundant supply even in the leanest endurance athletes. Carbohydrates are in much more limited supply and are needed not only as a direct fuel source but also because they allow fat to be burned effectively.

Although three different power systems supply your body with energy for training, ultimately only one source of fuel can be used for muscle contraction: adenosine triphosphate (ATP). You are constantly using ATP for both daily living and training, whether to simply breathe, go to school or work, or train in your sport. ATP is a high-energy chemical compound found in all muscle cells. When it is broken down, the energy released is used for muscle contraction. Because your muscles contain only a small amount of ATP, it must be steadily recharged for training to continue. The rate at which ATP is recharged in your body must meet the demands of the exercise you are performing. Low-intensity exercise requires a slow, steady supply of ATP, whereas high-intensity exercise requires a more rapid supply.

Because your body stores ATP in only small amounts, you need plenty of stored energy to recharge ATP and keep the energy flowing while you train. Body stores of carbohydrates, protein, and fat release varying amounts of ATP at varying rates when they are burned for fuel. Carbohydrates are stored in limited amounts in your blood as glucose and in your muscles and liver as glycogen. Blood glucose is your brain's sole source of energy at rest and during exercise. A steady supply of it keeps you focused while you perfect your swim stroke in the pool or negotiate a tricky turn on your bike.

However, your blood glucose levels can quickly run low and become unable to meet the energy demands of training. When this occurs, the liver breaks down its supply of glycogen into glucose and releases it directly into the bloodstream to maintain your blood glucose levels. The liver of a well-fed individual can store up to 400 calories worth of glycogen. But liver glycogen is a relatively short-lived fuel supply that fills up and empties depending on the timing and composition of your last meal. Depending on what you ate and how much you ate, liver glycogen stores generally last from 3 to 5 hours. You have likely experienced hunger and some of the symptoms that come with low blood glucose levels when you have not eaten for several hours, such as light-headedness, dizziness, and decreased mental focus. These symptoms, which signal the need for fuel, can occur 3 hours after breakfast, in the late afternoon, or anytime that your liver stores run low.

Clearly, your liver glycogen and blood glucose provide a limited supply of fuel. In fact, they can both become depleted fairly quickly during certain types of training sessions and during competition. In contrast to your liver glycogen stores, your muscle glycogen is a larger storage supply of energy, providing anywhere from 1,400 to 1,800 calories, depending on your body weight and the makeup of your diet. When you train at any intensity, from easy to hard and from steady to stop-and-go, this glycogen is converted to glucose and used by the muscle fibers for energy. When your muscle glycogen stores run low, as can occur during long training days and during hard high-intensity and interval training sessions, your muscles can also utilize the glucose in your bloodstream for fuel. You are constantly using your glycogen stores when training at most intensity levels, but how much carbohydrate you actually need, and the rate at which you burn carbohydrates (quickly, moderately, or slowly), depend on how hard and how long you train that day.

Endurance sport athletes benefit greatly from ensuring that their muscle glycogen stores are refueled after training sessions that significantly deplete these stores. Even if your training session does not fully deplete muscle glycogen stores, constant partial replacement of stores can drain your performance efforts. Several days of successive training without adequate glycogen replacement could ultimately result in poor energy levels and poor training.

Table 4.1 demonstrates that your body's supply of carbohydrates is relatively limited. These carbohydrate stores are easily depleted during very high-intensity exercise and long training sessions. You have probably experienced the symptoms of low body carbohydrate stores during one training session or another. When your blood glucose levels hit bottom during aerobic training,

TABLE **4.1**	CALORIES PROVIDED BY BODY-FUEL STORES

BODY-FUEL STORE	GRAMS	CALORIES
Carbohydrates		
Blood glucose	20	80
Liver glycogen	75–100	300–400
Muscle glycogen	300–450	1,200–1,800
Fat		
Blood fatty acids	< 1	7
Serum triglycerides	8	75
Muscle triglycerides	300	2,700
Adipose tissue triglycerides	9,000	80,000
Protein		
Muscle protein	7,500	30,000

NOTE: THESE VALUES CAN VARY DEPENDING ON THE SIZE OF THE INDIVIDUAL AND HIS OR HER BODY COMPOSITION, LEVEL OF FITNESS, AND DIET.

you may feel dizzy and be unable to focus and concentrate. You may have had to stop exercising altogether or slow down considerably in order to consume carbohydrates and get your blood glucose levels back up. Your legs may have felt heavy and sluggish, and normal training may have seemed harder than usual. You can avoid these energy-draining training experiences by simply starting your exercise session properly fueled and by consuming enough carbohydrates during the session to offset body-fuel losses.

Table 4.1 also shows that fat is the body's greatest source of energy even in the leanest athletes, providing more than 50,000 stored calories (though the exact amount depends on individual body composition). During exercise when your muscles require fat for fuel, the fat stored within your muscle cells, known as intramuscular triglycerides, is used for energy. Just like your muscle glycogen stores, intramuscular triglycerides must be replenished after training, though this fuel is not as easily depleted as muscle glycogen. Depending on the intensity and duration of the training session, you will also tap into the fat stored in adipose tissue and convert it to fatty acids that can be transported to your muscles. It is these more visible body-fat stores that provide a relatively unlimited supply of fat for fuel. These same stores often become the focus of weight-management efforts among both endurance athletes and members of the general public who exercise for their health. Some endurance athletes include specific training sessions in their program aimed at decreasing body-fat levels.

Muscle protein stores can also potentially supply several thousand calories worth of energy. However, breaking down your muscle protein for fuel is not ideal either for recovery or for health, and this process could be detrimental to your performance. Muscle tissue maintains your strength, and constant excess breakdown of this tissue places undue stress on your body and your immune system. Muscle tissue breakdown can best be avoided by maintaining optimal carbohydrate and calorie consumption.

Fat and glycogen are the main fuels that your body uses for energy during training. Exercise intensity, which can be measured in terms of VO_2max (see the sidebar "Heart Rate and Fuels for Training"), is particularly important in determining which of these two fuels your body prefers. Generally, the harder you train, the more carbohydrates you burn. Interval training or intermittent high-intensity training, in which you take your heart rate to higher intensities repeatedly, burns a significant amount of carbohydrates. Training itself activates the energy system that can best meet the fuel demands of the training session. It is your job to ensure that this energy system is well supplied.

Each of the three energy systems supplies the best type and amount of fuel to meet the energy demands of the training session that activates it. In other words, if your body needs carbohydrates quickly, then the glycolysis (lactic acid) system is activated. If your body requires a steady supply of fat, the aerobic system is activated. The phosphagen (creatine phosphate) system can be activated for an all-out sprint effort. Table 4.2 summarizes the characteristics of these energy systems. Besides showing the differences between the two anaerobic energy systems, the table subdivides the aerobic system into two types to distinguish the glycolytic process from the glycolytic/ lipolytic process. In reality, there is no strict division between the two

FIGURE **4.1** **FUEL SOURCES AT HIGH-INTENSITY EFFORTS**

TABLE **4.2**	THE BODY'S ENERGY SYSTEMS

ANAEROBIC SYSTEMS

ATP-CP System	Anaerobic Glycolysis (Lactic Acid System)
Highest rate of ATP production	High rate of ATP production
Very limited supply of ATP lasting 6–8 seconds	Limited supply of ATP lasting 2 minutes
Highest power output and intensity level	High power output and intensity level
Develops explosive power	Develops lactate tolerance
Uses ATP and creatine phosphate stored in body	Uses ATP, creatine phosphate, and muscle glycogen for fuel

AEROBIC SYSTEMS

Glycolytic (Aerobic Glycolysis) System	Glycolytic and Lipolytic System
15–90 minutes of exercise	Greater than 90 minutes of exercise
Low rate of ATP production	Lowest rate of ATP production
High supply of ATP	High supply of ATP
Low power production and low intensity	Lowest power output and intensity level
15–30 minutes of exercise: uses muscle glycogen and blood glucose for energy	Longer than 90 minutes of exercise: uses muscle glycogen, blood glucose, intramuscular fat, and adipose tissue fat for energy
60–90 minutes of exercise: uses muscle glycogen, blood glucose, and intramuscular fat for energy	

types of aerobic processes; rather, they occur along a continuum as low- to moderate-intensity exercise proceeds. It's also important to realize that although you may specifically train a selected energy system, most training sessions involve both aerobic and anaerobic metabolism. The energy systems do not work in an exclusive fashion, though one may predominate during a particular training session. These two metabolic pathways can work together and complement one another to meet the body's energy demands. Figure 4.1 illustrates the duration of exercise that is possible when maximizing the use of one energy system.

Exercise intensity and duration determine not only the predominant fuel system that your body will use to do the work but also the type of muscle fibers it will use to do the work. The three major fiber types, Type I, IIa, and IIb, all have specific training properties. Type I fibers are slow-twitch fibers that predominate in endurance activities. These fibers have a high capacity to produce aerobic energy and store fat for fuel. Type IIa and IIb fibers are fast-twitch fibers that can produce anaerobic energy but differ in some of their characteristics. Type IIa fibers are more of an intermediate fast-twitch fiber and also have the ability to produce energy aerobically. The type of training that you perform affects the aerobic capacity of this fiber, which can behave more like an endurance fiber with aerobic training. The IIb muscle fiber is purely fast-twitch and anaerobic and has a high capacity to produce power and store and burn muscle glycogen. The fat-burning, slow-twitch Type I fibers are larger and predominate in the larger muscle groups. Type IIa and IIb fibers are narrow and create speed.

THE PHOSPHAGEN SYSTEM (THE ATP-CP SYSTEM)

As its name indicates, the ATP-CP system consists of both ATP and another high-energy compound called creatine phosphate (CP). Because ATP is in such short supply, it must be continuously and rapidly resynthesized to provide energy. Like ATP, CP is an energy-rich compound. When it is broken down, it, too, supplies energy. However, CP's released energy does not directly fuel muscle contraction. Rather, the energy released by CP resynthesizes ATP. Like ATP and the energy released from it, CP is in short supply. Energy from the ATP-CP system can fuel high-intensity efforts for only 10 seconds. Even at 10 seconds' duration, only half of your energy needs come from ATP-CP. Fast-twitch muscle fibers use the ATP-CP system rapidly. This system fuels the initial seconds of sprint events and other events where maximal force is required. It is an important fuel source where single bursts of sustained high-intensity activity are completed. For endurance athletes, any type of workout that involves successive bursts of high-intensity activity intermingled with lower-intensity activity will also rely on the phosphagen system for fuel.

The endurance sport athlete who has the ability to store more creatine would have an advantage during this type of training. With enhanced storage of this important fuel, you can maintain a higher power output during successive bouts of very high-intensity activity. To improve the storage of creatine in your muscle, you must perform activities that focus on this energy system by performing high-intensity movements that are repeated multiple times during an exercise session. Consuming enough calories, carbohydrates, and protein for recovery also improves short-duration, high-intensity performance.

ANAEROBIC GLYCOLYSIS

Glycolysis is the second metabolic pathway within your muscle cells that is capable of rapidly producing ATP. As its name indicates, this production occurs through the breakdown of glycogen without the presence of oxygen. In glycolysis, a single glucose molecule is broken down from muscle glycogen to produce ATP. Anaerobic glycolysis provides energy for short-duration, high-intensity exercise lasting 10 seconds to several minutes. As exercise continues beyond 1 to 2 minutes, this system will taper off to provide less than half of your energy needs. Anaerobic glycolysis fuels activities such as high-intensity interval training sessions. At the onset of intense exercise, when oxygen cannot be delivered to your muscles quickly enough, this energy system is rapidly ignited to supply ATP.

The predominant source of energy during this type of activity is stored muscle glycogen. When this fuel runs out, your muscles cannot continue to perform at the same intensity and you become fatigued. This anaerobic energy source runs out quickly (after about 90 seconds) and must be followed by a period of rest of about 3 to 5 minutes for your muscles to become replenished with energy. This rest and recovery time is just as important as the high-intensity training time. If you need to run, swim, row, or cycle at full effort during training or competition, this anaerobic pathway is crucial.

AEROBIC METABOLISM

The aerobic pathway is the primary energy source for lower-intensity, prolonged exercise. This system is glycolytic and lipolytic, as it derives energy from both carbohydrates and fat, respectively.

This pathway provides half of the energy for exercise lasting longer than 1 minute and the majority of the energy for exercise lasting longer than 2 minutes. When you begin an exercise session, you initially use the anaerobic pathways for energy but then switch to a predominantly aerobic pathway. An adequate supply of oxygen must be delivered to the muscles in order for the oxygen system to release the energy stored in carbohydrates and fats. Protein is not normally used for energy production, but under certain conditions it may become a significant source of energy.

Although the aerobic system cannot produce ATP as rapidly as the two anaerobic systems, it can produce much greater quantities at a slower rate. The rate at which the oxygen system produces ATP also depends on whether *aerobic glycolysis* or *aerobic lipolysis* is taking place—that is, whether carbohydrate or fat is being burned for fuel. Figure 4.2 illustrates how carbohydrates, fat, and protein contribute at varying levels of steady-state exercise. Carbohydrates are a more efficient fuel than fat and constitute the

FIGURE **4.2**   **FUEL SOURCES DURING STEADY EXERCISE**

Rest
39%   3%   58%
FAT
CARBOHYDRATES
PROTEIN

Mild Intensity
49%   2%   49%

High Intensity
17%   8%   75%

HEART RATE AND FUELS FOR TRAINING

Without oxygen, training is not possible. The harder you exercise, the more oxygen your body requires to function. Eventually you will reach a level beyond which you cannot increase your oxygen use. This point where your oxygen consumption plateaus is called maximal oxygen consumption, or VO_2max. An athlete with a high VO_2max is considered to have a greater endurance capacity than an athlete with a lower VO_2max.

VO_2max is actually a measurement of your aerobic capacity, or the amount of oxygen your muscles can extract from the bloodstream. There are different ways of expressing VO_2max. It can be expressed in liters of oxygen used per minute (3.5 L/min.), or it can be expressed relative to body mass as ml/kg/min. (50 ml/kg/min.). Unfortunately, your ultimate aerobic capacity is mainly determined by genetics. But you can follow a training program that will enable you to reach your full oxygen capacity potential and subsequently perform at your best. Highly trained athletes can maintain maximal aerobic capacity for only several minutes. Most of the time, you are exercising at a percentage of your maximal aerobic capacity, often called "percentage of VO_2max." Because many athletes have not undergone the scientific testing available to determine VO_2max, exercise intensity is often expressed as a percentage of maximal heart rate. Many athletes are familiar with their maximal heart rate as they train with a heart rate monitor.

Lactate threshold is a related term. This measurement is usually expressed as a percentage of VO_2max but can also be expressed as a percentage of maximal heart rate. Like VO_2max, the level at which lactate threshold occurs varies among athletes. During exercise of increasing intensity, a by-product called lactic acid is produced. The point at which excess lactic acid begins to accumulate in your bloodstream is referred to as the lactate threshold. Every athlete has his or her own lactate threshold, and it is an important indicator of athletic performance. Basically, it measures an athlete's ability to sustain a high rate of energy expenditure without being limited by fatigue. An athlete with a lactate threshold at 75 percent of VO_2max should have better endurance potential than an athlete with the same VO_2max and a lactate threshold at 70 percent. This is because the higher lactate threshold allows the athlete to work closer to his or her aerobic capacity. In fact, lactate threshold is often a better predictor of endurance performance ability than VO_2max.

Genetics influences your lactate threshold, but so does training. Good training programs are designed to increase your lactate tolerance. Both your VO_2max and your lactate threshold can be

CONTINUES

measured from a graded exercise test on a bicycle or treadmill. Follow-up testing can determine how these performance measurements have responded to your current training program.

When you train with a heart rate monitor, it provides the feedback you need to perform the appropriate training session for that day while staying within a specific heart rate zone. A heart rate monitor can also provide you with feedback on the mix of fuels you burn during exercise. When you exercise at under 60 percent of your maximum heart rate, training is fueled mainly by your fat stores. As you become more highly trained, adaptations to training allow your fat tissue to release fatty acids into the bloodstream. These fatty acids and the fat stored in your muscle are seemingly in endless supply as they fuel your low-intensity efforts. However, muscle glycogen still provides some of the fuel supply during these low-intensity efforts, and eventually carbohydrate stores will run too low for training to continue.

At about 60 to 80 percent of your maximum heart rate, muscle glycogen and blood glucose stores supply about half of your energy needs. The other half of your energy needs comes from fat, and a small amount comes from protein. Your carbohydrate stores also limit exercise maintained at this level. Even at the lower end of moderate-intensity exercise, you eventually run low on glycogen. Depletion may not occur quickly, but it will happen.

As intensity increases, eventually your aerobic system cannot fully meet the demands of your training session. When you train at above 80 percent of your maximum heart rate, fat cannot be utilized as effectively as a fuel and provides less than 25 percent of your energy needs. This is because fat cannot be broken down quickly enough to fuel training. As would be expected, your production of lactic acid increases at this higher intensity. When you exercise at 90 to 95 percent of your maximum heart rate, your body essentially relies on glucose for energy.

The type of fuel you burn is also determined by your fitness level, and training has many benefits in terms of fuel usage. When you are fit, your body becomes more efficient at producing energy aerobically at a given intensity. Consequently, you burn more fat and less glycogen, sparing your much more limited glycogen stores for a while. This adaptation partly explains how elite athletes can tolerate intense exercise levels without "hitting the wall."

Adaptations in training can also occur with changes in lactic acid accumulation. For example, untrained individuals could begin to accumulate lactic acid at 50 to 60 percent of their maximal

HEART RATE AND FUELS FOR TRAINING	continued

aerobic capacity. Training can increase this lactate threshold to up to 70 to 75 percent, or even higher in elite athletes, allowing the well-trained athlete to use more fat and less glycogen at the same exercise intensity. Training programs are designed to increase your lactic acid tolerance in order to help you achieve your competition goals.

Endurance training has one other benefit. It increases your muscle storage capacity of glycogen. Your muscle glycogen is used at a slower rate when you are trained, and if you eat properly, you can begin exercise with higher glycogen stores. All these adaptations result in more stored fuel, more efficient use of fuel, and a higher fatigue threshold.

Regardless of the phase of training and type of training, for any endurance athletes, having adequate fuel stores for various types of training is crucial, and running low on fuel leads to fatigue and poor-quality training sessions. During any type of training session you benefit not only from the right nutrient mix in the daily diet but also from proper nutrient intake immediately before, during, and after training.

predominant fuel for steady exercise lasting more than 2 minutes and up to 3 hours. But one's storage capacity for carbohydrates in the muscles and liver is inadequate for certain endurance events, whereas fat stores are extensive. For the endurance athlete, glycogen depletion can occur during aerobic training as well as during sessions when aerobic training and anaerobic training are combined. For ultraendurance events lasting 4 to 6 hours and for long, low-intensity events, fat becomes the primary fuel source. This aspect of fuel burning applies to many endurance sport athletes during specific phases of their training, such as in long, low-intensity base training sessions or when preparing for specific events such as an Ironman triathlon, open-water long-distance swimming, or a long adventure race.

NUTRIENTS FOR ENDURANCE TRAINING

Chapter 2 outlines the health benefits of choosing high-quality, nutrient-rich food sources of carbohydrates, proteins, and fats. But how you time and portion these nutrients specific to your training schedule, for each training session, and within the context of your current training cycle clearly distinguishes your diet as an endurance athlete. Because nutrient timing and portioning are so essential to optimizing the energy available for training and your daily recovery, your nutritional program should be carefully planned each day. Though your nutrient requirements and food strategies can change throughout the season, and even from week to week, there are some essential fundamentals to the role that carbohydrates, proteins, and fats play in your training diet.

ENERGY

As an endurance athlete it is important that you appreciate just how much your daily training program affects your energy requirements. On very heavy training days, the number of calories you burn during exercise can easily exceed the number of calories your body requires for basic daily activity, more than doubling your energy needs. To excel at your sport—and to enjoy your training time—you must consume the calories your body needs for both everyday life and training. In short, eating enough food is essential to completing demanding training programs that test your endurance, power, and skill.

How many calories do you need? In some ways, we can only speculate about the answer to this question. Estimating energy needs is not a precise science, and although many formulas work fairly well, every athlete has a unique energy system with its own tally of energy use throughout the day. In addition, your ideal calorie intake depends on your training and body-composition goals. Your daily energy requirements are made up of the following components.

Resting metabolic rate (RMR), the amount of energy required to keep your body functioning while at rest. This energy keeps your brain functioning, maintains breathing, and keeps your heart beating. You also burn a small amount of energy when you digest food. For many North Americans, the RMR accounts for 60 to 75 percent of total energy expenditure for the day. However, this percentage can be far lower for serious athletes who burn a significant number of calories when training. RMR can be estimated using a number of validated formulas, which are used by health professionals such as sports dietitians when estimating your energy requirements. RMR calculators available online also use a standard formula of some sort to estimate this number. But metabolic rate can now be measured outside of strict laboratory conditions with a fair degree of accuracy, allowing athletes and others to more accurately predict their daily energy needs (but not their training needs). Many professional trainers and health-care specialists now provide the testing required to estimate RMR using new, portable versions of the RMR testing equipment. RMR can actually vary greatly from athlete to athlete, so this option of direct measurement can be very useful for some individuals, such as an endurance athlete struggling with weight-loss or weight-gain issues. RMR decreases with age, is greater in individuals with greater body mass, increases with greater muscle mass, and decreases with greater body-fat stores. These are only some of the factors that affect an individual's RMR.

Growth, the energy needed for physical growth among athletes who are still children or teenagers. This is a big factor for the high-school cross-country runner or swimmer. Pregnant and breast-feeding female athletes face similar energy needs (see the sidebar "Nutrition for Pregnancy and Exercise" in Chapter 6). Women need an additional 350 calories per day above their usual requirements during their second trimester of pregnancy and an additional 500 calories above their usual requirements during their third trimester of pregnancy.

Daily physical activity, the energy you burn to carry out your everyday activities—for example, the activity required of you at work or school. The number of calories needed for daily activity is generally small unless you have a physically demanding job that requires you to do a lot of walking or lifting, for example. For many individuals, this activity may constitute only about 15 percent of their energy requirements; others may have a higher daily energy expenditure.

Training expenditure, the calories you burn with exercise. This can be a large or small variable for the endurance athlete depending on that day's training intensity and duration. For example, you may have a light 4-mile run early in the week and a long 18-mile run on the weekend when you are preparing for a marathon. Triathletes and cyclists can burn thousands of calories on a long bike ride, whereas a 60-minute gym workout in the evening after a long workday burns significantly fewer calories.

Thermic effect of food, the calories required just to digest and absorb the food you consume. This number is always quite small but can vary with the type of meal or snack that you consume.

Although determining energy needs is not a precise science, some general indicators can help you to appreciate just how low, moderate, or high your calorie needs may be for daily recovery from one training session to the next. Of course, many athletes want to consider the proper calorie adjustments to be made for their body-composition goals, whether for muscle building, fat loss, or both. More specific nutritional information on changing body composition is provided in Chapter 6.

One method of estimating daily calorie needs is based on the amount of calories you require per pound of body weight as directly related to the amount of training you complete that day. These calculations take resting metabolic rate, daily energy needs, and energy for training into account. When in serious training mode and preparing for an important day of rowing, running, cycling, or swimming, it is best not to fall short on your calorie requirements. Several days in a row of not recharging your batteries fully may result in some unplanned rest days, days off, or poor-quality training sessions, all of which can hamper your competition goals.

The calorie descriptions listed here show how your activity can affect your total calorie needs for the day. Energy needs are not consistent every day. A 160-pound (73 kg) adult who trains for 90 minutes one day would require 18 to 24 calories per pound (40–53 kilocalories per kilogram [kcal/kg]) of body weight, or 2,880 to 3,840 calories, to meet his or her total energy needs, while that same adult completing 3 hours of training would require 24 to 29 calories per pound (52–63 kcal/kg) of body weight, or up to 4,640 calories for the day.

To estimate his or her caloric needs more specifically, this athlete could categorize the training sessions by intensity. On a day of mild activity, with no purposeful exercise or training, or even on a rest day from training, an athlete needs only 12 to 14 calories per pound (26–31 kcal/kg) of body weight. On days when you engage in up to 1 hour of moderate exercise, you need 15 to 17 calories per pound (33–37 kcal/kg) of body weight for the day. On a high-activity day, with 1 to 2 hours of moderate-intensity exercise, you need 18 to 24 calories per pound (40–53 kcal/kg) of body weight. Finally, on days when you have a very high level of activity, with several hours of training, you need 24 to 29 calories per pound (53–63 kcal/kg) of body weight.

You can also estimate the number of calories you need for a particular day by adding together the amount needed for your estimated or measured RMR, the amount needed for your daily activity when not training, and the amount needed for your particular sport for the amount of time that you train that day. Teenagers and pregnant women would also need to factor in the amount needed to meet their special requirements. RMR is generally estimated at 11 to 12 calories per pound (24–26 kcal/kg) of body weight, but it can be lower or higher in some individuals. You can fine-tune this number if you have your RMR tested by a professional. Daily calorie expenditures outside of training may add another few hundred calories. But clearly the amount of calories you burn can add up with heavy training.

For example, a female cyclist who weighs 140 pounds (64 kg) could estimate her RMR at 1,540 calories. She has a desk job and drives to work and may burn another 150 to 200 calories in her daily life. When she trains steadily on her bike for 2 hours she can burn 1,200 calories total. On a typical training day her energy needs will therefore require her to eat 2,890 to 2,940 calories. If she decides to complete 1 hour of weight training and 45 minutes of aerobic conditioning one day that week, the total calories burned would fall to 2,420 to 2,470 on that day, and she would have to adjust her intake accordingly.

The calorie expenditures supplied in Table 4.3 are listed per minute of activity for the endurance sports reviewed in this book. These figures represent averages, however. Seasoned athletes can become much more efficient in their sport—that is, they can move and use their muscles more efficiently than less experienced athletes, which results in conserving energy. They therefore burn fewer calories when training. Conversely, athletes who are new to an endurance sport are not as efficient in their movements and can burn more calories when training.

Endurance athletes now often train with a heart rate monitor to track the number of calories they are burning. When a heart rate monitor is used to measure energy expenditure, it is based

| TABLE **4.3** | CALORIE EXPENDITURE PER MINUTE OF ACTIVITY OF ENDURANCE SPORTS AND TRAINING ACTIVITIES |

	WEIGHT IN POUNDS (kg)										
	100 (45)	110 (50)	120 (55)	130 (59)	140 (64)	150 (68)	160 (73)	170 (77)	180 (82)	190 (86)	200 (91)
Swimming											
25 yards/min.	4.0	4.4	4.8	5.2	5.6	6.0	6.4	6.8	7.2	7.6	8.0
35 yards/min.	4.8	5.4	5.9	6.4	6.8	7.3	7.8	8.3	8.8	9.2	9.7
50 yards/min.	7.0	7.7	8.5	9.2	9.9	10.6	11.3	12.0	12.8	13.5	14.2
Running											
5 mph (12 min./mi.)	6.0	6.6	7.3	7.9	8.5	9.1	9.7	10.3	10.9	11.6	12.2
7 mph (8:35 min./mi.)	8.5	9.3	10.2	11.0	11.9	12.8	13.6	14.5	15.4	16.2	17.1
9 mph (6:40 min./mi.)	10.8	11.9	12.9	14.0	15.1	16.2	17.3	18.4	19.5	20.6	21.7
Cycling (flat road, no wind)											
15 mph (25 km/hr.)	7.3	8.0	8.7	9.5	10.0	10.9	11.6	12.4	13.1	13.8	14.5
20 mph (32 km/hr.)	10.7	11.7	12.8	13.9	14.9	16.0	17.1	18.1	19.2	20.3	21.3
25 mph (40 km/hr.)	13.5	15.0	16.3	17.7	19.0	20.5	21.8	23.0	24.5	25.9	27.2
Rowing, skull											
Leisure pace	4.7	5.0	5.4	5.9	6.3	6.8	7.4	8.0	8.6	9.2	9.8
Race pace	8.7	8.9	9.7	10.5	11.3	12.1	12.8	13.7	14.6	15.3	16.0
Hiking (3 mph)	4.5	5.0	5.4	5.9	6.3	6.8	7.3	7.7	8.2	8.6	9.1
Canoeing (5 mph)	5.7	6.3	6.9	7.5	8.1	8.7	9.3	9.8	10.4	11.0	11.6
Weight training	5.2	5.7	6.2	6.8	7.3	7.8	8.3	8.9	9.4	9.9	10.5
Aerobic conditioning	4.7	5.2	5.7	6.1	6.5	7.0	7.5	7.9	8.3	8.9	9.4

on an average linear relationship between heart rate and oxygen consumption. However, particular heart rate levels may not correspond to the same levels of oxygen consumption in every individual. Because of this individual variability, the monitor can provide only a rough estimation of calories burned. Even when you key your weight into the heart rate monitor and estimate your heart rate, you will receive only an estimate of the calories burned based on a one-size-fits-all equation.

CARBOHYDRATES: THE RECOVERY FUEL

You may or may not have experienced the symptoms of glycogen depletion during a single training session. It is possible, however, that you experienced it over a longer period without realizing it. The symptoms of gradual glycogen depletion can occur over successive days of training and can be much more subtle than simply "hitting the wall." Symptoms of glycogen depletion can creep up over a week's time or longer, producing feelings of sluggishness and heaviness. Besides experiencing general lethargy, you may not be able to put out an increased or even normal effort during training, or you may find it difficult to maintain your usual intensity and duration of training. The more muscle glycogen stored in your body, the better the quality of your interval training sessions and the better your energy levels during a long run or bike. Figure 4.3 illustrates how gradual glycogen depletion due to the combination of daily training and inadequate daily carbohydrate intake can occur slowly over a period of several days.

Numerous scientific studies have shown that a diet adequate in carbohydrates is superior for building, maintaining, and replenishing muscle glycogen stores. The amount of carbohydrate you consume in your diet directly affects the amount of glycogen you store in your muscles and liver. Inadequate intakes of carbohydrates will only lead to partial replenishment of muscle glycogen stores. If this incomplete replenishment occurs from one day to the next, your glycogen stores gradually become depleted over a period of a week or more, and your training will suffer. Adequate recovery allows you to start the next training session, whether it is 4, 8, 12, or 24 hours

FIGURE **4.3**	MUSCLE GLYCOGEN AND TRAINING

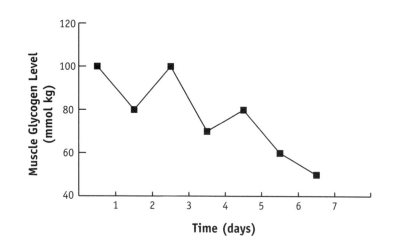

away, with optimal fuel to complete the exercise at the desired duration and intensity spelled out in your training program.

DAILY CARBOHYDRATE REQUIREMENTS: MATCHING INTAKE TO TRAINING

Carbohydrate recommendations are often expressed as a percentage of total calories. This is appropriate for general recommendations for nonathletes, when the goal is usually to decrease unwanted fat intake and increase wholesome carbohydrates from whole grains and fruits and vegetables. However, for endurance sport athletes, it is more appropriate to express carbohydrate needs as grams per pound (or kg) of weight based on the intensity and duration of the training session or sessions for that day. Regardless of the type of training session, your muscles require an absolute amount of carbohydrate to recover sufficiently, particularly after intense exercise sessions that are endurance based or that include plenty of high-intensity efforts, which can quickly deplete carbohydrate stores.

The ceiling for daily carbohydrate consumption—that is, the point at which your muscle storage capacity has been reached—is 4.5 to 5.5 grams of carbohydrates per pound (10–12 g/kg) of weight. Depending on the size of the athlete, this translates to anywhere from 500 to 700 grams of carbohydrates daily. Higher levels may not resynthesize muscle glycogen stores any faster, however. Most endurance athletes who meet both their energy and carbohydrate needs can average about 50 to 65 percent carbohydrate calories in their training diet. But depending on whether you are restricting calories for weight management or have very high energy needs, the percentage of carbohydrate consumed may vary. Typically, as an athlete you will have to consume greater quantities of carbohydrates than most people, including athletes participating in sports that do not have as high a fuel demand as endurance sports and individuals exercising for general fitness.

THE PHASES OF GLYCOGEN REPLENISHMENT

Because any cycle of your training program and every type of workout uses some amount of the more limited fuel supply of muscle glycogen, carbohydrate foods are the foods that you should focus on for recovery nutrition. There are actually several phases of glycogen repletion. If you train only every 24 hours, you simply need to consume the proper amount of carbohydrate between training sessions. However, many endurance athletes may train again in 12, 8, or even 4 hours. If training sessions are scheduled in these time frames, and if you have multiple workouts outlined in your training schedule, it is important that you take advantage of the early phases of muscle glycogen recovery. Initially there is a very rapid phase of recovery that lasts for the 30 to 60 minutes after exercise when muscle glycogen stores are very low. The rate of muscle glycogen resynthesis then remains somewhat elevated for the first 6 hours after training, after which it slows down. Specific nutritional strategies regarding food and fluid choices, portions, and timing presented in Chapter 5 are designed to maximize muscle glycogen resynthesis after training.

PROTEIN AND DAILY RECOVERY REQUIREMENTS

Although carbohydrate intake should receive the most emphasis in your endurance training diet, the demands of endurance training and training for power and strength also increase your need for protein. Protein needs are highest in endurance athletes who follow very intense training programs and who incorporate resistance training into their program. Intense training can also entail significant wear and tear on the muscles and ligaments, requiring protein for repair. Endurance sport athletes who engage in strength training can rely on glycogen for fuel during this mode of exercise and, most importantly, should consume enough carbohydrates so that protein is not utilized for fuel during training.

Your elevated protein requirements are easily met by a well-planned sports diet. What distinguishes a sports diet is how you time your protein intake, particularly around resistance training (see Chapter 5). Most North Americans consume a diet that easily meets the protein needs of an athlete participating in a demanding training program. Inadequate protein intake may be a concern only for athletes who follow a poorly planned vegetarian diet, who restrict their calories, or who have very specific food dislikes. Consider how easy it is to meet your daily protein requirements. Having some peanut butter and cereal with milk for breakfast, followed by a turkey sandwich for lunch and a stir-fry of lean red meat and rice for dinner will supply about 90 grams of protein. You will obtain additional protein from between-meal snacks. Foods such as whole grains and vegetables, which are not as concentrated in protein, still contribute to your total protein intake and can provide moderate amounts over the course of a day, supplementing your intake of more concentrated protein foods.

FAT REQUIREMENTS

Endurance athletes should consume approximately 0.5 gram of fat per pound (1 g/kg) of body weight to obtain adequate amounts of essential fatty acids. Fat can provide from 15 to 30 percent of the day's calories depending on the carbohydrate, protein, and especially energy needs for that day's training. Once carbohydrate and protein requirements are met for your training program and recovery, fat can make up the remainder of the calories appropriate for your weight and body-composition goals.

The most important strategy regarding fat intake is to consume enough healthy fats high in essential fatty acids, as outlined in Chapter 2. For athletes who need to monitor their weight closely to prevent unwanted weight gain, especially during specific training cycles when endurance athletes have lower energy needs, too much fat in the diet may present a problem. This is more likely to happen with athletes who frequently eat out or travel. Some athletes may be accustomed to eating out and frequenting fast-food establishments. A high-fat diet is often very calorie-dense and leaves less room for quality carbohydrates. Weight-conscious athletes should keep fat calories at 20 to 25 percent of total intake. (More on body-composition strategies is in Chapter 6.)

Emerging research regarding the fat requirements for athletes in ultraendurance training has shown that athletes who complete training sessions of more than 4 hours when preparing for an

TABLE 4.4   DAILY NUTRIENT REQUIREMENTS FOR TRAINING

TRAINING	NUTRIENT REQUIREMENTS	
Carbohydrates	**Grams per Pound**	**Grams per Kilogram**
3–4 hours moderate/high intensity	4.5–5.5	10–12
90 minutes to 3 hours moderate/high intensity	3–4.5	7–10
Under 1 hour moderate intensity/several hours low intensity	2.25–3	5–7
Protein		
GENERAL ENDURANCE TRAINING REQUIREMENTS:		
Moderate training	0.45	1
Heavy training	0.5–0.75	1.1–1.6
Very heavy training	0.8–0.9	1.8–2
SPECIAL CONSIDERATIONS:		
Growing teenage athlete	0.8–0.9	1.8–2
Athlete restricting calories	0.8–0.9	1.8–2
Strength training phase of training, experienced	0.5–0.7	1–1.5
Strength training phase of training, novice	0.8	1.8
Maximum recommended for extreme exercise loads	1	2.2
Fat		
Moderate training	< 0.5	1
Endurance training (training lasting over 4 hours)	0.5–0.55	1–1.2
Ultraendurance training	0.5–0.75	1–1.6

Ironman, ultrarunners, ultraswimmers, and ultracyclists can actually deplete their muscle stores of fat, or muscle triglycerides. While research regarding the fat requirements of ultraendurance athletes is still developing, it is speculated that a diet too low in fat could lead to inadequate replenishment of these intramuscular triglycerides. Just how much fat is needed for these long training sessions has not been definitely determined. But a diet with less than 20 percent of total calories from fat, or less than 0.5 gram of fat per pound (1 g/kg) of body weight, could be too low for replenishment purposes following these types of training sessions. Table 4.4 provides a summary of an endurance athlete's carbohydrate, protein, and fat requirements.

FLUID REQUIREMENTS

As explained in Chapter 1, water and fluid are essential components of your daily training diet. Thirst is not a good indicator of when you need to drink; it only signals that body fluid levels are already low. Significant weight fluctuations on the scale could signal inadequate daily hydration and poor rehydration efforts when not training. The color of your urine can also indicate the success of your daily hydration efforts: Pale or lemonade-colored urine indicates adequate hydration; darker urine indicates that you need to increase your fluid intake. Specific guidelines for hydrating during exercise and immediately post-exercise are reviewed further in Chapter 5.

PERIODIZING YOUR TRAINING DIET

Because training cycles vary in their specificity, volume, and intensity, general nutritional requirements for each training cycle can also vary. Each individual athlete also has unique nutritional needs throughout the season. Your nutritional requirements can vary with your individual training program, your body-composition goals, and your level of aerobic and anaerobic training as you fine-tune the program that best fits your sport and your goals for the season. There are some specific nutritional considerations for each training cycle, however, that should be helpful for many endurance athletes (see the sidebar "Training Periodization" and Table 4.5).

PREPARATION CYCLE
Because the preparation cycle is low to moderate in intensity and higher in volume as you build your training foundation, your body relies on a fairly even mix of carbohydrates and fat for fuel during training. During this training cycle, longer workouts tend to be lowest in intensity and consequently burn a greater percentage of fat. Strength training workouts in this phase of training also deplete muscle glycogen stores for fuel. Your protein requirements are only slightly higher

| TABLE **4.5** | **NUTRITIONAL PERIODIZATION** | | |

TRAINING CYCLE	NUTRITIONAL REQUIREMENTS	MALE, 160 lbs. (72 kg)	FEMALE, 140 lbs. (64 kg)
Preparation	3 g/lb. (6.5 g/kg) carbohydrates 0.5 g/lb. (1.1 g/kg) protein 0.5 g/lb. (1 g/kg) fat	2,960 calories 480 g carbohydrates 80 g protein 80 g fat	2,590 calories 420 g carbohydrates 70 g protein 70 g fat
Build	4.5 g/lb. (10 g/kg) carbohydrates 0.8 g/lb. (1.8 g/kg) protein 0.6 g/lb. (1.3 g/kg) fat	4,250 calories 720 g carbohydrates 128 g protein 96 g fat	3,725 calories 630 g carbohydrates 112 g protein 84 g fat
Transition	2.5 g/lb. (5.5 g/kg) carbohydrates 0.6 g/lb. (1.3 g/kg) protein < 0.5 g/lb. (< 1 g/kg) fat	2,700 calories 400 g carbohydrates 96 g protein 80 g fat	2,370 calories 350 g carbohydrates 84 g protein 70 g fat

TRAINING PERIODIZATION

Every endurance athlete, whether preparing for a marathon, looking ahead to a summer of bike racing, or building to a late-season half or full Ironman race, separates training into different phases, or cycles, each of which has a specific set of goals. This concept of progressive training cycles building to an important competition or event is referred to as *periodization*. Periodization is a training strategy designed to improve athletic performance by varying your training specificity, volume, and intensity, with rest and recovery incorporated at specific times during your training year to prepare you to do your best at an event or competition. More information about training periodization itself is available in books on the subject, through organizations and clubs, and through personal coaches who provide their athletes with highly personalized programs.

A *macrocycle* is the largest training cycle and typically lasts one full year. Looking at the macrocycle, an endurance athlete plots out his or her competition and events for the year. At the next level, the training program is broken up into four *mesocycles*, which can last several weeks or months depending on the athlete's goals, his or her strengths and weaknesses, and the number of events on the calendar. Each mesocycle, in turn, is broken down into smaller training cycles,

CONTINUES

TRAINING PERIODIZATION continued

or *microcycles*. These microcycles typically last 1 week but could last up to 4 weeks. They require the athlete to complete a specific daily training schedule. Though the terminology describing these cycles can vary somewhat, the mesocycles are commonly referred to as follows:

The Preparation Cycle *(also called a base cycle or foundation cycle):* This training mesocycle, which generally begins a macrocycle, is designed to develop aerobic endurance, muscular strength, and flexibility. An athlete in this phase attempts to overload the aerobic system in order to improve aerobic capacity and power. Endurance workouts are relatively long and of low to moderate intensity. This period generally lasts from 16 to 20 weeks and may consist of four or five 4-week training blocks. For athletes preparing for summer racing and events in the Northern Hemisphere, this training cycle typically begins in the late fall or early winter. However, it would take place earlier in the year for athletes living in a temperate climate who are preparing for an early-season race. As this training cycle nears completion, training intensity can increase, but the focus remains on the aerobic system.

The Build Cycle *(also called an intensity cycle):* In this cycle, intensity is increasing and volume is decreasing as an athlete builds power very specific to his or her sport, whether it is an individual sport like swimming, rowing, running, or cycling or involves a multisport focus, as in triathlons and adventure racing. This pre-race cycle typically lasts 8 to 12 weeks and focuses on improving VO_2max and lactate threshold. Training includes lactate-threshold and VO_2max-specific intervals, such as hill repeats for cycling and running, as well as strength training with heavier weights and fewer repetitions to emphasize explosive power. There is also an emphasis on sport-specific speed and technique. Your training volume can still remain fairly high. For summer racing, this period can take place during late winter and early spring. As your race or event day approaches, your training intensity increases, workouts are shorter, and overall training volume decreases. Both high-intensity training and adequate recovery from these workouts are essential. This training cycle also includes a decrease in training, or a "taper," before races and events that are of lesser importance to your season goals and simply a part of your training program.

The Race Cycle: This cycle includes a race taper, or specific decrease in training volume and intensity before a race, and the race itself. This type of cycle can be short, moderate in length,

TRAINING PERIODIZATION   continued

or long. For example, a taper for a sprint-distance triathlon would be short, whereas a taper for a marathon would be moderate and a taper in preparation for an Ironman triathlon might last several weeks. This race cycle focuses on the most important events or races of your season and demands very specific nutritional guidelines.

The Transition Cycle (also called an off-season cycle): The transition cycle is designed to provide 4 to 8 weeks of active recovery. Initially this period may require some real rest and recovery, which may last for 2 to 4 weeks after the last important race or event of the season. This mesocycle can then last another 4 to 12 weeks before another preparation cycle begins. The purpose of this training cycle is to maintain aerobic conditioning and to improve on your weaknesses and technique. The volume and intensity of exercise are lower in this cycle than in any other training cycle. This is a good time of year to work on your swim stroke or pedaling skills.

than normal at this point, though the timing of your protein intake around weight-training sessions is very important (for more information on nutrition for weight training see Chapter 6). Your energy needs are based on the volume of training, and fat can round out your caloric intake after you have consumed adequate carbohydrates and protein. The list below summarizes carbohydrate, protein, and fat needs for training:

CARBOHYDRATES	2.5 to 3 g/lb. (5.5–6.5 g/kg)	1 to 2 hours, low intensity
	3 to 4.5 g/lb. (6.5–10 g/kg)	3 to 4 hours
	Requirements can increase even more for the ultraendurance athlete.	
PROTEIN	0.5 to 0.6 g/lb. (1.1–1.3 g/kg)	
	Ultraendurance athletes can increase protein intake to 0.8 g/lb. (1.8 g/kg).	
	Proper timing of protein intake around weight training is very beneficial.	
FAT	0.4 to 0.5 g/lb. (0.9–1.0 g/kg)	
	Round out energy needs with healthy fats. Ultraendurance athletes require	
	a minimum of 0.5 g/lb. (more than 1 g/kg) to replace muscle fat.	

Calories can be adjusted down for weight loss or increased for a focus on muscle building. This is the best time in the training cycle to decrease weight and body fat without a significant compromise in recovery. Here's an example:

MALE TRIATHLETE, 170 LBS. (77 kg)
Training session: Cycling, 90 minutes, low intensity

Carbohydrate requirements	510 g (3 g/lb.) x 4 kcal/g	=	2,040 calories
Protein requirements	102 g (0.6 g/lb.) x 4 kcal/g	=	408 calories
Fat requirements	85 g (0.5 g/lb.) x 9 kcal/g	=	765 calories
Total caloric intake			3,213 (19 kcal/lb.)

Energy from fat can be decreased to 540 calories, or 60 grams, for weight loss or body-fat loss if this is the athlete's goal. If training is decreased to 1 hour on specific days, then the athlete's carbohydrate and protein intake can be shaved down slightly. A longer weekend training session of 2 hours would require a slightly higher carbohydrate intake. See the following two examples:

FEMALE RUNNER, 140 LBS. (64 kg)
Training session: Running, 75 minutes, 8.5 miles

Carbohydrate requirements	350 g (2.5 g/lb.) x 4 kcal/g	=	1,400 calories
Protein requirements	63 g (0.45 g/lb.) x 4 kcal/g	=	252 calories
Fat requirements	70 g (0.5 g/lb.) x 9 kcal/g	=	630 calories
Total caloric intake			2,282 (16 kcal/lb.)

MALE SWIMMER, 130 LBS. (59 kg)
Training session: Endurance workout, 90 minutes

20-minutes, warm-up

30–45 minutes at base/endurance pace

5 minutes, quick speed

5 minutes, cool-down

Carbohydrate requirements	358 g (2.75 g/lb.) x 4 kcal/g	=	1,432 calories
Protein requirements	78 g (0.6 g/lb.) x 4 kcal/g	=	312 calories
Fat requirements	52 g (0.4 g/lb.) x 9 kcal/g	=	468 calories
Total caloric intake			2,212 (17 kcal/lb.)

BUILD CYCLE

During this training cycle you will build your intensity, while overall volume will slightly decrease. Your calorie requirements will increase so that you can recover from the higher level of training, and strong attempts to decrease weight could result in insufficient recovery from training due to inadequate glycogen repletion, compromised lean body mass, and decreased energy. It is also important to take in adequate nutrition for recovery so that your body can meet the demands of the increased training and you can develop your ability to handle lactic acid. Speed sessions that take place at high intensity deplete muscle glycogen stores during training much faster than slow, steady training sessions. Your protein needs will also increase because of the stress placed on your muscles during higher-intensity training and the increased weights used during resistance training sessions.

CARBOHYDRATES	3 to 4.5 g/lb. (6.5-10 g/kg)	90 minutes to 2 hours, moderate to high intensity
	2.5 to 3 g/lb. (5.5-6.5 g/kg)	60 to 90 minutes, low to moderate intensity
	3 to 3.5 g/lb. (6.5-8 g/kg)	45 to 75 minutes, moderate to high intensity
	On specific training days, ultraendurance athletes such as Ironman triathletes may need to increase their carbohydrate intake to 5 to 5.5 g/lb. (11-12 g/kg).	
PROTEIN	0.6 to 0.8 g/lb. (1.3-1.8 g/kg)	
	Your increased protein requirements are easily met with a balanced diet. Protein should be timed properly before and after intense weight-training sessions. Very heavy training microcycles may require 0.9 g/lb. (2 g/kg) of protein.	
FAT	0.4 to 1 g/lb. (1-2 g/kg)	
	Higher fat intakes are related to increased energy requirements and are especially appropriate for ultraendurance athletes who are still experiencing fairly high training volumes.	

Caloric intake should be adequate to sustain energy levels for training. Even easy training sessions designed for recovery should be adequately replenished. Your body fat may decrease with training during this cycle, but you should not actively try to lose weight quickly. Even with your increased energy requirements you should focus on healthy food choices and keep treats to moderate levels. Here are two examples:

FEMALE CYCLIST, 150 LBS. (68 kg)

Training session: Interval session, 90 minutes

10-15 minutes, warm-up

5 minutes, short accelerations (20-30 seconds)

Intervals: 2 x 20 minutes tempo, with 5-10 minutes easy recovery

10-15 minutes, easy cool-down

Carbohydrate requirements	450 g (3 g/lb.) x 4 kcal/g	=	1,800 calories
Protein requirements	105 g (0.7 g/lb) x 4 kcal/g	=	420 calories
Fat requirements	90 g (0.6 g/lb.) x 9 kcal/g	=	810 calories
Total caloric intake			3,030 (20 kcal/lb.)

MALE RUNNER, 180 LBS. (82 kg)

Training session: Track workout, 60 minutes

10-15 minutes, warm-up

5-10 minutes, drills and short builds

Main set: 10-20 x 30 seconds to 2-5 x 4 minutes at high intensity

10-15 minutes, cool-down

Carbohydrate requirements	540 g (3 g/lb.) x 4 kcal/g	=	2,160 calories
Protein requirements	126 g (0.7 g/lb.) x 4 kcal/g	=	504 calories
Fat requirements	72 g (0.4 g/lb.) x 9 kcal/g	=	648 calories
Total caloric intake			3,312 (18 kcal/lb.)

RACE CYCLE

When you are preparing for a race or event that is the highlight of your season, there are specific nutritional strategies that you can follow to make sure you arrive with a full stock of stored muscle fuel for race day. Often referred to as your training taper, this structured decrease in training volume and intensity requires a decrease in energy intake while you consume enough carbohydrates to superload your muscles with glycogen. This training cycle may last several weeks when preceding a very long event such as an Ironman, or it can last just several days for a shorter triathlon. More on this training cycle and the required "carb-loading" is covered in Chapter 5.

TRANSITION CYCLE

Active rest and recovery are important parts of preparing for your next athletic goal. During this annual period of rest, you train to maintain your aerobic conditioning. The level of training might be just one-quarter of what you did during the preparation cycle. This is also a good time of year to try new activities and sports for fun and variety.

CARBOHYDRATES	2 to 2.5 g/lb. (4.5-5.5 g/kg)	Light to moderate intensity
	If you are going easy but still enjoy some volume, aim for 3 g/lb. (6.5 g/kg). Choose high-quality carbohydrates, as portions are lower.	
PROTEIN	0.5 to 0.6 g/lb. (1.1-1.3 g/kg)	
	These protein requirements are easily met on a well-balanced diet.	
FAT	Less than 0.5 g/lb. (1 g/kg)	

A decrease in calories is the biggest adjustment of this training cycle. Because you are used to eating ample calories during the periods of more structured training, it is easy to gain weight during this training cycle. Here are two examples:

MALE SWIMMER, 160 LBS. (73 kg)
Training session: Aerobic "dry-land" training in gym, 60 minutes

Carbohydrate requirements	400 g (2.5 g/lb.) x 4 kcal/g	=	1,600 calories
Protein requirements	96 g (0.6 g/lb) x 4 kcal/g	=	384 calories
Fat requirements	70 g (0.44 g/lb) x 9 kcal/g	=	630 calories
Total caloric intake			2,614 (16 kcal/kg)

FEMALE ADVENTURE RACER, 125 LBS. (57 kg)
Training session: Skill sets, 60 minutes

Carbohydrate requirements	250 g (2 g/lb.) x 4 kcal/g	=	1,000 calories
Protein requirements	63 g (0.5 g/lb.) x 4 kcal/g	=	252 calories
Fat requirements	63 g (0.5 g/lb.) x 9 kcal/g	=	567 calories
Total caloric intake			1,819 (14.5 kcal/lb.)

CREATING THE OPTIMAL TRAINING DIET: YOUR DAILY MEAL PLAN

As an endurance athlete who strives for optimal training and recovery, it is essential for you to translate sound scientific recommendations into everyday food choices that replenish your body's fuel stores and leave you feeling satisfied with your diet. Much of the success of your daily eating plan will hinge on consuming adequate calories and carbohydrates that match your training

WHAT ABOUT FAT LOADING?

The idea of fat loading is provocative, as the fat stored in your muscle and adipose tissue is an abundant supply of fuel. Even the leanest athletes have adequate fat stores to fuel low- to moderate-intensity training for several days, and endurance training enhances an athlete's capacity to burn fat at a given intensity.

Nutritional strategies that encourage athletes to "increase fat burning" are often promoted, but there are several problems associated with fat loading. Although following a fat-loading diet may sound like a tasty treat, it requires a level of meal-planning knowledge that is usually found only among sports dietitians. Training on a fat-loading diet can be extremely difficult. One study demonstrated that subjects responded poorly in training when following a low-carbohydrate, high-fat diet for several weeks. Diets that are very high in fat can also have detrimental health effects.

Several well-designed published studies on fat burning conducted by researchers at the Australian Institute of Sport in Canberra and other research laboratories have shed light on fat metabolism during exercise. These studies were designed to test the hypothesis that athletes may be able to adapt to a high-fat diet for three to five days prior to an event (thereby eliminating some of the risks associated with a long-term high-fat diet), followed by a carbohydrate load in the 48 hours prior to competition. The theory was that this technique would both maximize glycogen stores before competition and optimize the muscles' capacity for fat oxidation during endurance exercise. The studies concluded with a time trial performance test to better mimic real athletic conditions.

CONTINUES

program for that day (and the next day) and rounding out your meals and snacks with the correct balance of healthy proteins and fats.

Meal planning can seem complicated at first, but there are several strategies that can simplify this process. In fact, you will be amazed at how quickly you can adopt some new food strategies and incorporate them into your daily life of training and eating once you have a program and some structure in place. You will find that planning and organization make this part of your training program easier and more effective. Just as you plan ahead to ensure that all the necessary equipment and clothing are available for your workouts, you must also plan to ensure that the optimal foods and required sports nutrition supplements are available to support your training.

Table 4.5 lists the nutritional requirements of two athletes during different phases of their training—a 160-pound (73 kg) male and a 125-pound (57 kg) female. These two examples

WHAT ABOUT FAT LOADING? | continued

These studies indicated that several days on a fat-periodization diet could enhance an athlete's capacity for fat burning during exercise and that this effect could be maintained even after it was followed up by one day on a carbohydrate-loading diet, a high pre-exercise meal, and consumption of carbohydrates during exercise. However, the researchers did not detect measured benefits in endurance and ultraendurance performance. Fat loading also seemed to reduce the muscles' ability to break down glycogen during exercise that has high carbohydrate fuel demands. A more recent study measured the effects of the same fat-loading protocol on endurance exercise interspersed with periods of high-intensity exercise (as often happens in race and training situations). It revealed that there was no performance improvement and that the ability to complete sprints during the race was impaired.

Currently there is no justification for recommending fat-loading/glycogen-loading dietary protocols to improve endurance or ultraendurance performance, and it may even cause a performance detriment in situations where athletes need to sustain high-intensity exercise for brief periods.

demonstrate how nutritional requirements can vary from training cycle to cycle, and within a training cycle, as the types of workouts, the duration of the workouts, and the intensity of the workouts vary.

PRACTICAL CARBOHYDRATE ISSUES

Eating adequate amounts of carbohydrate at specific times in portions that allow you to prepare for training, recover from training, and arrive in good shape for competition can be a challenge. Obtaining wholesome carbohydrates conveniently is difficult enough in our society, but consuming them in the proper amounts at the right times takes a concerted effort. Some endurance sport athletes can easily meet their carbohydrate requirements on specific training days with plenty of well-chosen, wholesome carbohydrates. But on some training days the amounts required for fuel may exceed appetite. At these times, it is important to focus on carbohydrate-rich foods that are appealing, convenient, and easy on your stomach and digestive system.

Food tables that provide carbohydrate portions for 30-gram servings are provided to give you a framework for meal planning (see Table 4.6 and Appendix A). You can use such lists to make sure you are getting the correct total grams of carbohydrates required for training on a given day. A 180-pound triathlete training for 3 hours one day may require a full 700 grams of carbohydrates,

TABLE **4.6**	CARBOHYDRATE CONTENT OF FOODS

30 GRAMS CARBOHYDRATE SERVINGS FOR CEREALS, STARCHES, GRAINS		
	Food	**Portion**
Breads	Bagel	½ large, or 2 oz. (60 g)
	Bread	2 slices, or 2 oz. (60 g)
	Bread crumbs	½ c. (120 ml)
	Breadstick	2 oz. (60 g)
	Cornbread	1 square, or 2 oz. (60 g)
	Dinner roll	2 oz. (60 g)
	English muffin	1 whole, or 2 oz. (60 g)
	Hamburger bun	1 whole, or 2 oz. (60 g)
	Pita pocket	1 round, or 2 oz. (60 g)
Cereals	Bran cereal	⅔ c. (160 ml)
	Cereal, cold, unsweetened	1½ oz. (45 g)
	Cream of wheat, cooked	1 c. (240 ml)
	Granola, low-fat	½ c. (120 ml)
	Grape-Nuts	⅓ c., or 5 tbsp. (100 ml)
	Grits, cooked	1 c. (240 ml)
	Oatmeal, cooked	1 c. (240 ml)
	Puffed cereal	3 c. (720 ml)
	Shredded wheat	¼ c., or 1½ oz. (45 g)
Grains	Barley, raw	¼ c. (60 ml)
	Buckwheat, raw	¼ c. (60 ml)
	Bulgur, cooked	¾ c. (180 ml)
	Crackers	1½ oz. (45 g)
	Muffin, low-fat	3 oz. (90 g)
	Pancake mix, dry	⅓ c. (80 ml)
	Pancakes, 4-in. diameter	3
	Pasta, cooked	1 c. (240 ml)
	Pretzels	1½ oz. (45 g)
	Rice, cooked	⅔ c. (160 ml)
	Rice milk	1 c. (240 ml)
	Saltines	8, 1½ oz. (45 g)
	Tortilla, corn or flour	2

CONTINUES

TABLE **4.6**	CARBOHYDRATE CONTENT OF FOODS continued	

30 GRAMS CARBOHYDRATE SERVINGS FOR CEREALS, STARCHES, GRAINS		
	Food	**Portion**
Starchy Vegetables	Baked beans, cooked	³/₄ c. (180 ml)
	Corn, cooked	³/₄ c. (180 ml)
	Kidney beans, cooked	³/₄ c. (180 ml)
	Peas, cooked	1 c. (240 ml)
	Potato, baked	1 medium, or 5 oz. (150 g)
	Sweet potato, baked	4 oz. (120 ml)
Fruit	Apple	2 small
	Apples, dried	7 rings
	Applesauce, sweetened	¹/₂ c. (120 ml)
	Applesauce, unsweetened	1 c. (240 ml)
	Apricots, fresh	8 medium
	Banana	1 large
	Blueberries	1¹/₂ c. (360 ml)
	Cantaloupe, raw pieces	2 c. (480 ml)
	Dates, dried	1 medium
	Figs, dried	3 medium
	Fruit salad	1 c. (240 ml)
	Grapefruit	1 large
	Grapes	30, or 1 c. (240 ml)
	Kiwifruit	3 medium
	Mango	1 medium
	Nectarine	2 small
	Orange	2 medium
	Papaya	1 medium
	Peach	2 medium
	Pear	1 large
	Pineapple, fresh, pieces	1¹/₂ c. (360 ml)
	Plum	3 medium
	Raisins	¹/₃ c., or 3 tbsp. (60 ml)
	Raspberries	2 c. (480 ml)
	Strawberries	2¹/₂ c. (600 ml)
	Watermelon	3 slices, or 3 c. (720 ml)

CONTINUES

TABLE **4.6**	**CARBOHYDRATE CONTENT OF FOODS** continued

30 GRAMS CARBOHYDRATE SERVINGS FOR CEREALS, STARCHES, GRAINS		
	Food	**Portion**
Fruit and Vegetable Juices	Apple juice	8 oz. (240 ml)
	Carrot juice	10 oz. (300 ml)
	Cranberry juice cocktail	8 oz. (240 ml)
	Grape juice	8 oz. (240 ml)
	Grapefruit juice	8 oz. (240 ml)
	Orange juice	8 oz. (240 ml)
	Pineapple juice	8 oz. (240 ml)
	Vegetable juice cocktail	24 oz. (720 ml)
Sweets and Baked Goods	Angelfood cake	$1/12$ whole
	Cake, flour type	$1/12$ whole
	Chocolate milk	8 oz. (240 ml)
	Cookies, fat-free	4 small
	Fruit spreads, 100% fruit	2 tbsp. (40 ml)
	Gingersnaps	6 cookies
	Graham crackers	6 squares
	Granola bar, low-fat	1
	Honey	2 tbsp. (40 ml)
	Ice cream	1 c. (240 ml)
	Jam or jelly	2 tbsp. (40 ml)
	Pie	$1/8$ whole
	Pudding, regular	$1/2$ c. (120 ml)
	Sherbet	$1/2$ c. (120 ml)
	Sorbet	$1/2$ c. (120 ml)
	Syrup, regular	2 tbsp. (40 ml)
	Vanilla wafers	10 cookies
	Yogurt, frozen, fat-free	1 c. (240 ml)
	Yogurt, frozen, low-fat	$2/3$ c. (160 ml)

CONTINUES

TABLE **4.6**	**CARBOHYDRATE CONTENT OF FOODS** continued

10 GRAMS CARBOHYDRATE SERVINGS		
	Food	**Portion**
	Artichoke	1 medium
	Asparagus, boiled	1 c.
	Beans, green, boiled	1 c.
	Beet greens, cooked	1¼ c.
	Broccoli, boiled	1 c.
	Broccoli, raw	2 c.
	Brussels sprouts, boiled	¾ c.
	Cabbage, cooked	¾ c.
	Carrots, cooked	⅔ c.
Vegetables	Carrots, raw	2 medium
	Cauliflower, cooked	¾ c.
	Kale, boiled	1¼ c.
	Mushrooms, cooked	1 c.
	Mustard greens, cooked	1½ c.
	Peppers, sweet, raw	2 c.
	Spinach, boiled	1½ c.
	Summer squash, cooked	1 c.
	Tomato, raw	2 medium
	Milk, 1%	8 oz. (240 ml)
	Milk, 2%	8 oz. (240 ml)
	Buttermilk, 1%	8 oz. (240 ml)
Dairy Products	Milk, nonfat	8 oz. (240 ml)
	Yogurt, low-fat	8 oz. (240 ml)
	Yogurt, nonfat	8 oz. (240 ml)
	Yogurt, with fruit	8 oz. (240 ml)

PRACTICAL CARBOHYDRATE STRATEGIES FOR HEAVY TRAINING

On training days that demand a very high carbohydrate intake, timing and tolerance issues can complicate your efforts to meet specific nutrition goals. Consuming enough carbohydrates takes planning, as the amounts you require often exceed what is found in an everyday diet. But if you leave your diet to chance, your intake may be inadequate. Fortunately, it becomes easier if you follow some simple practical suggestions.

Sports bars and energy bars are a concentrated and convenient source of carbohydrates, supplying up to 50 grams per serving. They travel well and can be consumed quickly between training sessions or on the way back to class or work. But do keep in mind that these bars are often vitamin and mineral fortified. Make sure that you do not consume doses of these nutrients that are too high simply by overconsuming sports bars. Energy bars should not replace fruits, vegetables, and whole grains in your diet, but they can supplement a high-energy, high-carbohydrate diet based on fresh foods.

Moreover, getting too much fiber for your own personal tolerance could be hard on your digestive system on intense training days. Adding lower-fiber carbohydrate foods to the mix may be more practical when carbohydrates must be consumed in very large amounts. These foods can be consumed in combination with higher-fiber items and still be part of a diet that is adequate in fiber, vitamins, and minerals. Good choices include large bagels, calorically dense cereals, fruit juices, jams, honey, and syrup.

CONTINUES

whereas a runner of the same weight completing a shorter run may require only 400 grams of carbohydrates daily. Consuming 400 grams of carbohydrates in a given training day is much easier than consuming 700 grams—attaining the higher amount requires more structure and planning.

The food system outlined in this chapter provides you with the flexibility to emphasize various carbohydrate sources from one day to the next depending on your food preferences, fuel needs, training schedule, and training cycle. Food charts can be one of the most helpful tools you can employ as you strive to meet your carbohydrate requirements. They can make one of the most important nutrients in your training diet more accessible and manageable because they spell out precise daily servings and portions. During periods of high training volume and/or intensity, consuming adequate amounts of carbohydrate can be challenging. During lighter training cycles,

PRACTICAL CARBOHYDRATE STRATEGIES FOR HEAVY TRAINING   continued

A well-timed snack of yogurt with fruit, a low-fat milkshake, or a fruit smoothie can up your carbohydrate intake considerably and provide needed fluid, and these items also taste good. High-carbohydrate supplement drinks or meal replacements may also be a convenient source of carbohydrates and are easy to carry and quickly consumed. These products should not replace wholesome foods, however. Desserts can be part of a nutritious diet in reasonable amounts. Some carbohydrate-dense choices are sherbet, sorbet, and frozen yogurt topped with fruit.

Meeting your daily carbohydrate intake often requires consuming between-meal snacks and "grazing" throughout the day. Carbohydrate-rich foods should comprise at least half of your meals and snacks. Low-fiber choices may be tolerated better than high-fiber choices when you are eating close to the start of your training session.

Keep an eye out for carbohydrate foods that are also high in fat (often unhealthy fats), such as croissants, creamed or deep-fried vegetables, doughnuts, French toast, fried rice, muffins, pancakes, pastry, potato chips, snack crackers, and popcorn popped with oil.

downsizing your diet to more moderate portions can also be challenging because it requires a shift in meal planning. In practical terms, individualized plans can differ from athlete to athlete depending on medical history, food preferences, schedule, and culinary skills; the charts can help you to individualize the general recommendations to suit your unique needs and situation.

FOOD LISTS FOR PLANNING YOUR TRAINING DIET

Table 4.6 outlines the portion sizes of various foods that supply 30, 10, or 12 to 40 grams of carbohydrates per serving. If you are just learning to keep track of your carbohydrate consumption, using this list on a daily basis can simplify meal planning for your training diet and make it more effective. Make sure you choose carbohydrates from several food groups: the bread, cereal, and grain group; the fruit and fruit juice group; the vegetable group; and the milk, yogurt, and soy group. Then, supplement these on high-intake days with miscellaneous carbohydrate foods provided by snack items, desserts, and the like. On days when your carbohydrate needs are especially high, grains and starches are likely to make up a good portion of your diet because they are such concentrated food sources, providing 30 grams of carbohydrates per serving in the portion sizes supplied in the table. As discussed in Chapter 2, try to choose only lightly processed or whole-grain sources as much as possible. Many items from the grain group, such as pretzels and crackers, also make good snack choices.

Fruits, dried fruit, and fruit juices, which also provide 30 grams per serving in the listed amounts, are your next great source of carbohydrates. Because of the abundant nutrients they supply, they are excellent food choices for maintaining good health. Vegetables also provide carbohydrates—though, at about 10 grams per serving, not as much per portion as grains and fruits. However, few foods can match vegetables for their high nutrient content.

Dairy milk and yogurt, as well as other milks such as soy milk and rice milk, are also good sources of carbohydrates, ranging anywhere from 12 to 40 grams per serving in the amounts listed. Yogurts can be especially high in carbohydrates when they come mixed with fruit and sugars.

One last source of concentrated carbohydrates is sweets and desserts, which also supply 30 grams per serving in the portion sizes listed in the table. Sweets should not routinely replace more wholesome carbohydrate choices in your diet, but they are a source of additional carbohydrates. They offer the advantage of being more dense and less filling than some higher-fiber, more wholesome choices, and when your carbohydrate requirements are especially high, exceeding 500 grams daily, they do come in handy. For very heavy training days, you can also consider adding some sports nutrition products high in carbohydrates to your food plan.

Of course, endurance athletes cannot live—and should not live—on carbohydrates alone. Choosing quality proteins and healthy fats will provide you with essential nutrients and balance out your meals and snacks. Proteins and fats also keep you full longer and even out blood glucose levels during the day. The protein foods listed in Table 4.7 are ranked according to their fat content to aid you in making sure you do not exceed healthy limits of total fat and saturated fat in your diet. Plant proteins and milk and dairy sources should be emphasized for vegetarian athletes.

A well-balanced diet with adequate calories and with up to 15 to 20 percent of those calories from protein provides enough protein for the muscle growth and repair that endurance athletes engaged in hard training so need. It also should be enough for those who do strength training. Protein consumed in excess of your requirements is simply stored as fat—though, as explained earlier, it may also be burned for energy. Converting protein to fuel for exercise is inefficient, however, when compared with burning carbohydrates.

Consuming excess protein can result in other negative effects. Protein from both food and supplements increases your need for fluid, as your kidneys require more water to eliminate the end products of protein metabolism. A high protein intake should be accompanied by a high fluid intake. Individuals with liver or kidney problems are also susceptible to the negative effects of excessive dietary protein. Excess dietary protein leads to a short-lived increase in the urinary excretion of calcium, an important mineral for building healthy bone tissue. Thus, high protein

TABLE **4.7**	FAT CONTENT OF PROTEIN CHOICES

VERY LOW-FAT PROTEINS (< 2 g fat/oz., or 30 g)	LOW-FAT PROTEINS (3–4 g fat/oz., or 30 g)	MEDIUM-FAT PROTEINS (4–5 g fat/oz., or 30 g)	HIGH-FAT PROTEINS (6–8 g fat/oz., or 30 g)	VERY HIGH-FAT PROTEINS (> 8 g fat/oz., or 30 g)
Fish				
WHITE FISH Grouper Tuna Haddock Sole Halibut Bass *SHELLFISH* Crab Shrimp Lobster Clams	*DARK FISH* Salmon Mackerel Sardines	Tuna and salmon packed in oil		Any fried fish product
Cheese				
Fat-free cheeses Cottage cheese, 1% Cottage cheese, 2%	Low-fat cheeses	Feta cheese Mozzarella, part-skim Grated Parmesan	Mozzarella Neufchatel	American, processed Cream cheese Brie Cheddar Edam Monterey Jack Muenster Limburger Swiss
Beef				
Round, choice, 90% lean	Round, choice, 85% lean Rib-eye, choice Flank steak, choice Porterhouse, choice	Round, choice, 73% lean Round, choice, 80% lean	Roast beef Meat loaf	Short ribs Corned beef Prime cuts

CONTINUES

TABLE **4.7**	FAT CONTENT OF PROTEIN CHOICES continued			

VERY LOW-FAT PROTEINS (< 2 g fat/oz., or 30 g)	LOW-FAT PROTEINS (3–4 g fat/oz., or 30 g)	MEDIUM-FAT PROTEINS (4–5 g fat/oz., or 30 g)	HIGH-FAT PROTEINS (6–8 g fat/oz., or 30 g)	VERY HIGH-FAT PROTEINS (> 8 g fat/oz., or 30 g)
Pork				
Ham, lean, 95% fat-free Pork tenderloin Boneless sirloin chop Top loin chop	Sirloin roast Center loin chop Boneless rib roast Center rib chop Blade steak Canadian bacon	Pork butt	Italian sausage	Pâté Pastrami Bacon Pork sausage
Lamb				
Leg, top round Leg, shank, half	Loin chop Loin roast Rib chop	Roast lamb		Ground lamb
Legumes (per c.)				
Black beans Kidney beans Lentils Lima beans Pinto beans	Chickpeas	Tofu	Soybeans	
Poultry				
Turkey breast Chicken, white, no skin Turkey, dark, no skin	Chicken, dark, no skin Chicken, dark, w/skin Turkey, dark, w/skin Duck, roasted, no skin	Ground turkey, mixed meat/skin	Duck, roasted, w/skin	
Other				
95% fat-free luncheon meat Egg whites Egg substitute	86% fat-free luncheon meat Egg substitute	Eggs	Luncheon meat Bologna Turkey/chicken Hot dogs Salami	Knockwurst Bratwurst Beef/pork hot dogs Peanut butter

intakes should also be accompanied by adequate amounts of calcium. And although food sources of protein are best, they can contribute substantial amounts of fat and cholesterol to the diet. Consuming excess protein can therefore increase your risk of heart disease and other health problems. You should be selective regarding the type of protein foods you eat. There are plenty of low-fat animal protein food sources to choose from and plenty of healthy plant proteins as well. When planning meals, it is important to remember that the grains and vegetables that you consume also contribute to your daily protein intake.

Your protein needs for your daily training, muscle repair, and other important protein functions are easily met through a well-planned diet adequate in calories. The key is to obtain adequate amounts of quality lean or low-fat protein sources throughout the day and to consume enough calories so that protein is not burned for energy.

Table 4.8 outlines sources of fat in 5-gram servings according to the type of fat each food provides. Again, you can use the table as a guide in making your own individual food choices. Emphasize healthy essential fatty acids and foods high in monounsaturated fat. During periods of very high training volume, these healthy fats are a needed source of additional calories and add flavor and variety to your meals.

As you use these food tables—and the sample menus provided later in the book—you will discover how to follow my general guidelines while making adjustments to suit your own health goals and personal tastes. For example, if you do not like dairy products or are lactose-intolerant, you can easily emphasize other choices and keep dairy to a minimum. You could add servings of fruits and juices, or substitute soy milk for cow's milk. Or, on some training days you may wish to have fewer grain servings and increase the number of servings of fruits and fruit juices to match your carbohydrate requirements. On light training days, your carbohydrate needs may be lower than on others, and you can adjust your choices accordingly. The point is, these plans can and should be modified to suit your needs. However, regardless of your personalized food plan and preferences, for optimal performance and recovery you need to reach the recommended carbohydrate amounts in total grams. You should also keep in mind that your choices must also supply you with all the nutrients described in Part I.

FOOD JOURNALS: TRACKING YOUR INTAKE

Even with the food tables, some athletes may find it difficult to keep track of how many calories they have consumed throughout the day. By late afternoon, with all the distractions of everyday life, you may have forgotten how many grams of carbs you have taken in so far or how much protein you ate. Besides, most of your attention is being focused on the training itself. One useful tool for helping you to overcome this problem is a food journal. Keeping a food journal gives you a

TABLE **4.8**	SOURCES OF FAT

SOURCE		PORTION
Polyunsaturated Fat (5 grams per serving)		
Margarine	Stick, tub, or squeeze	1 tsp. (6 ml)
	Reduced-fat	1 tbsp. (20 ml)
Mayonnaise	Regular	1 tsp. (6 ml)
	Reduced-fat	1 tbsp. (20 ml)
Walnuts		4 halves
Oil: corn, safflower, soybean, flaxseed, walnut		1 tsp. (6 ml)
Salad dressing, regular		1 tbsp. (20 ml)
Sunflower seeds		1 tbsp. (20 ml)
Pumpkin seeds		1 tbsp. (20 ml)
Monounsaturated Fat (5 grams per serving)		
Avocado, medium		1/8 whole
Oil: Canola, olive, peanut		1 tsp. (6 ml)
Olives, black		8 large
Nuts	Almonds, cashews	6
	Peanuts	10
	Pecans	4 halves
Peanut butter		2 tsp. (12 ml)
Sesame seeds		1 tbsp. (20 ml)
Tahini paste		2 tsp. (12 ml)
Saturated Fat (5 grams per serving)		
Bacon, cooked		1 slice
Butter	Stick	1 tsp. (6 ml)
	Whipped	1 tsp. (6 ml)
	Reduced-fat	1 tbsp. (20 ml)
Cream, half-and-half		2 tbsp. (40 ml)
Shortening or lard		1 tsp. (6 ml)
Sour cream	Regular	2 tbsp. (40 ml)
	Reduced-fat	3 tbsp. (60 ml)

way to determine whether you are meeting your energy and nutrient requirements over the course of each day or week. To reap the most benefits, it is best if you write down your food choices and portions while you are still eating or immediately afterward. Don't forget to note snacks, supplements, and any fluids consumed. With help from the food lists provided, you can assess a number of items regarding your food intake:

- For starters, add up the number of carbohydrate grams you consumed during the day and determine whether your intake matches your training efforts. Note carbohydrate amounts from food labels, and use the food lists provided to estimate the amount of carbohydrate per serving. You can also tally your total serving intake from the carbohydrate-containing food lists and see how your choices match up with the meal plans provided. You can determine not only whether your daily totals are adequate but also whether the amount of carbohydrate you consumed before and after exercise was appropriate to support your training and recovery efforts.

- Record the amounts of fluids and carbohydrate that you consume before, during, and after your workout. By looking back over your records, you can learn whether you have been meeting the recommended fluid amounts and taking ample opportunity to consume fluids and carbohydrates during breaks in training. Note how your energy levels during training may fluctuate depending on your carbohydrate and fluid intake.

- Look through the day's intake to ensure that you are consuming the right amount of concentrated and high-quality lean protein. If you are vegetarian, check that your plant proteins are amply portioned so that your body receives all the required amino acids (see the sidebar "Protein and the Vegetarian Athlete"). Check that protein is included in your recovery foods and fluids and that you also consume high-quality protein before and after weight training.

- Determine whether the fats you consume are derived from healthy monounsaturated oil, liquid unhydrogenated polyunsaturated oil, and omega-3 fatty-acid food choices. Be sure to include good sources of essential fatty acids in your diet.

- Measure your intake of hydrating fluids for the day, including before and after training. Make sure that you are well hydrated before exercise and that you consume enough fluids to replace sweat losses after exercise.

- Check for hidden fats, such as those found in muffins, pastries, and high-fat crackers. Try to minimize your intake of these foods whenever possible.

- Pay attention to your eating patterns. Note if you become too hungry at some times during the day, and adjust your mealtimes accordingly. Pay attention to any eating that may occur due to boredom, stress, or other issues not related to hunger.

TABLE **4.9**	SERVING RECOMMENDATIONS FOR VARIOUS CALORIE LEVELS				

FOOD GROUPS	2,000 CALORIES	2,400 CALORIES	2,900 CALORIES	3,400 CALORIES	4,000 CALORIES
Grains	6	7	8	10	12
Fruits	3	3	4	5	6
Vegetables	2	3	3	3	3
Milk/yogurt/ soy milk	2	2	2 (milk) 1 (yogurt)	2 (milk) 1 (yogurt)	3 (milk) 1 (yogurt)
Protein	6	6	6	7	8
Fats	3	4	5	6	8
Menu breakdown	315 g carbohydrates 84 g protein 45 g fat	350 g carbohydrates 112 g protein 60 g fat	450 g carbohydrates 114 g protein 70 g fat	550 g carbohydrates 120 g protein 80 g fat	650 g carbohydrates 150 g protein 89 g fat

Finally, see Table 4.9 for examples of the number of servings of each food type that can combine to make up a well-balanced sports nutrition diet at different levels of calorie intake. Then, check your food journal to see if any adjustments should be made to improve your overall mix.

LABEL-READING TIPS

Nutritional information on labels can help you determine the nutritional breakdown of foods. First check the ingredient list. You may want to include more whole-wheat flours and other whole grains in your diet. Ingredients are listed on the labels by weight, from the item weighing the most to the one weighing the least.

Pay attention to the serving size on the label and compare it with the amount that you actually eat. Portions you consume may be double those on the package, and you should adjust the nutrition information accordingly. You can also use the label to evaluate if a food will significantly impact your carbohydrate intake by checking the total grams of carbohydrates listed. You can then determine what portion of that particular food would provide 30 grams or more of carbohydrates to help you meet your training requirements.

Total fat grams, as well as calories from fat, are also listed. To determine the percentage of calories from fat, divide the fat calories per serving by the total calories per serving and multiply by 100. Keep higher-fat foods in perspective. Your fat intake needs to be considered in the context of an entire day. Your total day's intake should provide 20 to 25 percent fat calories, which allows

PROTEIN AND THE VEGETARIAN ATHLETE

Vegetarianism and veganism can certainly provide a basis for a healthy diet, and many athletes are successful in their sport while maintaining a vegetarian diet. However, endurance athletes do have increased protein requirements, and vegetarian athletes should appreciate that a quality plant is not as concentrated a source of protein as an animal protein. It is possible, however, to compensate for the reduced number of protein grams in vegetable sources. The first key for vegetarian endurance athletes is to consume enough carbohydrate calories so that the protein they do consume is not processed for energy. Second, vegetarians should emphasize high-quality and concentrated plant protein sources. Certain grains, dried peas and beans, lentils, nuts, and seeds are some of the best sources. Soy products such as tempeh and tofu are almost equivalent to animal protein in quality.

Although it is not necessary to combine or complement various plant proteins at the same meal, as was once thought, vegetarians should make a concentrated effort to obtain an adequate combination of plant proteins in their diet throughout the day. Your body will make its own complete proteins over the course of the day if you consume enough calories from a variety of sources. If your calorie intake falls short, some of the protein you consume may be processed for energy rather than utilized for important functions that only protein can accomplish.

Protein Tips for Vegetarians

- Include a protein-rich food at all meals and snacks.
- Add milk or a fortified soy milk or yogurt equivalent to every meal and snack.
- Use nut butters, hummus, and low-fat cheeses (soy or regular) for toppings on breads, bagels, and crackers.
- Add nuts and seeds to a fruit and yogurt snack.
- Eat tofu and tempeh—both make good elements of a stir-fry.
- Experiment with quick and easy bean recipes such as burritos, casseroles, and salads.
- Make thick soups and stews with beans and lentils.
- Experiment with various meat-replacement products on the market, such as tofu dogs and burgers.

CONTINUES

PROTEIN AND THE VEGETARIAN ATHLETE   continued

Meal-Planning Tips for Vegetarians

- Health-food stores provide a wide variety of vegetarian food choices and convenience items; more and more supermarkets are now broadening their selection of these items as well, and some have special health-food sections. Take the time to browse these markets and discover new products.
- The number of textured vegetable protein products has increased significantly. You can now buy high-protein products that resemble and taste like hot dogs, burgers, and breakfast sausages. These can be used to make quick and easy lunches.
- Tofu can be substituted for chicken in most recipes. Seasoned tofu is available, and you can also season the recipe to spice up the tofu's milder taste.
- Substitute vegetable broth when recipes call for beef or chicken stock. Vegetable broth is available in many supermarkets and health-food stores.
- Canned lentils, chickpeas, and beans are a quick and nutritious vegetarian option. Many bean and lentil recipes can be batch-cooked and frozen for later use.
- Purchase calcium-fortified soy and rice milks if you drink these products instead of dairy milk.
- Purchase iron-fortified cereals, and consume them with products high in vitamin C such as orange juice.

for some healthy foods that may be a bit higher in fat. Some foods, such as dried pasta are low in fat, while others, such as margarine, provide a high amount of fat.

The Daily Values (DV) for various vitamins and minerals provided on the nutrition label are based on a 2,000-calorie intake. The percentage of DV can tell you whether a food is high or low in a nutrient such as calcium, fiber, iron, or vitamin C. A food is considered to be a good source of a nutrient if it provides 20 percent of the DV. Besides increasing your intake of foods high in specific nutrients, you can use the DV to avoid excess fat, saturated fat, and cholesterol.

5

TIMING FOOD AND FLUID INTAKE FOR
TRAINING AND COMPETITION

Fine-Tuning Your Food Plan for Optimal Performance

THINK OF YOUR DAILY TRAINING DIET as a 24-hour outline of your carbohydrate, protein, and fat requirements. The guidelines described in Chapter 4 tell you how to determine how much fuel your body needs each day and what types of fuel it needs. These amounts and types of fuel will change from day to day depending on your daily training session and your training cycle. You can fine-tune your diet even more, however, through specific timing of your food and fluid intake. Matching your intake patterns to the specific fuel demands of your training schedule optimizes your energy for training, enhances your recovery from training, and helps you to meet your body-composition goals. Timing is especially important for endurance athletes who have a full schedule of training built around work or school. One of the biggest nutritional mistakes an athlete can make is to undermine his or her own performance by not taking in enough of the foods needed to provide fuel for training. But not timing this fuel intake properly is also a mistake. The wrong timing can definitely have a detrimental effect on your performance. This conclusion is backed up by plenty of solid research that has paved the way for specific nutritional strategies that endurance athletes can practice in the hours before, during, and after training.

Ideally, your training and recovery diet will take you in top nutritional form from one training session to the next. However, real life can sometimes (or perhaps often) get in the way of recharging your fuel stores to the optimal levels required for quality training. A hectic training schedule, especially when combined with work or school, often leaves limited time for meals and snacks, let alone meal preparation. Daily training sessions and other life commitments can easily get in the way, leaving only brief windows of time for meal preparation and eating the recommended amounts of fuel. Nevertheless, it is safe to say that all athletes can benefit from careful timing. Even an athlete with an ideal daily training diet can obtain a clear performance boost from paying attention to the foods and fluids he or she consumes during the 4-hour period before training and the 4-hour period after training.

Our bodies run well on a steady supply of fuel throughout the day. Each time you consume a meal or snack, you add some carbohydrate stores to your liver and ensure optimal blood glucose levels for the next several hours. When we overconsume fuel at any given meal or snack, the excess—whether from carbs, protein, or fat—is simply sent to our fat stores (though carbs and proteins must be converted to fat first, of course). For this reason, eating several times daily seems to work well not only from a weight-management perspective but also from a fueling perspective. As we consume foods and fluids throughout the day, we allow our bodies to both prepare for and recover from training, often more than once daily.

What you consume in the hours before, during, and after training should match up with the fuel depletion that occurs during the training session. When training for your endurance sport, the longer and harder your training session, the greater the risk of developing glycogen depletion and dehydration. Remember that a full supply of glycogen stores provides anywhere from 1,400 to 1,800 calories' worth of fuel. During steady exercise at a moderate to high intensity, you burn through this fuel in less than 90 minutes. During high-intensity training, such as when completing a session focusing on speed work and interval training, you can burn through fuel quickly and experience significant glycogen depletion in less than 1 hour. Once you experience muscle glycogen depletion, fatigue sets in and you cannot respond to the demands of training. Even with plenty of fat stores remaining, you may need to decrease your exercise intensity. In fact, you may not even be able to complete the training session. Your fat stores cannot supply fuel quickly enough to sustain the high intensities in some types of workouts, and consequently your muscle fibers don't receive the fuel they need to contract during exercise.

How quickly you deplete your body-fuel stores depends on the nature of your training. When you bike at a steady, moderate rate, you steadily burn both fat and carbohydrates. Speed workouts at the track can deplete your carbohydrate stores in under an hour. Indoor gym workouts that incorporate cardiovascular work and resistance training are also glycogen depleting. Glycogen depletion from just one training session can be significant. But glycogen depletion can also occur gradually over several days' time or even over one or several weeks' time.

Blood glucose provides a very limited amount of fuel during exercise. It is your brain's only fuel source and is supplied and maintained by your liver glycogen stores. When you run low on blood glucose, you cannot focus on the exercise task at hand. You may experience light-headedness, poor concentration, and irritability, and you may not perform the skills for your sport as easily as you know you can. Exercise will seem much harder, and coordination will suffer. Your judgment can also become impaired, and this can affect your technique. You may have to slow down considerably or stop exercising altogether, because the blood glucose supplied by your liver is also an important fuel source for your muscles when they become depleted of glycogen.

Other body nutrient stores can also become depleted. Fluid depletion is an important concern and can impede your training efforts. Dehydration can slow down both moderate- and high-intensity efforts, impair your mental concentration, decrease muscular endurance, and result in overheating, possibly to dangerous levels in hot weather. Excess sodium losses can also adversely affect your performance and increase health risks during exercise.

NUTRITIONAL STRATEGIES BEFORE TRAINING

Endurance sport athletes who want to complete their training program or compete at their best can benefit from several pre-exercise nutrition strategies designed to minimize the fuel, fluid, and electrolyte depletion that can occur during training. Making the most of specific food and fluid choices before training or competition offers several important performance advantages:

- It allows you to start training or competition with optimal fluid levels, helping to delay or at least minimize dehydration.
- It refills liver glycogen stores and decreases your risk of developing hypoglycemia during exercise.
- It tops off your muscle glycogen stores and delays glycogen depletion while training and competing.
- It provides you with fuel and fluid during the early part of exercise.
- It ensures that your stomach is settled and prevents hunger pains during exercise.
- It provides a psychological edge and certain level of comfort to know you've consumed a well-tested pre-competition meal.

Clearly, stocking your liver and muscle glycogen stores before exercise is essential prior to demanding training sessions. The nutritional strategies recommended below are specific about how to time your pre-exercise meals and snacks. The guidelines are flexible enough, however, to allow some variations due to schedules dictated by work, school, and practice times. Often an appropriately portioned and timed pre-exercise meal is just what an endurance sport athlete needs to fuel his or her training session, restore fuel depleted from a previous training session, and replenish fuel stores after the overnight fast that takes place during sleep. The recommended portions and suggested foods and fluids to be consumed are directly related to the timing of your pre-exercise meal. Meta-bolically speaking, there are two distinct time periods for pre-exercise eating: 2 to 4 hours before exercise, and 30 to 60 minutes before exercise. When you eat is often a matter of practicality and scheduling. What you eat is truly a matter of metabolic, gastrointestinal, and personal tolerances.

3 TO 4 HOURS BEFORE EXERCISE

Many seasoned athletes have identified the window of time occurring 3 to 4 hours before training as an optimal period for pre-exercise eating. During this time, you can consume a moderate to large meal and still have plenty of digestion time. The main focus of this pre-exercise meal should be to replenish your liver glycogen stores and to store fuel in your gastrointestinal (GI) tract for later release. With the right timing and portions, eating 3 to 4 hours before exercise will provide the following benefits:

- It restores liver glycogen to normal levels.
- It enables your body to store carbohydrates in the muscle to be used as needed, if portions are large enough.
- It allows you to store some carbohydrates in the gut for absorption and release during exercise.
- It prevents you from feeling hungry during training.

Metabolically and physically, you can consume a substantial amount of carbohydrate in the 3- to 4-hour period prior to training. Consuming carbohydrates within this time frame does elevate blood insulin levels and favor the use of carbohydrates as a fuel. But because you can consume a good amount of carbohydrate during this time, blood glucose levels remain nice and steady. Research indicates that eating during this period enhances performance. Not eating during this period before training could put a drain on your training sessions.

Pre-exercise eating portions should be appropriate for your tolerances, but try to consume the upper limits for a fuel and performance benefit. For every hour that you allow yourself some di-gestion time, consume just under half a gram of carbohydrates for every pound (approximately 1 g/kg) of body weight. Using this formula, you can safely consume 2 grams of carbohydrates per pound (4 g/kg) 4 hours before exercise and 1.5 grams per pound (3 g/kg) 3 hours before exercise.

For example, if you decide to eat a large meal or snack 4 hours before a long run or hard train-ing ride, 2 grams of carbohydrates per pound (4 g/kg) for a 160-pound (73 kg) athlete would translate to 320 grams of carbohydrates. It would probably be easiest on your stomach if a portion of this fairly substantial meal consisted of dense, low-fiber foods and even some liquid carbohydrate sources. The more intense the workout, the more carefully you want to pay attention to specific food tolerances and timing.

For easy digestion, you can obtain 300 grams of carbohydrates by consuming one large bagel topped with 2 tablespoons of jam, followed by a fruited yogurt and 32 ounces of a sports drink. With the full 4 hours of digestion time, you may also find that 1 cup of granola, 8 ounces of skim milk, one large banana, and 12 ounces of juice accompanied by two slices of toast and 2 tablespoons of jam, all providing 200 grams of carbohydrates, is also well tolerated. This pre-exercise meal could be topped off with 12 ounces of a high-carbohydrate energy drink to provide a total of close to 300 grams of carbohydrates. Of course, some athletes can only tolerate smaller meals even with 4 hours of digestion time. Every athlete needs to iron out his or her individual tolerances in regard to foods and portions when eating in the 3- to 4-hour period before training.

Eating a few hours beforehand can be ideal for several exercise start times. An early-morning breakfast can be consumed at 6:00 to 7:00 for a 9:00 to 10:00 a.m. start time. For a later start time, such as 2:00 p.m., you may want to consume a larger breakfast of easily digested foods at 10:00 a.m. An evening workout at 6:00 p.m. could easily be preceded by a large afternoon snack at 2:00 to 3:00 p.m.

2 HOURS BEFORE EXERCISE

Consuming food 3 to 4 hours before training may not always be possible because of scheduling conflicts and very early start times (rising at 5:00 a.m. to eat prior to an 8:00 a.m. workout does not sound very appealing). Because of timing constraints, eating 2 hours before training may be your preferred choice. One good rule for pre-exercise eating is that the closer to exercise you plan to eat, the smaller the meal you should consume. Try to keep your intake of carbohydrates to 1 gram per pound (2 g/kg) of body weight in this time interval. For example, a 160-pound (73 kg) athlete could consume up to 160 grams of carbohydrates.

With this close timing, liquid carbohydrate choices become even more attractive because they are more quickly digested. Breakfast shakes, liquid meal replacements, smoothies, and sports supplements often provide more than 50 grams of carbohydrates per serving. A juice smoothie may work well, as do easily digested energy bars.

Eating 2 hours prior to exercise could be the best timing for an early or mid-morning training start time. It can also work well for tricky early-afternoon training times. Following a large breakfast that is well digested, a small to moderate snack 2 hours before training works well for many athletes who plan ahead for afternoon or evening start times.

1 HOUR BEFORE EXERCISE

A variety of scenarios could necessitate the need for food 30 to 60 minutes prior to exercise. Rising in the extreme early hours of the morning simply to eat food and fuel up for an early training time may not be feasible or desirable. Other scheduling scenarios could result in a large time gap between the last sizable meal and the start of a training session, and hunger and limited fuel during training can become a significant issue. You may also find it helpful to eat closer to longer training sessions because the added fuel can provide a performance benefit.

Whether or not you should consume carbohydrates 30 to 60 minutes prior to exercise depends on your tolerances and training schedule. You are most likely to benefit from ingesting fuel 30 to 60 minutes prior to exercise when the carbohydrates you consume replenish compromised fuel stores. So consider consuming carbohydrates within an hour before exercise if you have not eaten for 4 hours or more before training, or prior to early-morning training when liver glycogen is low. Eating an hour before intense training sessions can prevent hunger and provide needed extra calories for endurance athletes who have very high energy requirements.

Consuming carbohydrates just 30 to 60 minutes prior to exercise will have different metabolic results than consuming them several hours before exercise. When you eat at the later time, there will be marked increases in your blood glucose and blood insulin levels prior to training. A decline in blood glucose during training follows, and your liver decreases the amount of glucose it sends into your bloodstream.

Owing to these metabolic effects, some controversy has surfaced over the years in athletic circles regarding carbohydrate consumption in the hour before exercise. The concern has been that carbohydrate consumption at this time can result in hypoglycemia, or a decrease in blood glucose levels, during exercise, which produces negative symptoms and can have an adverse effect on performance. In fact, however, many studies have confirmed that consuming carbohydrates in the hour before exercise does not impair performance and can actually help performance. These studies used exercise test protocols that mimicked steady-state endurance training, not the high-intensity, moderate-intensity mix that would have better mimicked some of your training sessions. But what was also interesting about these studies was the variation in individual blood glucose responses seen in the test subjects. Results showed that although blood glucose may drop during the early part of training, it quickly corrects itself to normal levels, and the majority of athletes experience no adverse symptoms or performance effects. A small number of subjects, however, did experience some hypoglycemia and a negative effect on performance.

If you are concerned that you may be a carbohydrate-sensitive athlete during the hour prior to training, you may find a few sensible strategies useful. Consuming a high enough number of carbohydrates may simply offset any lowered blood glucose levels and hypoglycemic symptoms. Amounts of 70 grams or more seem to maintain blood glucose levels in individuals susceptible to exercise hypoglycemia. Individuals not susceptible to hypoglycemia can consume only 50 grams of carbohydrates and still obtain a performance benefit, but they may be able to consume more than 70 grams just as well. Athletes can often tolerate up to 100 grams of carbohydrates in the hour prior to training. Choices and amounts are a matter of preference and GI comfort. Practical choices include carbohydrate gels, energy bars, and carbohydrate or sports drinks, which often provide 30 to 50 grams of carbohydrates per serving. Endurance athletes can choose one of the items or any combination of them in portions that are tolerated.

Regardless of your training schedule, a pre-training meal or snack can provide some performance benefit. While the main part of your nutritional intake will be carbohydrates, small amounts of protein, and perhaps fat, may be tolerated if appropriately timed. Determine your optimal pre-exercise meal through experimentation during training. The recommended carbohydrate amounts for various pre-exercise meal times is summarized later in this chapter (see Table 5.5).

THE GLYCEMIC INDEX

Some endurance athletes may choose to incorporate foods that are low to moderate on the glycemic index scale into their pre-training meal in order to maintain steady blood glucose levels over the next few hours and through training. Although research regarding pre-exercise eating and low-glycemic foods does not fully back this strategy, choosing low-glycemic foods in the several hours before training certainly does not hurt performance. Often the decision to choose these lower-glycemic foods is a matter of personal preference and tolerance; athletes can find what works best for them through experimentation. As you experiment with consuming low- to moderate-glycemic-index foods (see Appendix A), you will be able to determine what choices work best for you.

As discussed in Chapter 1, adding protein and a small amount of fat to a meal can blunt the glycemic effect of the meal. Small amounts of lean protein and easily digested sources of fat can help to maintain steady blood glucose levels and prevent hunger during exercise, and these foods are often well tolerated when consumed 2 to 4 hours prior to training. Many low-glycemic carbohydrate options, such as unprocessed grains and fruits, are also good sources of fiber, and timing can be an important issue for these foods before training. However, in the 30 to 60 minutes prior to training, many well-tolerated options are not likely to be whole, unprocessed foods but rather sports nutrition supplements. Frequently these products have a higher glycemic index than whole foods, though as new products become available this may change.

TABLE **5.1**	PRE-EXERCISE MEAL SUGGESTIONS

		2 slices toast or small bagel (60 g) 1 large banana 2 tbsp. jelly (40 ml) 8 oz. juice (240 ml)
1½ c. concentrated carbohydrate beverage (360 ml) 1 slice of toast **90 g carbohydrates** **380 calories**	1 carbohydrate gel 24 oz. of sports drink (720 ml) **95 g carbohydrates** **380 calories**	**120 g carbohydrates** **520 calories**
Chicken, 2 oz. (60 g) Bread, 2 slices (60 g) Fruit juice, 16 oz. (480 ml) Pretzels, 2 oz. (60 g) Carbohydrate supplement, 16 oz. (480 ml) **220 g carbohydrates** **1,030 calories**	Fruit smoothie: 8 oz. yogurt (240 ml) 8 oz. milk (240 ml) 8 oz. juice (240 ml) 1 c. fruit Bagel, 1 large (120 g) Jam, 2 tbsp. (40 ml) Energy bar, 1 whole **225 g carbohydrates** **1,185 calories**	Pasta, 2 c. cooked (480 ml) Marinara sauce, 1 c. (240 ml) Bread, 2 slices (60 g) Frozen yogurt, 12 oz. (360 ml) Fruit juice, 8 oz. (240 ml) Margarine, 2 tsp. (24 ml) **235 g carbohydrates** **986 calories**
Pancakes, 4 medium Fruit topping, ½ c. (120 ml) Syrup, ½ c. (120 ml) Fruit juice, 8 oz. (240 ml) **270 g carbohydrates** **1,200 calories**	Cooked cereal, 2 c. (480 ml) Instant breakfast drink, 1 serving Banana, 1 large Orange juice, 8 oz. (240 ml) Carbohydrate beverage, 24 oz. (720 ml) **300 g carbohydrates** **1,410 calories**	Rice, 3 c. cooked (720 ml) Cooked vegetables, 1 c. (240 ml) Shrimp, 4 oz. (120 g) Sorbet, 1 c. (240 ml) Soft drink, 12 oz. (360 ml) Oil, 2 tsp. (14 ml) Carbohydrate beverage, 16 oz. (480 ml) **300 g carbohydrates** **1,600 calories**

Athletes should also consider that consuming a carbohydrate source during training (more on that strategy later in this chapter) can easily offset any drop in blood glucose, making the types of carbohydrates that you consume before exercise less important.

The bottom line is that you should focus on pre-training nutrition strategies that are appropriate for your training times, schedule, and tolerances and that are based on smart experimentation. Table 5.1 offers some pre-exercise meal suggestions in various carbohydrate amounts.

HYDRATION BEFORE TRAINING

Dehydration is one of the most significant performance-related problems that can occur during training (and competition). It can put a halt to your training long before you feel the effects of fuel depletion. Despite your best attempts to keep up with your sweat losses during training, it is possible that you are not going to match 100 percent of your fluid losses. Depending on the type of training session, you may have ample or limited opportunity to drink during training.

Just as strategies to maximize muscle and liver glycogen stores offer a performance advantage, so do techniques for maximizing fluid stores before training. Pre-hydrating is not considered to be as effective as drinking during exercise to offset dehydration and its detrimental performance effects. However, if you anticipate that it may be difficult to drink plenty of fluids during training, either because there is no way to carry enough fluids with you or because there will be little opportunity to drink during the training session, pre-hydrating could be a very important and practical strategy. Even when training sessions allow time and opportunities for replenishing fluids and replacing sweat losses, and an athlete is consciously making an effort to hydrate during exercise, only up to 80 percent of sweat losses are usually replaced.

At all costs, avoid starting training in a dehydrated state. Your goal during training is to keep up with sweat losses as much as possible, so starting out dehydrated already puts you behind on your fluid-intake efforts. It is important to plan ahead and begin your next training session as well hydrated as possible. To prepare for the next day's training, consume 16 ounces (480 ml) of fluid before bedtime. Your early-morning intake should then consist of 16 to 24 ounces (480-720 ml) of fluid. Prior to training, you should attempt to consume another 8 to 10 ounces (240-300 ml) of fluid every hour during the day. About 1 hour before training, you can consume 16 to 32 ounces (480-960 ml) of fluid. At this time, fluids providing carbohydrates and small amounts of sodium, such as sports drinks, are likely to be the best choice and may have some hydration advantages over water. You can fill your fluid stores further by drinking another 8 to 16 ounces (240-480 ml) 20 minutes prior to training. You should be adequately hydrated in preparation for training if you focus on these simple guidelines.

NUTRITIONAL STRATEGIES DURING TRAINING

Even when you start training well fueled, you can significantly drain your fluid stores, carbohydrates, and even electrolytes during moderate- to high-intensity training and during very prolonged training sessions. That's why consuming adequate fluid, carbohydrates, and electrolytes during training and competition is beneficial to your performance. This practice can bring you these benefits:

- It delays and minimizes dehydration.
- It maintains blood glucose levels.
- It offsets muscle and liver glycogen depletion.
- It provides fuel for your brain.
- It offsets electrolyte losses, particularly sodium.

FLUID REQUIREMENTS DURING EXERCISE

Dehydration can develop when you train both indoors and outdoors, and it can negatively affect your performance long before fuel depletion begins to drain your efforts. In cold and hot weather, during the peak of the racing season or during the off-season months, it can develop sooner than you might think and can affect you in ways you may not realize.

When you train, heat is a major by-product of your working muscles. As this heat builds up, your body temperature rises. Water then acts as a coolant to keep the body from overheating. During exercise, sweating is the body's primary mechanism for getting rid of excess heat. Sweat losses can easily reach anywhere from 16 to 32 ounces (500–960 ml) and sometimes even 48 ounces (1.5 L) or more per hour depending on environmental conditions, exercise intensity, and the sweat rate of the individual athlete. Sweat losses can reach over 64 ounces (approximately 2 L) or more per hour in some endurance athletes, especially during hot-weather training.

Even losing as little as 2 percent of your body weight through sweating can impair your ability to exercise. When you sweat, your blood volume goes down and stress is placed on your cardiovascular system, which reduces your ability to take in and utilize oxygen. Muscular endurance ability is also impaired with dehydration, and your heart rate may increase at a given level of intensity. When fluid losses through sweat are not replaced, your body temperature rises further and exercise becomes harder. Clearly, not meeting your fluid needs hinders your athletic goals.

Unfortunately, thirst is not a very good indicator of the amount of fluid that your body requires, either during exercise or at rest. Some early signs and symptoms of dehydration are lightheadedness, headaches, decreased appetite, dark-colored urine, and fatigue. By the time you are thirsty, you have already lost 1 percent of your body weight through fluid loss. Even fluid losses of 1 to 2 percent of your body weight can adversely affect performance. When fluid losses reach more than 2 to 4 percent of your body weight, increased thirst and symptoms such as irritability and nausea may occur. Dehydration can also result in GI upset. Consequently, when you make the effort to drink more after you have become dehydrated, your rehydration efforts can result in stomach discomfort. At losses of 5 to 6 percent of body weight, there will be an increase in heart rate and breathing regulation, and body temperature regulation will be significantly impaired. Remember, too, that dehydration can affect your mental concentration and ability to perform the skills required for your sport. Clearly, dehydration does not support your top performance if it affects movement control, decision making, and concentration.

The longer and harder you train, the greater the risk that your sweat losses will impair your performance. Your sweat losses are also affected by your genetic makeup, fitness level, and acclimatization to the temperature in which you are training. Although you will have greater sweat losses in the heat than in cooler weather, your hydration can also be compromised in the cooler weather because you are working so hard. By preventing dehydration, you will likely avoid the following detrimental physiological effects:

- Increased heart rate
- Raised body temperature
- Decreased blood volume
- Decreased cardiac output
- Decreased skin blood flow
- Heightened perception of effort
- Compromised mental concentration
- Compromised fine-motor skills
- Delayed stomach emptying of fluids
- Greater risk of gastrointestinal upset

Of course, dehydration can result in serious health risks, including heat exhaustion and even heatstroke. Those suffering from heat exhaustion may feel weak, may have cold and clammy skin, may have a weak pulse, and may experience faintness, fatigue, and nausea. When depletion of body fluid is severe, an athlete may even stop sweating; in this case, his or her skin may feel cool and dry. The athlete may be semiconscious and have reduced blood flow to the brain. This condition requires immediate medical attention. Heatstroke is an even more serious condition and is characterized by hot and dry skin and a very high body temperature. Heatstroke is most likely to occur from overexertion in extreme heat accompanied by poor hydration strategies. Previous illness, poor preparation for training in the heat, and even certain medications can increase risk of heat illness.

It is important to gauge your sweat losses during various types of training sessions in a number of environmental conditions. Athletes cannot train themselves to adapt to or tolerate dehydration. Preventing or minimizing it as much as possible is therefore essential. Just as sweat rates vary greatly among athletes, however, there is also much variability in efforts to replace fluids during exercise. Ideally, endurance athletes should try to match their fluid intake to their fluid losses; most athletes fall short of this goal, however, replacing only 50 to 80 percent of their fluid losses during their training sessions even under the best of conditions. Even if you do make a strong effort to match your fluid losses, your gastrointestinal system can only absorb a certain volume of fluid per hour. Practical considerations, however, may be the main obstacle to adequate fluid replacement during exercise. Consuming the recommended amounts can be challenging because of the logistics of obtaining fluid when training and competing, limited opportunities to drink, taste preferences, and GI tolerances.

When you regularly train in the heat, your body does adapt, or acclimatize. As your conditioning improves, your sweat rate increases and there is greater blood flow to your muscles and skin. Your heart is able to pump more blood, and sweating begins at a lower core body temperature. Your core temperature will not rise as quickly or increase to as high a level when you are in an acclimatized state. Thus, when you are acclimatized you actually sweat more, not less. It is best if your skills at hydrating during exercising keep pace with your adaptation to heat so that you are adept at replacing these increased fluid losses.

At any level of training and in any environmental condition you need to assess drinking opportunities and fluid availability. Training and preparing for your sport in the gym simply require that you bring fluids with you. Matching fluid intake to sweat losses should not be a problem in most indoor training situations. Outdoor workouts may prove more challenging. Clearly, it is much easier to drink fluids when you are on your bike than when you are on a run. During swim practices you can keep a bottle of fluid at the end of your lane, and during rowing practice you can have a water bottle within reach (though getting a moment with your hands free to drink it may be challenging). Refer to the sidebar "Estimating Your Sweat Losses" for guidelines on estimating your fluid losses during training and gauging your efforts to rehydrate. Once you have come up with the best fluid strategies for the various types of training sessions that you engage in, it is up to you to make the most of your opportunities to drink during training. Regardless of your fluid-replacement strategies, you are more likely to consume fluids that taste good and are the proper temperature for your training conditions.

Not only do you need to focus on how much fluid to consume, you should also be aware of the most optimal and appropriate fluid choices for training in various environments and conditions. Commercial sports drinks are often used by endurance athletes not only because of their flavor but also because they provide fuel and electrolytes in the form of carbohydrates and sodium chloride.

FUEL REQUIREMENTS DURING EXERCISE

Due to the sheer length of many endurance sport workouts, and the high-intensity, intermittent nature of speed and interval training, fuel replacement can be an important consideration. Carbohydrates consumed during training can maintain blood glucose levels and provide fuel to glycogen-depleted muscles. In addition, carbohydrate consumption during interval training may allow your body to store glucose in the muscle fibers during the time those fibers are at rest. For example, as you exercise at low intensity between hard efforts, the muscle fibers that fuel the high-intensity efforts can be replenished.

Your brain can also benefit from carbohydrate intake during long, intense training sessions, as consuming only water can result in lowered blood glucose levels. Because your brain counts on glucose for fuel, lowered blood glucose can have some negative effects on your central nervous system. Having adequate blood glucose to fuel your brain helps you maintain the high level of skill required by your endurance sport. Carbohydrate intake can prevent or reverse symptoms of glucose deprivation such as fatigue, perception of increased effort, and poor coordination. Carbohydrates are thought to prevent the increase in brain serotonin levels that can occur during prolonged exercise. Serotonin produces feelings of drowsiness and fatigue and is helpful at bedtime, but not in the middle of a workout when you want to make the most of the time available to reach your fitness goals.

Much of the research on carbohydrate intake during exercise has centered on steady-state endurance activity. But studies also demonstrate that besides providing performance benefits for exercise lasting 90 minutes or longer, carbohydrates may improve performance during high-intensity exercise lasting about 60 minutes. Several studies over the past decade measured the performance effects of consuming a sports drink during exercise performed at 80 to 90 percent VO_2max and lasting about 1 hour. Results indicated that the sports drink provided a performance benefit.

Several additional studies measured the performance effects of carbohydrates on intermittent, high-intensity exercise lasting about 1 hour. These workouts more closely resembled the type of training conducted in interval or speed workouts. The bottom line was that athletes who consumed a sports drink at rest intervals were able to work out longer than those who consumed

ESTIMATING YOUR SWEAT LOSSES

This technique for estimating sweat losses is fairly accurate, especially in warm-weather training. Use it to check your sweat losses for various types of training sessions, whether indoors or out, to better estimate fluid needs.

- Check your weight on the scale before and after training. Because you will want to know your actual weight without shoes and clothing, both weigh-ins should be done in the nude, and after training be sure to towel dry to eliminate most of the sweat on your body. Then, calculate your weight loss from the exercise session by subtracting the post-training weight from the pre-training weight. For example, an athlete who started a workout session at 160 pounds and ended it at 158 pounds (going from 73 to 72 kg) has experienced a 2-pound (0.9 kg) loss of water weight during training. This is not the final answer, however, because the athlete may have taken in fluids by drinking during your workout or lost fluids through urination. To account for these factors, follow the steps outlined below.
- Keep track of the amount of fluid that you consumed during a training session. Fifteen ounces of fluid weigh about 1 pound (1,000 ml of fluid equal 1 kg). You can also weigh the bottle before and after your training session to determine the actual weight of the fluid you consumed during training. You can use a graduated water bottle during these workouts for more precise calculations.

CONTINUES

a placebo. Researchers speculated that the carbohydrate drinks provided fuel for the fast-twitch muscle fibers, which operate at high intensities, by replenishing them during the rest intervals between high-intensity efforts. Although these results are not conclusive, and more research of this type is needed, consider consuming a sports drink during long training sessions, and even during short sessions if they are high in intensity, to both meet the demands of reduced muscle glycogen and boost fluid reserves.

SPORTS DRINKS

Much research has gone into the development of sports drinks in an effort to come up with the ideal fluid for athletes to consume during their workouts. The basic theory—that athletes need a convenient way to take in both fluids and carbohydrates in order to maintain hydration and

ESTIMATING YOUR SWEAT LOSSES   continued

Let's say the hypothetical athlete mentioned above consumed 60 ounces (1,800 ml) of fluid during a 2-hour training session, and this fluid weighed 4 pounds (1.8 kg).

- Add the amount of weight lost to the amount of fluid consumed. For example, the athlete who had a 2-pound weight loss during training and drank 4 pounds of fluid during training would add 2 and 4. Since 2 plus 4 equals 6, this means he lost 6 pounds of fluid (or 0.9 + 1.8 kg = 2.7 kg).
- Record any urine volume that occurred between the weigh-ins and subtract this number (translated into pounds or kilograms) from the result obtained in step 3.
- Divide the weight of total fluid lost by the exercise time. For example, 6 pounds, or 90 ounces of fluid, divided by 2 hours equals 45 ounces per hour for sweat losses (2.7 kg equals 2,700 ml fluid, divided by 2 hours equals 1,350 ml lost per hour).

This procedure can be translated into a formula:

Sweat rate = (body weight pre-training – body weight post-training
+ fluid ingestion – urine volume) ÷ exercise time

Sweat rates in athletes can vary from 24 ounces, or 3 cups (720 ml), of fluid per hour to 80 ounces, or 10 cups (2,400 ml) or more.

fuel stores during exercise—is sound. Sports drinks can deliver the right ingredients to your body in a timely and well-tolerated manner. A high-quality sports drink passes easily through the digestion and absorption process, emptying from your stomach quickly, entering your small intestine, and then getting absorbed into the bloodstream. The carbohydrates from the drink are then available to maintain blood glucose levels, supply energy to exercising muscles, and replenish muscle fuel stores. The fluid from your sports drink also maintains blood volume and offsets sweat losses.

In an effort to develop scientifically sound formulations, sports drink researchers have looked at each of the steps in digestion and absorption to see where the flow may actually slow down or speed up. If your sports drink gets bogged down in any one of these steps, it takes the fluid and carbohydrates that much longer to reach your bloodstream and muscles. Consequently, the sports drink is not as performance enhancing as it could be. Researchers have concluded that two main factors determine how quickly a drink leaves your stomach: the concentration of carbohydrates in the drink and the volume of fluid in your stomach.

Concentration

It has not proved easy for researchers to find the ideal formulation for a sports drink. It involves striking a delicate balance. Although researchers agree that carbohydrates are essential ingredients, they have had to experiment to determine how many carbohydrates to include in the mix. On one hand, a higher concentration of carbohydrates provides more fuel than a lower concentration; on the other hand, the greater the concentration, the longer it takes for the fluid to empty from an athlete's stomach. Research has determined that a concentration of about 4 to 8 percent carbohydrates empties from the stomach very efficiently. Thus, most sports drinks fall into this range. This drink concentration allows fluid to reach your bloodstream pretty much as quickly as water but still deliver performance-boosting carbohydrates. Drinks of this type also seem to be well tolerated by most athletes, and tolerance to these products can improve with practice. In contrast, drinks of 10 to 12 percent carbohydrates, such as soft drinks and fruit juices, empty more slowly from the stomach. Although they do provide carbohydrates and energy, these drinks are not as hydrating as sports drinks and should be diluted if they are consumed during exercise.

Volume

The volume of fluids in your stomach affects the degree of stomach distention and consequently affects gastric emptying. Increased stomach distention will result in liquids emptying from your stomach more quickly, with about 50 percent of stomach contents being emptied every 10 minutes. To maximize emptying, try to start exercise with a comfortably full stomach and drink at regular intervals of about 10 to 15 minutes, if possible. How much fluid an athlete can empty from his or her stomach is highly variable. However, emptying rates of 24 to 40 ounces, or 3 to 5 cups (720–1,200 ml), per hour are commonly seen. The most important strategy is to consume fluid whenever the opportunity presents itself. Aim to consume at least one 20-ounce (600 ml) squeeze bottle for every hour of a workout. Refill your bottle as needed whenever possible, depending on the duration and nature of the training session.

Intestinal Absorption

Studies measuring intestinal absorption rates have determined that sports drink solutions are as readily absorbed as water. Different forms of carbohydrates are absorbed across the intestinal wall via various transport mechanisms. Although the majority of research has demonstrated that the maximum amount of carbohydrate that an athlete can comfortably absorb is about 1 gram per minute, some newer research is looking at the effect of two or three sources of carbohydrates on intestinal absorption. Mixing carbohydrate sources could allow for faster absorption rates, so that the carbohydrates could become available as fuel for training and competition rather than sitting in the gut and causing GI problems. This strategy could be especially important in events that require the athlete to maximize fuel absorption in order to keep up with the fuel burned during competition, such as ultraendurance runs. Improved absorption should translate into improved performance. More research is needed, however, before more definitive recommendations can be supported. For now, individual athletes simply need to experiment with different brands or mixes of brands to determine which sports drinks and carbohydrate concentrations they tolerate best for different types of training sessions.

Brands that provide at least two sources of carbohydrates are worth trying. Carbohydrate sources can include glucose polymers, glucose, sucrose, and fructose. Some drinks have a mix of these, allowing various carbohydrate types to be transported simultaneously. These carbohydrate mixes all appear to have a moderate to high glycemic index, which gives them the ability to quickly raise blood glucose levels and supply a quick burst of both brain power and energy.

Glucose polymers do not seem to offer any absorption advantages over glucose, but they are popular because they have a milder taste. Glucose may seem overly sweet to some athletes. Fructose is the only type of carbohydrate not used in high amounts or by itself in a sports beverage. Large amounts of fructose are not well absorbed and can lead to GI upset. But drinks that contain some fructose should provide easily tolerated concentrations and additional flavor. Some sports drink advertisers have made claims concerning their product's effect on blood glucose levels and insulin, touting the type of carbohydrate used and the glycemic index of the drink. These claims are usually unsubstantiated. There is virtually no research comparing the performance effects of sports drinks with various glycemic index levels. But the high-glycemic effect of most sports drinks quickly raises blood glucose levels to provide quick fuel for serious athletes during training and competition. The number of sports drinks with a lower glycemic index is limited, and the glycemic index of many sports drinks is not available.

Just as with various food choices, the glycemic index of a sports drink is not necessarily related to whether the drink is a "simple" or "complex" carbohydrate. Maltodextrin, which is often promoted as a complex carbohydrate source, has a high glycemic index, whereas the simple sugar fructose has a very low glycemic index. Often, the choice of a sports drink comes down to personal tolerances and preferences and what products are most accessible to the athlete or team. Appendix C provides a listing of the glycemic index of various sports drinks and carbohydrate sources currently on the market.

Temperature

During exercise, cooler fluids empty from your stomach more quickly than warmer fluids. Of course, during training sessions in hotter weather, cooler fluids are more palatable and appealing as well. You are more likely to drink greater volumes of fluid if it is cool. Prepare bottles ahead of time and make sure that you start with a cold drink.

Amount and Timing

General guidelines for the consumption of sports drinks during exercise are the same as the water-intake guidelines described previously, or about 4 to 8 ounces (120–240 ml) every 15 to 20 minutes. Drink at regular intervals during training or whenever there is adequate opportunity to drink. Performance benefits occur when an athlete takes in about 30 grams of carbohydrates per hour. However, 50 to 60 grams may be even better during high-intensity exercise, particularly after some muscle glycogen depletion has already occurred. Every athlete has his or her own personal tolerances and carbohydrate requirements that maintain optimal energy levels during training.

Check the labels and instructions of your sports drinks. Then determine what volume you would need to consume to obtain 30 to 60 grams or more of carbohydrates per hour. Experiment to determine what consumption volume best enhances your performance and hydration levels.

As far as timing is concerned, large single feedings and smaller, regular intakes of a sports drink are both beneficial. Basically, drink whenever possible, as the nature of your training session permits. Consuming carbohydrates after depletion has set in can help, but it is more prudent to consume the carbohydrates early on in order to prevent fatigue. Don't wait until the signs and symptoms of a low fuel tank register before consuming your carbohydrate sports drink.

Other Factors

Athletes may sometimes consume slightly carbonated beverages. As long as carbonation does not create the sensation of being too full, a drink that is of the proper carbohydrate concentration should empty from the stomach easily. Many ultraendurance athletes consume cola in the defizzed and perhaps slightly diluted state toward the end of long events for a welcome flavor change and a caffeine pickup. An athlete's own state of hydration can also affect his or her ability to tolerate fluid. As longer training sessions and races progress, the level of dehydration progresses as well. Ironically, the more dehydrated an athlete becomes, the slower the rate of gastric emptying. Once an athlete reaches a very slow rate of gastric emptying, attempting to drink more fluid only exacerbates the condition and can even result in nutritional upheaval, such as vomiting, particularly during very demanding races like the Ironman. Of course, mental stress can have a significant impact upon the gastrointestinal system. Being keyed up for an important training session or race can also slow down the rate of gastric emptying.

Other Sources of Carbohydrates

In recent years the sports nutrition industry has developed new options for refueling. In addition to sports drinks, which offer carbohydrates in liquid form, there are products that offer carbohydrates in semiliquid and solid form. These sports supplements may be consumed before, during, and/or after exercise. Tolerances to these products can vary, however, depending on the intensity of exercise and the timing of the carbohydrate supplement. Obviously, carbohydrate drinks offer the advantage of supplying both hydration and fuel, and for this reason they are more practical than the supplements. But many endurance athletes may appreciate the more concentrated carbohydrate gels, especially in situations where energy needs outweigh the desire for fluid. They are a convenient carbohydrate source. Nevertheless, these products should be consumed with some fluid. More solid items, such as energy bars, may take the edge off hunger during training, though most athletes prefer to avoid solid items during high-intensity training sessions.

Basically, fluid and carbohydrate choices can be somewhat individualized. Keep in mind that your body may need fluids much more than it needs carbohydrate supplementation when training outdoors in hot weather. However, your carbohydrate needs may be a greater priority at the end of an intense workout. At that point, a gel taken with water or a more concentrated sports drink may provide the shot of energy you need to maintain performance.

Protein During Training

Some sports drinks now on the market contain small amounts of protein. Several studies have attempted to evaluate whether these drinks offer any advantage over more traditional sports drinks. As is often the case in sports nutrition research, the studies have had conflicting results due to variations in research design and testing protocols. In the case of endurance exercise, particularly ultraendurance exercise, some athletes may add in small amounts of protein into their race nutrition plan. It is not recommended, however, that you consistently consume a protein-containing product during training and competition. Rather, focus on products and strategies that replace fluid, carbohydrate fuel, and sodium. Research does indicate that protein stores and muscle are less likely to be utilized as a fuel source if carbohydrate intake is optimal. Researchers are also looking at how protein intake during exercise may or may not affect markers of muscle damage.

The Electrolyte Edge

Though your sweat consists mainly of water, it does contain a number of electrolytes, including sodium, potassium, and calcium. A quart of sweat (960 ml) can contain 500 to 1,800 milligrams of sodium, 700 to 2,100 milligrams of chloride, 150 to 300 milligrams of potassium, and 40 milligrams of calcium. Clearly, the main electrolyte lost in sweat is salt, or sodium chloride, though electrolyte losses in sweat can vary widely among individual athletes. Because electrolytes are the major solid component of sweat, much research has focused on the replacement needs of these nutrients during exercise. Sodium and potassium have been the most frequently studied electrolytes, though chloride is also a consideration. Sodium is an important consideration for athletes who train in the heat and humidity. Those who are prone to developing low blood sodium levels, or hyponatremia, and muscle cramping are especially interested in the subject because sodium levels seem to be related to these conditions. Some athletes continue to have high losses of sodium in their sweat even when they are acclimatized to warm weather. This may be due to genetic or other influences.

At the same time, we often hear about the dangers of consuming high levels of sodium in our society. While restricting sodium may be a useful health strategy in sodium-sensitive and sedentary individuals and in anyone susceptible to high blood pressure, it may not be the best strategy for the endurance athlete susceptible to muscle cramping or prone to moderate to high sodium losses through sweating. Several hours of sweating daily during training can add up to significant sodium losses in some athletes, particularly ultraendurance athletes. These sodium losses need to be replaced with a diet adequate in salt. Sports drinks have varying levels of sodium, and athletes prone to high sodium sweat losses and cramping can choose those higher in sodium. Some physiology laboratories can measure sodium losses in individual athletes, but determining whether you have high sodium content in your sweat does not have to be expensive or difficult. Often there are clear markers to indicate high sodium sweat losses, such as salt rings and marks on your skin and workout clothing. Acclimatization to heat should result in a decrease in the salt content of sweat, though as mentioned above, this may not occur as efficiently in some salty sweaters.

Preventing Hyponatremia

You may already be familiar with the term *hyponatremia*, or abnormally lowered blood sodium levels. This condition can develop during and after long training sessions, and particularly during competition. Many endurance athletes experience mild or moderate lowered blood sodium from time to time. But severe hyponatremia can be dangerous and even fatal. The lower the blood sodium level drops, the more serious and life-threatening the symptoms. Symptoms of hyponatremia include headache, confusion, nausea, cramping, bloated stomach, and swollen extremities. At the very least, this condition can slow down your competitive efforts and is best prevented.

There are multiple causes of hyponatremia. The main instigators, however, are excess fluid intake, in which the blood sodium is diluted, and a high rate of sodium loss from sweating. Endurance athletes who naturally have a high concentration of sodium in their sweat, or who simply sweat a lot, are especially susceptible to the condition. But usually when athletes develop hyponatremia during an endurance event, it is because they were drinking too much water. In addition, for reasons that have not been clearly defined, there seems to be a higher incidence of hyponatremia among female athletes. The condition also seems to be particularly common in marathon running. Drinking excessively during a race taper in the two to three days before competition may set the stage for hyponatremia. Drinking in excess of fluid needs during the race can lower blood sodium levels further, and replacing sweat losses with plain water, rather than a sodium-containing sports drink, aggravates the condition even more. Slower finishers are likely at increased risk for developing hyponatremia because of the relative ease with which they can consume excess fluid, and athletes who are not well prepared for an event and poorly acclimatized are also at increased risk.

Although fluid overload often characterizes hyponatremia, restricting water intake is not the answer—athletes competing in ultraendurance events who do this will end up finishing their event both dehydrated and sodium depleted. Thus, unless it is medically contraindicated, endurance athletes should consume some salt in their diet. Athletes with special health considerations—for example, older athletes who may have questions about how salt intake may affect their blood pressure or heart health—should consult with a physician on these matters. In addition, although it is best to maintain good hydration levels prior to competition, athletes should be sure not to overhydrate. During a race taper, sweat losses from training decrease considerably. Drink regularly, and monitor your urine color to assess your hydration status. During a race it is important to match your fluid intake with sweat losses and not overdrink. Athletes who know they are prone to hyponatremia because of their sweat rate or content should always consume sports drinks that contain sodium, and these athletes can reach for sports drinks with higher sodium levels. Endurance athletes with exceptionally high sodium requirements may even take salt or electrolyte tablets during training to offset high sodium sweat losses. These tablets should not be consumed in excess, however, and they should be taken with fluid. High-sodium foods such as pretzels and chicken broth are often offered on ultraendurance racecourses such as an Ironman or ultramarathon.

Fluid, Fuel, and Electrolyte Replacement Strategies

Obtaining adequate fuel and fluid during training sessions, and replacing high sodium losses if needed, takes practice, experience, and experimentation. Here are some practical tips for making the most of your fuel and fluid intake during exercise:

Have a plan and drink on a schedule. Have a squeeze bottle of fluid ready and available for training so that you can consume fluid during breaks or regular intervals during training. Check your intake every hour to determine whether you are keeping up with the required fluid amounts.

Consume 4 to 8 ounces (120-240 ml) of fluid during every 15 to 20 minutes of exercise. Practice drinking at regular intervals so that you become highly skilled at consuming enough fluid during training. Take big gulps, as larger volumes empty from your stomach more quickly. For many athletes this fluid intake is a good starting point for minimizing dehydration.

Know your sweat losses by monitoring your weight before and after training. It is not necessary to consume more fluid than your body requires, but do try to consume adequate fluid during practice to minimize sweat losses. If you lose more than 2 pounds (approximately 1 kg) during a workout lasting an hour or more, you need to drink more. Gaining weight during workouts indicates that you are consuming too much fluid relative to your sweat losses.

Start exercise well hydrated. Drink 16 to 20 ounces (480–600 ml) of fluid in the hour before exercise, and start your training with a comfortably full stomach. This will speed up gastric emptying, as will drinking fluid every 15 to 20 minutes.

Start drinking early. This strategy is especially important if the nature of your training session will not allow for frequent drinking breaks and opportunities. Even if you start training adequately hydrated, it does not pay to practice "catch-up" drinking. Once you are dehydrated, fluids empty from your stomach more slowly. In extreme situations, dehydration may lead to GI upset, including a bloated stomach. Because fluids are emptying slowly, you will feel dehydrated and compensate by attempting to drink more, further aggravating stomach upset.

Develop a taste for various sports drinks. Although you likely have a favorite sports drink brand and flavor that you prefer during training, practice with products and flavors that are also available during competition and get used to their taste and feel during training. This allows for greater flexibility and improved drinking on competition day.

Fluids should be accessible. Ensuring that you have adequate fluid available is fairly simple during an indoor training session. Keeping a squeeze bottle on hand should allow you to drink an ample amount of fluid whether you are training indoors or out.

Use a sports drink during moderate- to high-intensity workout sessions lasting longer than 60 minutes. Research indicates that this combination of fluid and carbohydrates improves performance by replacing sweat losses and providing carbohydrate fuel for your muscles.

Consume at least 30 to 60 grams of carbohydrates per hour from a sports drink during moderate- to high-intensity training. This will ensure that you do not become dehydrated and will also provide fuel as glycogen stores become depleted. Optimally, you can absorb about 0.5 gram of carbohydrates for every pound (1 g/kg) of body weight over a 1-hour period. Most sports drinks provide 14 to 20 grams of carbohydrates per 8-ounce (240 ml) serving. One full 20-ounce (600 ml) squeeze bottle will provide 35 to 50 grams and should be consumed over a 1-hour workout.

Experiment carefully with other sources of carbohydrates. During intense training sessions or sessions where carbohydrate requirements outweigh fluid considerations, a more solid form of carbohydrates, such as a gel, may be appealing and provide needed carbohydrate fuel to prevent depletion. Gel servings usually provide up to 50 grams of carbohydrates per gulp. Just remember to consume gels with plenty of water; otherwise they empty from your stomach slowly because they are so concentrated.

Know your sweat losses in different environmental conditions and at different times during the season. Monitor your weight before and after training in various temperatures and types of training sessions and at different times of the year. Condition yourself to drink the proper volumes to replace sweat losses in various situations. As your conditioning improves, your sweat rate will actually increase. Sweat rates also increase with acclimatization, though the sodium concentration of sweat should decrease.

Have a squeeze bottle or even a back-mounted hydration system at each training session, and consume fluids from it regularly. Whenever appropriate, the coaching and training staff should have policies in place that make fluids readily available.

Drink during the warm-up. Have a regular fluid intake when preparing for your workout. Start exercise with fluid in your stomach to encourage gastric emptying.

Pay attention to signs of dehydration. Frequent gastrointestinal problems may indicate that you are not drinking enough. Gastric emptying is delayed when you are dehydrated. It may appear that you do not tolerate a particular product, when what is actually occurring is that the product is unable to empty from your stomach, and further drinking causes bloating.

Note the signs and symptoms of hypoglycemia. If you feel dizzy or light-headed, or experience an inability to focus, your blood glucose levels are probably running low. Be proactive and try to increase your intake of carbohydrates with sports drinks or gels.

Refine your drinking technique. Practice drinking in all types of training situations. Know your limits regarding exercise intensity and your ability to tolerate certain volumes of fluid ingestion. Push your limits and maximize your fluid intake to maintain fluid balance.

Pay attention to your sodium intake if you are susceptible to muscle cramping or are a salty sweater. Emphasize salty foods, and salt your foods to taste during periods of heavy training, particularly in hot weather. Choose higher-sodium sports drinks for training and competition. If you plan to use electrolyte replacement tablets in competition, experiment with them first in training and consume them with plenty of fluid.

SWEAT AND HYDRATION DURING COLD-WEATHER TRAINING

During cold-weather training, those nice warm and insulating clothes you wear to keep warm contribute to a rise in body temperature that promotes sweating. Your hydration can become compromised in cold weather through several physiological mechanisms. One is cold-induced diuresis. When you exercise in the cold, the blood vessels that carry blood to your skin, feet, hands, and ears all constrict in order to conserve heat and maintain body temperature. When your blood vessels constrict, your blood pressure increases and the blood pressure specifically in your kidneys rises, which causes you to urinate and lose fluid and sodium. Water loss also occurs when you breathe cold air. Your lung passages warm the air and saturate it with water, and when you exhale this water-saturated air, there is fluid loss. Fluid losses from your lungs can add up to more than 1 quart (about 1 L) daily when you are outdoors for a day of training in the cold. These losses increase with intense exercise. Moreover, even in the cold air, an increase in your body temperature during exercise can result in sweat losses. And even without the adverse effects of dehydration, training in the cold can adversely affect your coordination, fine-motor skills, strength, power production, and aerobic power.

Dehydration levels of over 2 percent body weight can reduce mental concentration in cold weather. The negative effects of dehydration can be as significant in cold weather as in warm weather when the training is long and intense. Fluids may be less readily available at cold-weather events. Even if fluids are available, when the temperature is below 32° Fahrenheit (0° Celsius) they will begin to freeze. Drinking in the cold may also be uncomfortable owing to the logistics of keeping your hands warm and wanting to avoid pit stops. You are also not as thirsty in cold weather and may not so readily crave fluids.

Very little information is available on sodium losses when training in cold weather. It is possible that some athletes still have high sodium losses and could develop sodium problems during very long training sessions or ultraendurance competition. This is most likely to occur with excess intake of plain water and inadequate replacement of sodium.

Although optimal hydration can be a challenge in cold weather, you can follow a few warming strategies to keep the fluids flowing. Sports drinks can be heated before training and placed inside a bottle or thermos covered with an insulating layer. Experiment with drinks and flavors that appeal to you when heated. Warm sports drinks should be easier to down on a cold winter day than cold drinks, and they can help to maintain your core body temperature.

CONTINUES

Newer tube-fed winter hydration systems are available for training in the cold. Hydration systems are handy, as they do not require that you reach for your bottle with cold fingers and thick gloves. To prevent the drink tube from freezing, there are now products with an insulated hose as well as bite valves covered with insulating caps. In full-blown winter weather, make sure that you fill the fluid reservoir with warm or hot fluid. You should also blow back into the drink tube after you have taken a hydrating gulp to prevent fluid from sitting and freezing in the drink tube. Also, keep the fluid reservoir and hose as close to your body as possible so that your body heat can keep the system warm.

NUTRITIONAL RECOVERY STRATEGIES AFTER EXERCISE

What you eat and drink from one training session to the next has a very significant impact on your nutritional recovery. Consuming the total amounts of carbohydrate, protein, and fat that you require for your 24-hour nutritional recovery is essential. But for up to 4 to 6 hours after moderate to hard training, you can make the most of your nutritional recovery because the rate at which you can replace muscle fuel, specifically muscle glycogen, is accelerated at that time. Making the most of this accelerated recovery window is especially important when you need to train again in less than 24 hours. Paying attention to recovery nutrition in the hours after training can also improve rehydration efforts.

CARBOHYDRATES AND IMMEDIATE RECOVERY

Because of the daily demands placed upon muscle glycogen, carbohydrate intake should be one of your primary nutritional considerations immediately after training. Delaying your carbohydrate intake after a tough training session by even 2 hours can slow down the replenishment process. Several scientific studies have concluded that athletes should consume anywhere from 0.5 to 0.7 gram of carbohydrates per pound (1–1.5 g/kg) of body weight within 30 minutes of completing intense exercise to take advantage of the optimal time for muscle glycogen replacement. One study demonstrated that subjects fed carbohydrates a full 2 hours after exercise synthesized the carbohydrates into glycogen 45 percent more slowly than subjects fed carbohydrates immediately after exercise. It appears that muscle glycogen storage is slightly enhanced for up to 2 hours after exercise, during which time the muscle has a greater capacity to take up blood glucose.

Studies have also shown that both liquid and solid carbohydrates are adequate in refueling the body after hard exercise. However, emphasizing higher-glycemic carbohydrate foods that elicit a higher insulin response, such as sports nutrition supplements and breads and cereals, may enhance glycogen resynthesis. A list of high-glycemic foods is provided in Appendix A.

Besides consuming carbohydrates immediately after hard training, you should consume the same recommended carbohydrate amount (following the grams-per-pound formula) again in 2 hours. This allows you to continue to take advantage of the recovery process and stimulate muscle glycogen resynthesis. Glycogen resynthesis does slow down over time, but it is still relatively elevated in the 5 to 6 hours after training.

For the rest of the day, carbohydrates can be consumed as a series of snacks or a few larger meals, depending on your training schedule, food preferences, and total daily carbohydrate requirements. Both eating styles will promote glycogen recovery if the total amount of carbohydrate consumed is adequate. Eating a balanced mix of low-, moderate-, and high-glycemic carbohydrates throughout the day will support the glycogen recovery process. But consuming an adequate amount of total carbohydrate grams over the 24-hour period is a very important carbohydrate recovery strategy.

PROTEIN AND IMMEDIATE RECOVERY

A fair amount of debate has focused on the benefits of adding protein to the recovery carbohydrate snack immediately after exercise. In some studies, the results could be invalid because any benefit seemingly derived from the protein may have been due to the fact that the protein simply provided additional calories over the foods given to the carbohydrate-only group. Studies where researchers provided the same amount of calories when comparing a carbohydrate-only dose to a carbohydrate-and-protein combination dose indicate that carbohydrates alone can promote optimal recovery. What is certain is that having protein contribute about one-fourth of your recovery snack will not compromise your muscle glycogen recovery, and it may well contribute to muscle glycogen recovery. Consuming some protein immediately after exercise may also speed up the repair of muscle tissue and provide important nutrients for your immune system. It will also send you on your way to optimizing your protein intake until the next training session, whether that session is the next day or even later the same day.

Whether you consume carbohydrates alone or a carbohydrate-and-protein combination may be a matter of convenience. Packing and transporting high-carbohydrate items may be easier than including items containing protein. But if you do wish to include protein in your post-training snack, keep in mind that recovery protein should be from high-quality sources such as whey, dairy and soy milk, yogurt, and lean meats. A variety of commercial recovery products are also available. Although these are not necessary, they can be very convenient for replenishing your body immediately after training. Experiment with your own low-fat shake and smoothie recipes made from cow's milk, yogurt, soy milk, or juice and fresh or frozen fruit for a hydrating carbohydrate-and-protein combination. Ten to 20 grams of high-quality protein is more than adequate for your immediate protein intake.

FLUID AND IMMEDIATE RECOVERY

Rehydration is a top priority after moderate to hard training, as athletes typically replace only three-fourths of their sweat losses through drinking during exercise. Your goal is to fully restore fluid losses from one training session to the next, while keeping in mind that thirst is not a reliable indicator of fluid losses. Not only are you already dehydrated by the time you feel thirsty, the thirst mechanism will shut down before you have sufficiently replaced all your fluid losses. Try to consume 20 to 24 ounces (600–720 ml) of fluid for every pound (0.5 kg) of weight lost after training. Sixteen ounces (480 ml) actually replaces a fluid loss of 1 pound (0.5 kilogram), but the higher volume of 24 ounces (720 ml) should be sufficient to replace both sweat and urine losses.

Pay attention to what stimulates your desire to drink. You may prefer a sweet product or something a bit salty. The temperature of the drink may also affect the volume of fluid you consume. It makes sense that a cool drink would be more palatable, particularly in hot weather, but it may be difficult to drink large amounts of a very cold beverage.

Some athletes may feel reluctant to weigh themselves before and after every training session. You may also not have a scale available every time you train or would prefer not to get overly focused on a weight number. What you can do is obtain pre- and post-exercise weights after specific types of training sessions. These weight checks will provide you with valuable data. For example, you may discover that you replace only 50 percent of your fluid needs during hard training sessions, but meet 80 percent of your fluid requirements during less demanding exercise when it may be easier to consume fluid. Once you have established the replenishment levels of your best drinking efforts, you can develop a system for rehydrating after exercise. You may want to determine what your typical fluid losses are for specific types of environmental conditions, both indoors and outdoor, and for both hot- and cold-weather training. You can also check the color of your urine to evaluate your hydration efforts.

On days when you know you are to train or compete in extreme conditions, you may want to check your weight before and after exercise carefully. During intense training times and in hot-weather training, you can perform a daily check on your hydration status. After urinating in the morning, check your weight. If your usual weight is down by more than 1 pound (0.5 kg), you may not be keeping up with your usual fluid requirements.

Limit caffeine-containing beverages for several hours after exercise to optimize fluid replacement. Consume alcohol only after your fluid balance has been restored, if at all.

SODIUM AND IMMEDIATE RECOVERY

Sodium not only may stimulate your drive to drink but also can enhance the rehydration process. In most athletes, sweating results in large fluid losses and relatively small sodium losses. When you finish exercise, your blood volume and total body water are reduced, but there is a mild increase in blood concentration and its sodium content. When you consume large amounts of plain water after exercise, you dilute your blood before your full blood volume has been restored. This dilutional effect shuts down the thirst mechanism, and you will urinate to bring the concentration of the blood to a normal level. The end result is that you have produced a large amount of diluted urine before you are fully rehydrated.

You can offset this negative effect by consuming some sodium after exercise. One series of studies determined that rehydrating with drinks containing sodium produced significantly lower urine losses than low-sodium drinks, indicating that more of the fluid consumed was retained and therefore that better hydration occurred. Therefore, it is recommended that when your fluid losses are significant, you replace sodium losses as well. It appears that some individuals may have greater sodium sweat losses than others, so consuming sodium after exercise may be prudent unless medically contraindicated. Some athletes may actually require up to several grams of sodium over the course of the day, especially when training in extreme conditions.

If your fluid losses exceed 1 to 2 pounds (0.5–1 kg) during exercise, you should make a focused effort to drink fluids on a schedule and incorporate fluids into your recovery nutrition strategies. Products that contain sodium can also be integrated into your food and fluid choices to facilitate rehydration. If your recovery time is short, and the next training session is to take place in several hours, it makes sense to actively include sodium in your fluid and food choices.

Sports drinks are formulated for tolerable consumption during exercise, not after exercise. Post-exercise, a 150-pound (68 kg) athlete requires 75 grams of carbohydrates, which translates to 40 ounces (1,200 ml) of a sports drink. Sports drinks are relatively low in sodium, though higher-sodium formulas are available. You may consider adding 0.25 to 0.5 teaspoon (575–1,150 ml) of salt to your total fluid intake. However, consuming a sports drink rather than a recovery drink may not be your most effective recovery fluid strategy, though it is preferable to plain water when rehydration is important.

Although the recovery process is a continual effort that takes place from one training session to the next, you can get off to a good start by paying close attention to what you consume immediately and within the 2 hours after exercise. Then follow these post-exercise nutrition practices with food

TABLE **5.2**	IMMEDIATE NUTRITIONAL RECOVERY GUIDELINES	
TRAINING PROGRAM	**POST-TRAINING NUTRITIONAL STRATEGIES (within 30–60 minutes)**	**ONGOING RECOVERY STRATEGIES**
High-intensity training greater than 60 minutes	Consume 50–75 g carbohydrates Choose high-glycemic carbohydrates Consume 10–15 g high quality proteins (optional) Drink 20–24 oz. (600–720 ml) for every pound of weight lost Consume sodium-containing fluids in hot weather	Consume another 50–75 g carbohydrates in 2–3 hours Continue rehydrating to baseline weight Include sodium in meals and snacks in hot weather
Moderate- or high-intensity training greater than 90 minutes	Consume 50–75 g carbohydrates Choose high glycemic carbohydrates Consume 10–15 g high quality proteins Drink 20–24 oz. (600–720 ml) fluid for every pound of weight lost Consume 250 mg sodium with rehydration	Consume another 50–75 g carbohydrates in 2–3 hours Continue rehydrating to baseline weight Include sodium in meals and snacks
Aerobic conditioning less than 60 minutes	Rehydrate with liquid supplement containing carbohydrates and sodium Consume light carbohydrate snack of up to 50 g	Monitor weight and return to baseline with fluid intake Regular intake of meals and snacks to meet nutritional needs

and fluid choices that match your daily training requirements. Table 5.2 outlines the principles of immediate nutritional recovery. Some practical guidelines for post-exercise recovery are:

- Be organized. Many of your meals and snacks are likely to be consumed away from home. Prepare foods and fluids the night before for the next day's training as needed.
- Plan your food and fluid choices so that you can consume the optimal amounts of carbohydrate, protein, fluid, and sodium for your immediate recovery nutrition needs.
- Use the food list provided in Chapter 4 to consume enough carbohydrates—0.5 gram per pound (1.2 g/kg) of body weight.
- After moderate to hard training, be prepared to consume the same nutrient amounts again in 2 hours.
- If your appetite is suppressed after hard training, focus on liquid choices such as high-carbohydrate supplements, commercial or homemade smoothies, yogurt drinks, or sports recovery drinks.

- Avoid foods with a low glycemic index or that are very high in fiber immediately after training. These foods may not result in as speedy a recovery and may not be as well tolerated after training.
- Don't consume excessive amounts of protein immediately after training. Animal foods and high-protein supplements are very concentrated proteins, and often only small portions or doses are required for your nutritional recovery mix.
- Fat does not play an important role in the immediate recovery nutrition mix. Consuming fat immediately after training could delay gastric emptying and crowd out more important nutrients such as carbohydrates and protein.
- After training, drink on a schedule rather than according to thirst.
- Check labels to ensure that the foods and fluids you consume after training contain some sodium.

IMMEDIATE POST-TRAINING FOOD AND FLUID CHOICES

Practice to determine what post-training food and fluid choices are best for your preferences, tolerances, and schedule. Recovery products concentrated in carbohydrates, providing anywhere from 50 to 100 grams per 16-ounce (480 ml) serving, are available. Some of these products also provide up to 25 grams of protein per serving. Sports tubes that provide only protein are also available and can be consumed with a high-carbohydrate food or fluid source. Aim for recovery products that have a higher sodium content. Some favorite food choices among endurance athletes are:

- Cereal, dairy or soy milk, and fruit. High-glycemic cereals are good choices.
- Bagel with peanut butter, jam, and orange juice.
- Smoothie made with soy or dairy milk, yogurt, and frozen fruit.
- Yogurt, granola, and fruit.
- Energy bar and fruit.
- Baked potato with yogurt topping.
- Pancakes with syrup.
- Pasta salad with low-fat cheese.
- Turkey sandwich with pretzels.

NUTRITIONAL STRATEGIES FOR COMPETITION

Fine-tuning your food and fluid strategies before, during, and after training can also set the stage for competition day. Although the meals and snacks that you consume on race day are important,

PRACTICAL USES OF SPORTS NUTRITION PRODUCTS

Endurance athletes can't avoid the intense marketing of various sports drinks, gels, energy bars, recovery drinks, sports shakes, and high-energy drinks. While Appendix C presents a comparison chart of many of these products, a summary of some practical uses of these products is provided below. When you consume a wide variety of sports nutrition supplements over the course of a day or even a week, it is important to consider the other nutrients they provide, such as vitamins and minerals. Consider your intake in the context of your entire day's diet plan and be careful not to get too many vitamins and minerals through use of these products and supplements in combination.

Sports Drinks

Consume 16 to 24 ounces (480–720 ml) in the hour before exercise.

Consume 4 to 8 ounces (120–240 ml) every 15 to 20 minutes as your training session allows, or drink to match your sweat rate as much as possible.

Consume after exercise with high-carbohydrate foods and supplements.

Gels

Consume one packet in the 30 to 60 minutes prior to training and competition.

Consume during training with 16 ounces of water.

Consume as part of a recovery nutrition snack.

Energy Bars

Consume in the 30 to 60 minutes prior to training and competition.

Consume during training with fluid when a solid carbohydrate source is appropriate or desired.

Consume as part of a recovery snack after training.

Consume as part of a high-energy meal plan during heavy training cycles and for carbohydrate loading.

High-Energy Carbohydrate Drinks

Consume as part of a pre-training and pre-competition meal or snack.

Consume as part of immediate post-exercise recovery nutrition.

Consume as part of a high-energy meal plan.

CONTINUES

PRACTICAL USES OF SPORTS NUTRITION PRODUCTS   continued

High-Carbohydrate Protein Drinks

Consume before and after resistance training for quality protein combined with carbohydrates.

Consume as part of a pre-training and pre-competition meal.

Consume as part of your immediate recovery nutrition plan.

Consume as part of a high-energy training meal plan.

Sports Shakes

Use as a pre-exercise snack for an easily digested carbohydrate and protein source.

Include in a carb-loading meal or competition morning meal for easily digested nutrients.

Drink as a recovery snack after training.

Include in a high-energy nutrition plan.

Use as a quick meal or snack for convenience.

---

specific nutrition strategies in the days and hours leading up to competition can also benefit your performance. Many endurance athletes taper training before an important event, and this period of relative rest presents an important opportunity to fuel up. Adjusting your pre-race meal to account for race-day nerves and the hard effort ahead is also an important consideration. Having a specific plan for your nutritional strategies during endurance competition events—for example, the multiple heats that swimmers may need to complete over the course of a competition lasting several days—can give you that extra boost you need to do your best.

ONE WEEK PRIOR TO COMPETITION: CARBOHYDRATE LOADING

When you have the luxury of tapering for an important competition such as a triathlon, marathon, adventure race, or full day of swimming or rowing competition, you are presented with a prime opportunity to maximize your carbohydrate fuel stores. The combination of not dipping into your muscle glycogen as deeply as you would with regular training and maximizing your carbohydrate intake is known as "carbohydrate loading." Although this process traditionally takes place over the course of a week, some athletes adapt it to their needs by lengthening or shortening the carb-loading period. An athlete facing a short race or competition may load carbohydrates over just a 24- to 48-hour period before competition, whereas an athlete preparing for an ultraendurance event, such as an Ironman triathlon or ultramarathon, may taper for several weeks and then load carbohydrates for the last week of his or her taper.

Research indicates that muscle glycogen stores return to normal with 24 hours of rest and a high-carbohydrate diet if there is no significant muscle damage. However, it may be ideal to rest and eat up for an additional 24 hours to bring muscle glycogen levels from the normal full level of 100 to 120 millimoles per kilogram (mmol/kg) to the supercompensated level of 150 to 200 mmol/kg. Carbohydrate loading will allow you to perform at your desired pace for a longer period of time and is especially useful for competitions where you anticipate that your time will be longer than 90 minutes. During longer race tapers designed for a longer event, focus on reaching a full recovery so that your muscles are rested and fueled for the big day.

Sports dietitians currently recommend the "modified" carbohydrate-loading regimen because it is gentler than but just as effective as the old strategy, which contained a stringent "depletion" phase. Devised in the 1960s, this depletion phase started a week before competition and lasted about three to four days. It involved depleting glycogen stores through a combination of hard training and a low-carbohydrate diet. This was followed by three to four days of combined rest and a high-carbohydrate diet to glycogen load the muscle. Athletes often complained of feeling and training poorly during the depletion phase. This difficult strategy was phased out after research in the 1980s showed that it was unnecessary to achieve the high levels of muscle glycogen that the technique produced. A three- to four-day taper combined with a high-carbohydrate diet was found to be sufficient to achieve the same glycogen-loading levels. Below are a few guidelines to consider when carbohydrate loading:

- Gradually taper your training for 1 week prior to the event (longer if that is outlined in your training program). Eat your normal training diet that matches your intake with your training during days 7 to 4 of the 1-week taper countdown. You should consume at least 3 grams of carbohydrates per pound (6.6 g/kg) of body weight.
- For the last few days of the week, taper your training further, or even rest completely on days 3 to 1 of the countdown. Consume a high-carbohydrate diet providing from 4 to 5 grams of carbohydrates per pound (9–11 g/kg) of body weight.
- The carbohydrate amounts required for an athlete to glycogen load can vary from the above recommendations. Ideally, on days 7 to 4 you will consume more total carbohydrates than previously in your training, or in excess of what a particular training session normally requires, and on days 3 to 1 you will "carb-load."
- Your caloric needs may decrease during this time because of the marked decrease in training. You can lower both your protein and fat intake in the 72 hours before the race, as requirements for these nutrients are decreased.
- If you cannot taper for a full week, reduce your training for 3 days and load up on carbohydrates.

- Exercise lightly the day before the competition to relieve any muscle stiffness and to keep your muscles "sharp" for competition.
- Have a food plan laid out ahead of time that ensures that you consume enough carbohydrates to glycogen load. Carbohydrate loading is not synonymous with "pigging out," nor is it a food free-for-all. You don't want high-fat foods to replace those precious carbohydrates.
- You may want to emphasize low-fiber and compact carbohydrate food sources to minimize any gastrointestinal upset and to ensure that you consume the prescribed carbohydrate amounts.
- Be aware that for every gram of glycogen you store in your body, you also store up to 3 grams of water. This effect can result in a weight gain of several pounds. This extra fluid will help delay dehydration during the event.
- Pay close attention to what you eat the day and night before the competition and the day of the competition. Specific guidelines will be provided later in this chapter.
- Monitor your urine color to determine if you are adequately hydrated. Pay attention to daily hydration needs, but keep in mind that you may not be creating as large a fluid deficit as you would during periods of heavier training.
- If you are competing in an event lasting longer than 6 hours, or if you are a heavy and salty sweater, be generous with the salt shaker and consume salty foods such as pretzels, tomato juice, and salty soups.
- Don't try any new or unusual foods or spicy items that may not agree with you in the days leading up to a race.

Having a sound menu plan in mind can take some of the stress off of carbohydrate loading. Table 5.3 provides a list of some high-carbohydrate, low-fiber foods that should be well tolerated and that provide 30 grams of carbohydrates per listed serving. Starches, breads, and cereals that are low in fiber are fairly concentrated sources. Fruit and fruit juices are also good sources of carbohydrates. Sports nutrition supplements such as energy bars, gels, concentrated carbohydrate drinks, and high-carbohydrate meal replacements may also fit nicely into your meal plan for their predictability and easy digestion.

The food lists in Chapter 4 provide an extended list of 30-gram carbohydrate servings. You have to consider how you will prepare and portion foods as you decrease your intake of proteins and fats during this carbohydrate-loading phase so as not to overeat calories and shut out the carbohydrates required for full replenishment of stored fuel. Many meals and snacks can be fat- and protein-free, with just enough consumed for satiety and fullness. Consuming between-meal snacks is another strategy for obtaining the recommended carbohydrate amounts. Buying sports supplements and

TABLE **5.3**	LOW-FIBER, HIGH-CARBOHYDRATE FOODS

30 GRAMS OF CARBOHYDRATES PER SERVING

Bagel, 2 oz. (60 g)

Bread, white, 2 slices

Pita pocket, 1½ rounds

Dinner rolls, 2

English muffin, 1

Muffin, low-fat, low-fiber, 3 oz. (90 g)

Tortillas, 2

Cooked cereal, 1 c. (240 ml)

Apple, 1½ medium

Applesauce, sweetened, ½ c. (120 ml)

Grapefruit, 1 large

Canned fruit, 1 c. (240 ml)

Cold cereal, low-fiber, 1½ oz. (45 g)

Graham crackers, 6

Saltines, 8

Rice, cooked, white, ⅔ c. (200 ml)

Pasta, cooked, 1 c. (240 ml)

Pretzels, white flour, 1½ oz. (45 g)

Potato, baked, no skin, 1 medium

Sweet potato, no skin, 4 oz. (120 g)

Apple juice, 8 oz. (240 ml)

Carrot juice, 10 oz. (300 ml)

Grape juice, 6 oz. (200 ml)

Cranberry juice cocktail, 8 oz. (240 ml)

Milk, skim, 20 oz. (500 ml)

Yogurt with fruit, 1 c. (240 ml)

TABLE **5.4**	HIGH-CARBOHYDRATE, PRE-COMPETITION MENU

BREAKFAST

Orange juice, 1 c. (240 ml)

Cornflakes, 1 c. (240 ml)

Banana, 1 large

Skim milk, 1 c. (240 ml)

Toast, 2 slices

Margarine, 1 tsp. (8 ml)

Jelly, 2 tbsp. (40 ml)

147 g carbohydrates, 750 calories

SNACK

Yogurt with fruit, 6 oz. (200 ml)

20 g carbohydrates, 150 calories

LUNCH

Lean turkey, 3 oz. (90 g)

White bread, 2 slices

Pretzels, ¾ oz. (20 g)

Pear, 1 large

Apple juice, 8 oz. (240 ml)

105 g carbohydrates, 585 calories

SNACK

Energy bar, 1 medium

40 g carbohydrates, 200 calories

DINNER

Cooked rice, 2 c. (480 ml)

Ground turkey, 3 oz. (90 g)

Cooked peas, 1 c. (240 ml)

Bread, 2 slices

160 g carbohydrates, 961 calories

SNACK

Frozen yogurt, 12 oz. (360 ml)

Fig Newtons, 2

102 g carbohydrates, 460 calories

TOTAL: 574 G CARBOHYDRATES, 3,100 CALORIES

commercial products may make life simpler during carbohydrate loading. Table 5.4 provides a sample menu for a very high-carbohydrate-loading day at more than 700 grams of carbohydrates. If this level exceeds your carbohydrate needs, simply trim back on some of the carbohydrate portions or one or more of the listed snacks.

48 HOURS BEFORE THE EVENT

This is really your big day to load up on carbs, for several reasons. You are not likely to have much of any type of activity on this day, so it is truly a rest day, and you still have one more day of your taper after consuming a large dose of carbohydrates. This allows for plenty of digestion time after a few substantial high-carbohydrate meals. Good carbohydrate choices on this day include white rice, bread, bagels, low-fiber cereal, fruit, juice, a variety of sports nutrition supplements such as high-energy drinks and bars, and small amounts of very lean protein such as poultry or fish. Minimal oils should be used in food preparation. A large carb-loading meal with pasta, rice, or potatoes can be used as a base for this meal, but a 3-ounce portion of protein would also be fine. Stick with cooked, easy-to-digest vegetables; you should probably skip the salad. Drink plenty of fluids (but don't overhydrate), and include fluid choices that also provide carbohydrates. You may need to eat five or six times on this day to get in the total grams of carbohydrates required. Carry high-carbohydrate snacks and fluids with you wherever you go so that you can continue to steadily fuel and hydrate your body. A light evening snack can top off your carbohydrate intake for the day.

THE DAY BEFORE THE EVENT

The day before the event, your nutritional focus should be on consuming adequate carbohydrates but also sticking to very simple and easy-to-digest foods. Only minimal amounts of fats and proteins are required the day before the event. Make sure that you have your large meal consumed by 5:00 p.m. or even earlier if you expect a very early morning start. Since most races and events do start early in the morning, the last thing you want to do is to feel groggy and full from consuming a large dinner late in the evening the night before a race. Also, your pre-race meal on the morning of the event is an essential component of your nutrition plan. It is important that you wake up that morning feeling hungry and ready to eat. The day before and especially the night before the event, you do not want to try any new and unusual foods that could result in gastrointestinal upset. Be especially careful to limit fiber-containing foods, gassy foods such as broccoli and beans, and alcohol. Practice having various meals the night before an important morning training session to see what works best for you. Make simple meals that can be ordered in most restaurants when traveling. Pasta dishes low in fat are a common favorite among athletes, but other choices also work well. Try rice-based dishes, baked potatoes, and white breads. You will probably want to avoid salads and other raw vegetables and raw fruits the night before an important training session or race. Again, carry carbohydrate-containing foods and fluids to keep the fuel supply steady. Sports drinks and high-carbohydrate drinks that contain sodium provide a great way to hydrate the day before the race. Continue to go heavy on the salt as needed by salting your food and consuming salty items.

RACE MORNING

Depending on your race time, personal tolerances, and experience, you should consume a light to large meal 3 to 4 hours before competition. Many seasoned endurance athletes have identified this time period as optimal for pre-race eating, as you can achieve a good balance between optimal food consumption and adequate digestion time. Hopefully you will greet the morning well hydrated and with muscle glycogen stored at peak levels by practicing proper nutrition techniques for several days before the race. The main focus of this pre-race meal should be to replenish your liver glycogen stores. This valuable fuel falls to low levels overnight, especially if you spend your night tossing and turning from pre-race nerves. With the right timing and portions, eating 3 to 4 hours before exercise will allow you to:

- Restore liver glycogen to normal levels.
- Store carbohydrates in the muscle as needed, if portions are large enough.
- Have some carbohydrates stored in the gut for absorption and release during exercise.
- Avoid feeling hungry during longer events and competitions.

On the morning of competition, it is especially important to choose foods that you enjoy and tolerate and that also provide both a physiological and a psychological edge. For every hour you allow yourself to digest, consume just less than half a gram of carbohydrates for every pound of body weight. For example, if you decide to eat a large meal 4 hours before a triathlon or swimming competition, you can consume 2 grams of carbohydrates per pound. For a 150-pound (68 kg) athlete, this translates to 300 grams of carbohydrates (and 1,200 calories). It is probably easiest on your stomach if a good portion of this fairly substantial meal consists of dense, low-fiber foods and some liquid carbohydrate sources. You can obtain 300 grams of carbohydrates by consuming one large bagel topped with 2 tablespoons (40 ml) of jam, followed by a fruited yogurt and 32 ounces (960 ml) of a concentrated sports drink. The small amounts of protein in the yogurt may help keep you full a bit longer. You can also add peanut butter or cream cheese to your bagel if a small amount of fat is well tolerated. Of course, some athletes can only tolerate smaller meals close to exercise, particularly competition. Every athlete needs to iron out individual tolerances in terms of foods, portions, and timing. Table 5.5 provides pre-competition meal suggestions.

TABLE **5.5**	**MEAL TIMING BEFORE TRAINING AND COMPETITION**

TIMING	CARBOHYDRATE/FOOD RECOMMENDATIONS	SAMPLE FOODS	START TIMES
Night before	High-carbohydrate meal (300 g carbohydrates) Low in fiber Easy on fat Plenty of fluids	Pasta dishes Rice dishes Lean protein Cooked vegetables	Essential for early starts Helpful for any start time
3–4 hours prior	Carbohydrates: 1.5–2 g/lb. wt. (3–4 g/kg) Low-fat proteins in moderate amounts Low to moderate amount easily digested fat Low fiber Plenty of fluids	150-pound (68 kg) athlete: 225–300 g carbohydrates Cereals, bread, crackers, milk, yogurt, fruit, juices, jelly, muffins, bagels	*FOR MID-MORNING STARTS:* Eat at 7:00 a.m. for 10:00 a.m. start *MID-AFTERNOON STARTS:* Eat at 10:00 a.m. for 2:00 p.m. start *FOR EVENING STARTS:* Eat at 4:00 p.m. for a 7:00 p.m. start after adequate carbohydrate meals
2 hours prior	Carbohydrates: Up to 1 g/lb. wt. (2 g/kg) Minimal low-fat protein Low fat and fiber Plenty of fluid	150-pound (68 kg) athlete: 130–150 g carbohydrates Cereals, bread, milk, yogurt, fruit, juices, jelly, crackers	*FOR MID-MORNING STARTS:* Eat at 8:00 a.m. for 10:00 a.m. start *FOR MID-AFTERNOON STARTS:* Eat at noon for 2:00 p.m. start after a large morning breakfast *FOR LATE STARTS:* Eat at 6:00 p.m. for 8:00 p.m. start after adequate carbohydrate meals throughout the day
1 hour prior	Carbohydrates: 0.5 g/lb. wt. (1.0 g/kg) Emphasize liquids 50 to 100 g easy-to-digest carbohydrates in the form of liquid or gel, solid if tolerated Limit or avoid protein, and limit fat and fiber	Sports drinks, concentrated carbohydrate drinks and gels, sports bars, tolerated fruits	*FOR EARLY STARTS:* Eat at 6:00 a.m. for 8:00 a.m. start *FOR MID-MORNING STARTS:* For 10:00 a.m. start, have snack/liquid at 9:00 a.m. in addition to 6:30–7:00 a.m. meal
Immediately prior	Carbohydrates	Sports drinks Energy bars if exercise starts at moderate intensity for at least 30 minutes	For any start time

In the hours leading up to the race you can also continue to hydrate with a sports drink. These drinks can provide easy-to-digest carbohydrates and sodium as well as fluid. You may want to stop drinking, however, 30 minutes or more before the start of the race to allow your stomach to empty comfortably and to empty your bladder. Some athletes even like to top off their carbohydrate intake in the 90 minutes before the start of competition with an energy bar or gel. You can practice this strategy in training and determine if it works well for you.

Obviously, meal timing and portioning are especially important the day of competition. Make sure that you have a well-thought-out and thoroughly rehearsed game plan for eating times and portions on the day of the event. Experiment with meal and snack timing in training, and try to mimic the schedule of an upcoming competition. For earlier start times, you may want to consider one moderate-sized meal several hours beforehand. If you do not want to rise as early as this strategy requires, however, a smaller meal can be consumed closer to the event.

Later start times may necessitate eating one large meal earlier in the day, followed by a series of snacks as the start of competition approaches. On competition day, you can enjoy sports nutrition supplements that are easily digested and well tolerated. Liquid meal replacements, high-carbohydrate energy drinks, and sports drinks and gels can be consumed leading up to the start time. Refer to Tables 5.4 and 5.5 for pre-competition meal and snack timing suggestions.

6

WEIGHT, MUSCLE BUILDING, AND
CHANGING BODY COMPOSITION

Boosting Your Strength-to-Weight Ratio

ENDURANCE ATHLETES COME IN A VARIETY of shapes and sizes. Some began participating in sports in grade school or high school when their bodies were developing and growing and their body composition was still in flux. Others participate in their chosen sport well into their years as masters athletes. Some may be genetically blessed with a physique that is well suited to their sport and attain their body-composition goals easily, while others need to work hard to achieve these goals. Whichever category you fit into, you may find that focusing on body composition can improve your strength, fitness, and performance. Building muscle and strength and decreasing body fat can also help you build a good foundation for optimal health as you age. This focus can be particularly helpful after age thirty-five, when loss of a small amount of muscle mass is a normal part of the aging process.

There are smart and sensible ways to attain a lean and strong body. However, some athletes resort to destructive methods of manipulating their body composition in an attempt to attain an overly idealized body that may not be realistic for their age, growth and development, level of training, body type, or genetic tendencies. It is easy to assume that dropping a few "extra" pounds will improve your performance and that intense training builds muscle strength. But athletic success is not always that simple. Examples abound of athletes at all levels who have restricted their diet or increased their training in an attempt to improve body composition, with the end result being a decrease in energy levels and performance. It is important that you keep an open mind regarding your "best weight." Don't compromise your recovery and energy to build a few pounds of muscle or lose a few pounds of fat.

Optimal performance in endurance sports depends on a number of interrelated factors, including the ability to sustain power near your anaerobic threshold, a high VO_2max, efficient technique, a high power-to-weight ratio, and a low level of body fat. The last two factors mean that an endurance athlete carrying excess weight or lacking in muscle strength can be at greater risk for injury when performing the skills required for his or her sport. Of course, being overweight or ignoring the strength-training component of your program will also have adverse performance effects.

But less is not necessarily better. When striving to make body-composition changes, athletes need to realize that they will perform their best when they reach and maintain their own optimal body composition, not some idealized body composition that would require excessive training efforts and restrictive food strategies. Severe food restriction and excessive training can result in low energy levels and poor-quality training sessions, increase the risk of injury, and pose both short- and long-term health risks.

Reaching body-composition goals for optimal performance can go hand in hand with strength training, or resistance training, a common element of endurance training programs. The high levels of muscle mass and strength that can be achieved with resistance training are important factors in athletic performance whether it is on the road or in the pool. Optimal and effective methods for gaining muscle mass have long intrigued sports nutritionists and the industries that pay for heavy marketing and promotion of muscle-building products. However, the keys to maximizing strength include your genetic potential, an appropriate resistance training program, and specific muscle-building nutritional strategies supported by solid scientific research.

Clearly, many endurance athletes can benefit from building muscle and maintaining optimal levels of body fat. Let's take a look at some strategies for doing just that.

BUILDING MUSCLE

Hormones—specifically growth hormones, testosterone, insulin, and insulin-like growth factor—largely control muscle growth. Nutrition can very effectively support your efforts to increase lean body mass by affecting these hormone levels and providing your body with the nutritional tools required for optimal muscle building. Many of the nutritional strategies for muscle building center not only on your daily training diet but also on the intake of certain nutrients timed specifically around your weight-training sessions to optimize your muscle-building efforts.

The keys to optimizing muscle-building efforts include the following:

- Attaining enough calories so that your body has the energy required to build muscle
- Consuming enough carbohydrates so that you meet the fuel demand for both resistance training and training for your sport

- Having enough protein in your daily diet
- Timing your nutrient intake before and after resistance training, particularly for protein
- Consuming fluids and carbohydrates during your workout

NUTRITIONAL REQUIREMENTS FOR BUILDING MUSCLE
Calories and Carbohydrates

When you strength train, you likely are also participating in regular training for your sport and could be burning significant amounts of stored body fuel from various types of exercise sessions. During weight training, the stored fuels of creatine phosphate and muscle glycogen serve as important energy sources. When combined with other components of your endurance training program, resistance training can provide a further drain on your body's carbohydrate fuel stores. Although you may typically think of increased protein intake in relation to strength training, one main goal should be to consume adequate energy to build muscle tissue.

One of the most important nutrition guidelines for effectively building muscle is to consume enough calories. Because of the increased energy it takes to build body tissue, falling short on your calorie requirements will impair your rate of muscle building. An additional 350 to 500 calories daily are needed to gain 1 pound of muscle mass per week. Further increases in muscle building require additional calories. Once you gain the muscle and strength that you desire for your sport and performance, it also takes an adequate amount of energy to maintain this increased weight. Keep in mind that these additional calories are the calories required above your energy needs for training and recovery in your sport. The combination of your endurance training program and your weight training can have a significant impact on your energy needs.

Often the perception is that extra calories consumed to build muscle should be protein calories. Although protein is required to build muscle tissue, it is only one of the ingredients needed for the tissue-building process. The amount of protein that you require as an endurance athlete should be adequate to cover your daily needs for muscle building; your protein needs may increase only slightly, if at all, when you are adding resistance training to your day. In fact, many of the extra calories needed for muscle building should come from carbohydrates in your diet. The most important factor in your protein intake is not amount, but timing.

Muscle glycogen is an important fuel source during weight training, and an intense session may deplete 30 percent of your muscle glycogen stores. When this type of training is combined with your endurance training, muscle glycogen stores can become significantly depleted in a day or over several days. Regardless of how quickly you deplete these stores, it is important that you replenish glycogen stores adequately after training, whether in the weight room at the gym, after a workout in the pool, or after a bike or run.

Protein

Although large amounts of protein are not necessary, protein is still important for the repair and growth of muscle fibers. Strength training causes the breakdown of muscle fibers, which respond by making bigger and stronger muscle fibers to protect against further stress. Protein is one of the main construction materials needed for this repair process to take place. Athletes who strength train do have higher protein requirements than sedentary individuals, but the amount of protein they consume for endurance training is likely more than adequate to put them in positive protein balance. *Positive protein balance* means that you consume enough protein to meet all the protein-requiring processes and functions in your body, including the synthesis of new muscle tissue.

If you do consume protein in excess of what is required for both your strength training and endurance training, this extra protein is burned for energy, which is not a very efficient process, or simply stored as fat, which may not be desirable. More is not better, and eating twice as much protein as your body requires won't make your muscles twice as big. Strength training also makes your body more efficient at utilizing the protein in your diet.

Real foods can easily be part of a well-balanced diet that meets your protein requirements for both weight training and endurance training. Stick with the high-quality sources of protein mentioned in Chapter 2, such as lean red meat, poultry, fish, skim milk dairy products, and soy products. You will also obtain protein from some plant foods, all of which contribute to your total protein intake. Fat in your diet should continue to round out your calories just as it would for your regular training diet.

TIMING YOUR NUTRITIONAL INTAKE

After weight training, your body synthesizes new muscle protein and replenishes muscle glycogen. Several studies have indicated that an athlete's nutritional intake in the hours before and after weight training can have a significant impact on his or her muscle-building efforts. Consuming a combination of carbohydrates and protein both before and after weight training is more effective in promoting muscle building than just increasing your overall daily protein intake.

Consume protein prior to and after your resistance training efforts. Aim for about 15 to 20 grams of protein in the meal or snack that you eat in the 1 hour before strength training, emphasizing high-quality sources such as skim milk dairy products, whey protein, and protein from animal foods, as essential amino acids are the most potent stimulators of muscle protein synthesis. Combine this protein with 35 to 50 grams of carbohydrates. Go for the higher carbohydrate amount if your resistance training session is followed by an endurance workout.

You can also include both carbohydrates and protein in the next snack or meal that you consume after weight training to continue to facilitate the recovery and muscle-building process. Aim for some recovery nutrition foods and fluids within the 1 to 2 hours after weight training. Carbohydrates and protein consumed after resistance training should also stimulate both muscle glycogen and protein synthesis. This form of supplementation increases blood levels of insulin and growth hormone, both of which are tissue-building agents. High-glycemic carbohydrates can be emphasized after resistance training, just as they can after your regular training sessions. Aim for 15 to 20 grams of protein and 50 grams or more of carbohydrates in your recovery snack or meal.

Often your nutritional choices before and after weight training will, out of necessity, depend on practical considerations. Keep snacks on hand to consume both before and after resistance training. Aim for convenience choices, such as low-fat shakes or smoothies. Pack protein-containing snacks such as yogurt with fruit, a peanut butter and honey sandwich, or low-fat cheese and crackers to take with you to the gym. A commercial sports supplement containing a mix of carbohydrates and protein is convenient and meets your nutritional requirements in the hour before and after weight training.

What you consume during resistance training may be beneficial to your recovery and the quality of your training sessions. Although adenosine triphosphate (ATP) and creatine phosphate in the muscle are your primary fuel sources during weight-training sessions, muscle glycogen can become depleted to varying degrees between training sets, depending on the intensity and duration of your training. Between sets, your muscle will use the glycolysis energy pathway to regenerate ATP stores. Consuming a sports drink for the carbohydrates it provides can help you maintain muscle glycogen stores and provide energy during your workout. These drinks also provide fluid and assist you in maintaining adequate hydration levels. Of course, consuming plain water during resistance training is also recommended. As with any training session, try to start your workout well hydrated.

PROTEIN SUPPLEMENTS AND WEIGHT TRAINING

Athletes who become serious about strength training inevitably wonder whether they should take protein supplements. Those who decide to try them may be bewildered by the number of choices—there are many products on the market containing protein from a variety of sources. These products can optimize muscle building, but again, the timing of the protein intake is the key. The protein in the supplements is not necessarily any better than the protein contained in foods; however, the supplements are convenient and may make your protein consumption at the right times easier to accomplish when you are not at home. The supplements can be consumed with moderate amounts of carbohydrate, so follow the recommendations described above for your diet on a day that includes strength training.

Which of the protein sources used in these supplements is best? Basically, there are several sources that provide high-quality protein. Whey protein is an increasingly popular protein supplement.

Whey is the component of milk that is separated out when making cheese and other dairy products. It is a high-quality protein and easy to digest. Whey protein can also be lactose-free in the form of whey protein isolate. Soy protein is also an excellent source of protein, especially soy protein isolate. It is a high-quality protein choice for vegetarians and is lactose-free. Casein is another protein obtained through cheese production. It does not have as strong of an amino acid profile as whey protein but is still a good protein source. Egg protein is obtained from egg whites and is considered the standard against which to compare other proteins—though consuming real eggs may not be as convenient a protein source as supplements, depending on the timing and location of your training.

Like many other sports nutrition strategies and choices, use of protein supplements rather than real food before and after resistance training is a matter of what is most convenient for you. These products should be taken with a carbohydrate source such as juice. Often, only a small scoop of the protein supplement is needed to provide 15 to 20 grams, though higher doses may be encouraged on the label.

But the supplements can also be expensive and they do not necessarily offer any muscle-building advantage over real protein foods. High-quality protein can be obtained from milk and yogurt, tofu and other soy products, and poultry and lean meats. Practical protein and carbohydrate combinations for your pre- and post-weight-training meals or snacks would include homemade smoothies that use a variety of quality protein ingredients such as soy milk, yogurt, and/or cow's milk. Fruit juice or fruit can be added for carbohydrates. A generous serving of yogurt with fruit can make a good protein and carbohydrate combination. Low-fat cheese is also a high-quality protein source that can be consumed with fruit or a granola bar.

YOUR WEIGHT-TRAINING DIET

The nutritional strategies for optimizing muscle building and increasing strength are complex and interrelated. Consuming adequate calories is a key to providing your body with the energy to build muscle. However, your daily protein needs must be met, and the timing of your protein intake is also important, particularly before and after training. Weight training, like your regular training for your sport, is a fuel-depleting exercise. Consuming carbohydrates with your protein both before and after training can facilitate energy and recovery, and consuming carbohydrates during training itself can also fuel your efforts.

To gain muscle mass while following a strength training program, you need an additional 350 to 500 calories daily for a muscle gain of 1 pound per week. These additional calories can come mainly from carbohydrates and some protein. Here are some strategies for obtaining additional calories:

- Add a bit more protein to sandwiches and dinners.
- Top carbohydrate foods such as bagels with jams and honeys.
- Add another snack to your meal plan.
- Add a fruited yogurt, fruit smoothie, low-fat shake, or instant breakfast drink to your meal plan.
- Add a pasta or rice salad side to your lunch.
- Consider a high-calorie shake or meal replacement.
- Make oatmeal and soups with milk.
- Add wheat germ, sunflower seeds, and dried fruit to cereals.
- Choose higher-calorie juices such as apple, cranberry, nectars, and blends.
- Choose calorie-dense cereals such as muesli, granola, and Grape-Nuts.
- Have the higher-calorie starchy vegetables such as peas, corn, and winter squash.

Table 6.1 summarizes the nutritional strategies for building muscle mass.

TABLE 6.1   NUTRITIONAL FACTORS IN DAILY DIET FOR MUSCLE BUILDING

NUTRIENT	ROLE OF NUTRIENT
Calories	Provide additional 350–500 calories in daily diet to build 1 pound of muscle per week.
Carbohydrates	Fuel source during weight training. Required in diet to replenish glycogen stores for comprehensive training program that includes aerobic and anaerobic conditioning.
Protein	Required for muscle building. Protein needs are easily met on a well-planned diet for a comprehensive training program that includes weight training and aerobic and anaerobic training.
Fat	Adequate amounts needed to maintain hormone levels, including testosterone. Healthy fats should be emphasized for cardiovascular health.

ONE HOUR BEFORE WEIGHT TRAINING	DURING TRAINING	AFTER TRAINING
Consume 10–15 g high-quality protein from whey, dairy, or soy sources. Consume 25–50 g carbohydrates. Pre-hydrate with 16–24 oz. (600–720 ml) fluid.	Consume 16 oz. (600 ml) of carbohydrate electrolyte beverage, if desired. Consume gel and water for carbohydrate and fluid sources, if desired.	Consume 10–15 g high-quality proteins from whey, dairy, or soy sources. Consume 25–50 g carbohydrates. Rehydrate with 20 oz. (600 ml) of fluid per pound (0.5 kg) of weight lost during session.

NUTRITIONAL REQUIREMENTS FOR INJURY RECOVERY

You may at some point in your career as an endurance athlete suffer from strains, abrasions, bruising, or fractures. Most likely the speed at which your injury heals is of concern to you. While you may have a rehabilitation program mapped out, the calories and nutrients that you require for this program may differ from your usual eating. What is clear, however, is that protein, fat, carbohydrates, and vitamins and minerals are essential for timely and complete healing of injuries. Weight-management issues may also present themselves at the time of an injury due to a marked decrease in energy expenditure.

Nutritional considerations can vary among specific situations and athletes. But often during rehabilitation an athlete fears putting on body fat. The injury often results in significant changes in energy expenditure as a result of changes in an athlete's training program. For a period of time, the volume and intensity of training will decrease, and the type of training may temporarily change. Endurance athletes become accustomed to eating enough to support a demanding training program, and when an injury occurs, it may be difficult to know how and when to cut back on this caloric intake to achieve the proper caloric balance. Muscle mass may also decrease during the recovery period, depending on the type of rehabilitation program that is prescribed. Depending on the type and extent of the injury, an athlete's caloric expenditure may decrease by several thousand calories per week. An athlete who decreases training volume by just 4 hours a week could experience a weekly 1-pound weight gain if he or she continues to follow his or her usual eating habits.

At the other extreme, an athlete who cuts back too much on calories may not be eating enough to support the healing process. When recovering from an injury, it is best not to undereat protein and calories. Protein is necessary for the growth and repair of body tissue, supports healthy immune function, and is required for the synthesis of enzymes and hormones. Undereating calories can also lead to increased incidence of infection and slower wound healing.

Regardless of the type of injury, it is important to maintain energy balance. Injured athletes can keep a food record and determine their normal caloric intake. They then can trim anywhere from 200 to 500 calories or more daily to prevent weight gain if needed. Sometimes the intake of carbohydrates and protein needs to be decreased slightly to prevent a gain in body fat. Excess dietary fat that was easily burned off in training should also be shaved down. But if you are recovering from an injury, avoid drastic dietary restrictions so that you don't miss out on needed nutrients. Often some personalized guidance from a sports dietitian can be helpful when you are injured.

CONTINUES

NUTRITIONAL REQUIREMENTS FOR INJURY RECOVERY continued

In many instances, starting a good resistance and rehabilitation program provides a big advantage. Building muscle takes work and energy, allowing you to consume more calories than you would be able to consume if you simply cut back on training or stopped for a time altogether. A good rehabilitation program can thus somewhat offset the decreased caloric expenditure that typically occurs during recovery from an injury. If these weight-training sessions are intense, consuming carbohydrates during training can facilitate recovery and muscle repair.

After an initial period of healing, athletes often engage in rehabilitation programs that are just as demanding as their usual training, though the program may differ in scope and timing. Your usual meal plan may need to be adjusted to support energy levels at specific training times and encourage tissue repair and muscle-building efforts.

When you are injured, increasing your intake of certain nutrients and perhaps even supplementation may support the healing process. One of the principal functions of vitamin C is collagen synthesis, a core component of scar tissue. Collagen is also required for the formation and maintenance of connective tissue such as cartilage as well as tendons and bones. Vitamin C plays a role in red blood cell synthesis, too. Load up on some of the good vitamin C sources listed in Chapter 2. Fruits and vegetables are abundant in vitamin C and are also low-calorie foods. Increasing your intake of fruits and vegetables will also provide antioxidants and bioflavonoids that can protect your muscles against damage during exercise and further support the healing process.

Other important vitamins for a recovery nutrition plan are vitamin A, which supports collagen formation and the immune system, and the B vitamins, especially if there has been trauma and stress associated with the injury.

Several minerals, including iron and zinc, play important roles in the recovery process as well. Zinc is a component of many enzymes involved in energy metabolism and is required for protein synthesis and wound healing. Zinc from animal protein is best absorbed. Iron, of course, is needed for oxygen transport and the formation of hemoglobin and myoglobin, processes that enable the athlete to maintain a high level of rehabilitation training. Good sources are listed in Chapter 2.

Your protein and calorie requirements can change at specific phases of the rehabilitation process. However, a nutrient-dense diet is a plus at any time after an injury. A good multivitamin and mineral supplement high in antioxidants and bioflavonoids can also be useful at this time for the extra insurance it provides that you are getting all the nutrients you need for recovery.

LOSING FAT

Some endurance athletes monitor their weight and attempt to become leaner in hopes of improving their performance. Often, their efforts to manipulate their body composition result in frequent weight checks on the scale. It is important that you keep the scale in perspective, however, as it provides only a rudimentary measure and tells you little about body-fat levels or changes during the training season. There are other methods of estimating body fat that are much more useful for training purposes.

The scale obviously weighs all of you—muscle, fat, bone, water and fluid fluctuations, and body organs—and does not differentiate among these body tissues. For this reason, highly muscular athletes may weigh at the high end of their "ideal" weight. Conversely, thin, small-boned people weigh less. Your body weight is influenced by much more than what you eat and how much you train. Many of the factors that affect your weight are determined by genetics and are often out of your control.

The best use of a scale is to monitor long-term changes over time as they coincide with monitored body-composition changes and to measure short-term changes related to your hydration status. As mentioned previously, weight loss after a hard training session provides feedback regarding your level of hydration. It is recommended that for every pound (0.5 kg) of weight lost during exercise, you rehydrate with 24 ounces (720 ml) of noncaffeinated fluid.

Long-term weight changes as measured by a scale can provide you with a crude indicator regarding changes in body composition over time or even help you determine whether you are keeping up with or exceeding your energy needs. Chronic, unwanted weight loss can indicate that you are not meeting your caloric requirements, and perhaps that you are pushing yourself to an overtrained state. It is also important not to get overly focused on an idealized weight obtained from a height and weight chart, or on the weight and body-fat levels of the top athletes in your endurance sport. Although certain body-fat averages have been measured for specific sports, a number of interconnected factors other than body fat affect an athlete's performance. Athletes can be successful at varying degrees of reasonable body-fat levels, with some competitors at the low end of the body-fat range and others at the high end. Top athletes do not always fit the lean and muscular ideal for their sport, and a low body-fat level does not guarantee success.

TECHNIQUES FOR MEASURING BODY-FAT LEVELS

Regardless of the body-fat measurement technique that you employ, keep in mind that they all measure your body fat indirectly. When choosing a body-fat measurement technique, consider the following guidelines:

- The technique and formula used to estimate your body fat should be valid for athletes in your sport, for your gender, and for your age range.
- A reliable technician should perform the technique.
- The same technique should be repeated over time to obtain long-term data and to measure progressive changes.
- The results should be interpreted by a knowledgeable expert who is aware of the limitations of the technique and can advise you appropriately.

Clearly, the measurement of body composition is far from an exact science. One commonly utilized technique, for example, skinfold testing, has a standard error of 3 percent. This means that if an athlete tests at 15 percent body fat, his or her actual body-fat level could range from 12 to 18 percent. Body-fat assessments provide a possible range of body fat rather than an absolute number. When monitoring your body composition over time, it is very important that you do not try to compare the results you obtain via different techniques and technicians. Table 6.2 provides a perspective on body-fat measures for male and female endurance athletes in various endurance sports. But no individual athlete should feel pressured to meet a certain body-fat number: Each

---

TABLE 6.2   **BODY-FAT LEVELS FOR HEALTH AND ENDURANCE SPORTS**

RATING	BODY-FAT LEVELS	SPORT	MEASURED BODY-FAT LEVELS
At risk (low levels)	Males: < 5% Females: < 9%	Running	Males: 6–13% Females: 10–19%
Very low	Males: 6–10% Females: 10–15%	Cycling	Males: 8–10% Females: 12–18%
Below average	Males: 11–14% Females: 16–19%	Triathlon	Males: 5–11% Females: 7–17%
Average	Males: 15–18% Females: 20–25%	Swimming	Males: 7–12% Females: 14–24%
Above average	Males: 19–24% Females: 26–29%	Rowing	*HEAVYWEIGHT* Males: 6–10% Females: 19–25% *LIGHTWEIGHT* Males: 6–9% Females: 16–18%
At risk (high levels)	Males: 25% or more Females: 30% or more		

athlete is unique and performs best at a body-fat level appropriate to his or her own genetic in-
heritance and training level, among other factors.

The body-fat measurement techniques listed below are the ones most commonly used. They
all contain some inherent range of error, and they all provide only an estimate of body composition rather than an exact figure derived from a direct measurement of body fat. Accuracy also can
vary among technicians. If you decide to obtain a body-composition assessment, find an experienced technician who works with athletes regularly.

Hydrostatic Weighing

The hydrostatic method, a water-displacement technique, is often cited as the "gold standard" of
body-fat assessment, despite having a standard error of at least 2 percent. Hydrostatic weighing
involves being weighed underwater after expelling as much air from your lungs as possible. Your
body density is estimated from the difference between your weight on land and your weight under
water. Your body fat is then extrapolated from this information.

Like all methods, hydrostatic weighing is not error-free. This method assumes a constant fat-free
body density and may not be appropriate for all population groups. There is some potential error related to your hydration status and how much air is actually left in your lungs when you are weighed.
In addition, the procedure for underwater weighing can be a bit uncomfortable. The method can be
useful, however, and is offered at some sports medicine centers and universities. Health clubs may
offer it as a special service several times throughout the year. This technique, when administered by
a skilled technician over time, can help you to gauge body-composition changes.

Air Displacement

Also known as *body plethysmography,* this technique measures body density through air displacement rather than water displacement. Your body-fat percentage is calculated based on standard
equations. This technique provides body-fat estimations similar to underwater weighing, though
more data are needed on the results obtained from this method for competitive athletes. To complete the procedure, you sit in an enclosed capsule (a Bod Pod) while a computer measures the
amount of air displaced.

This is an expensive system, but it is less inconvenient than underwater weighing. In addition,
it is not yet widely available, though some universities and health clubs do offer it.

Bioelectrical Impedance Analysis (BIA)

Use of bioelectrical impedance analysis has markedly increased over the past ten years because it
is relatively inexpensive, portable, and convenient. BIA is based on the conductive property of dif-

ferent tissues within the body. Because muscles contain a high percentage of water, they conduct current more quickly than fat stores. The BIA machine passes a small and undetectable current through the body and analyzes the resistance to the flow of the current. The slower the signal, the more body fat you have.

Although BIA is relatively quick and simple, it may overestimate body fat in lean individuals, and the results can be affected by hydration levels. If you are not well hydrated, you will appear to have a higher level of body fat than you actually have. You should be well hydrated for the test, but you should not drink fluids for 4 hours before the test so that you will have an empty bladder. It is also best not to exercise within 12 hours of the test. Alcohol, diuretics, and caffeine should be avoided prior to this procedure as well.

Many individuals are now purchasing a home scale (Tanita brand) that measures body fat with this technique. To use the scale effectively, you should take the readings at the same time of day each time, be well hydrated, and have an empty bladder. Avoid early-morning readings when you are most likely to be dehydrated.

Skinfold Calipers

The skinfold caliper technique is the most widely used and the most inexpensive and convenient method of measuring body fat. For this procedure, a technician uses calipers to indirectly measure the double thickness of subcutaneous fat underneath the skin. Several standard skinfold sites have been identified on the body: abdomen, arm, thigh, hip area, and back of shoulder. They must be accurately marked, and the skinfold is then pinched and gently pulled away from the body. The sum of several skinfolds (anywhere from three to seven sites) is plugged into a formula that is then used to estimate total body fat.

This technique has several disadvantages. It requires a skilled technician, and it assumes that subcutaneous fat is proportional to total body fat. Moreover, the formulas for skinfold measurements are based on body-composition measurements from underwater weighing. The formulas used for skinfold measurements should be appropriate for athletes and their sport. When formulas for the general population are used, body fat is often underestimated in athletes. Skinfold measurements may also underestimate body fat in very lean athletes.

However, when kept in perspective, this technique can be useful. Besides calculating the body-fat percentage, you can use it to obtain a number that is the sum of all the skinfolds measured. This absolute number is not formula dependent and can be monitored over time. For example, a twenty-year-old male cross-country runner may have a three-site skinfold sum of 40 millimeters and an estimated body fat of 11 percent. A follow-up measurement several months later may show an increase in body weight along with a decrease in the total skinfold sum to 36 millimeters.

These results would indicate a probable loss in body fat and increase in muscle mass. This trend can be monitored every several months and over a year's time to provide useful feedback regarding training and diet.

Tape-measure readings can also be combined with skinfold assessment, with measurements taken at thigh, arm, and abdominal sites. The more skinfold measurement sites required by the formula, the better—you should never compare body-fat estimations made over time using different formulas.

CHANGING BODY COMPOSITION

Because body composition is the result of genetics as well as training and diet, some athletes may naturally have a body composition considered optimal for their sport, while others have to struggle to stay within a preferred range. Extreme efforts to maintain a set body composition may not be worth the energy it takes, as it may compromise the quality of your diet and training. It is also important to keep a healthy perspective on body fat. Aim for an appropriate range rather than a specific number. Body-fat levels may change over the course of a season—and over the course of your life—depending on the phase of your training, your age, and the stage of your competitive career.

If you are considering trying to improve your body-fat composition, have it assessed by a skilled technician. An optimal goal for weight can be determined, but it is important to be realistic regarding how much body fat you want to lose and how quickly you should try to reach your goal. This may require some professional advice and some realism on the athlete's part.

First, consider your genetics. Experts suggest that genetics strongly influences the amount of fat your body stores. If you have a history of struggling with body fat and can say the same of your family members, consider a moderate and gentle weight-loss goal. Next, look at your lifestyle. Food choices are heavily influenced by your schedule, commitments, environment, and stress levels. It is important for your weight-loss and body-fat goals to be reasonable, as you have to meet the energy demands not only of training but of life in general—and work or school—as well.

Dieting Pitfalls

Dieting certainly presents several pitfalls for the endurance athlete. An athlete who is glycogen depleted, electrolyte depleted, low on protein, and dehydrated from dieting will not perform at his or her best and likely will perform poorly. Rigid dieting and too much calorie restriction can deplete body-fuel stores. Intense weight-loss efforts can also result in hormonal imbalances, iron-deficiency anemia, compromised bone health, and loss of muscular strength and power. Severe dieting can make you crabby, tired, and obsessive. Dieting just isn't fun.

Food is fuel for your hardworking body, and your body does not respond positively when fuel runs low. A low fuel gauge sends out a slew of appetite-triggering brain chemicals that drive you to eat. What many dieters perceive as a lack of willpower is really the body's drive for self-preservation. Restricting foods can lead to overeating and even binge eating, thwarting weight-loss efforts. Besides playing games with the body, dieting wreaks havoc with the mind. Restrictive eating can lead to feelings of deprivation and a preoccupation with food.

Besides triggering overeating, drastic calorie reduction can break down body protein stores for energy. This muscle loss not only hinders your strength and power but also negatively impacts your metabolism. Muscle is what keeps your furnace burning. Your body responds to calorie restriction by lowering its resting metabolic rate. Eating normally can restore your metabolism, though this may take time if you have a history of repeated dieting. With repeated dieting, your body may become more efficient at utilizing calories and storing body fat.

Healthy Weight-Loss Guidelines

A healthy weight for an athlete is about how you feel and perform, not just about how you perceive how you look or what the scale is telling you. It can be difficult in our society to keep a healthy perspective on weight. The ideal has become more muscular and leaner than ever, while as a whole the population is gaining weight. Often the ideal portrayed in the media is unhealthy and unrealistic and can only be attained through excessive exercise and overly restrictive eating.

Healthy weight loss starts with setting a realistic goal and avoiding quick, unbalanced, and extreme weight-loss approaches. Try to accomplish your goal in a reasonable amount of time and during the off-season for your sport. Let's take a look at some sensible weight-loss guidelines.

Set a realistic body-composition and weight-loss goal. It is very likely that your training program emphasizes both muscle building and maintaining a low level of body fat. Often, real body-composition changes do not result in drastic body-weight changes, as the scale measures all body tissue, not just fat. Elicit the advice of a qualified professional who can assess your body-composition results and recommend changes in body composition that are appropriate for your age, gender, growth and development, current training program, and sport.

Set a realistic calorie deficit. Keep in mind that when you attempt to lose body fat, you have to restrict calories; however, when you desire to build muscle, you need to consume adequate calories. It is important to find a balance between your body-composition and strength-development goals. Females should not exceed a weight loss of 1 pound weekly, and males, 2 pounds weekly, especially during heavy training periods. Losing 1 pound weekly requires a deficit of 500 calories daily. Greater weight loss requires even more restriction. Losing 2 pounds weekly requires a daily

1,000-calorie deficit, clearly calling for some intense calorie-cutting and calorie-burning efforts that are not always appropriate during periods of growth and/or heavy training cycles.

Remember that trimming no more than 200 to 300 calories daily may be the safest and most effective long-term weight-loss approach. This mild reduction should have no metabolism-lowering effects and will not precipitate feelings of hunger and deprivation. However, if you are stepping up your muscle-building efforts, your best results may be obtained by following the proper training program and the nutrition program that is optimal for building muscle mass.

Keep a food journal to assess your current eating habits. Write down your food intake, the times of your meals and snacks, and your portion sizes for 1 week. Record your training sessions as well, noting the duration and intensity of training in conjunction with your food intake. You can also record your moods, thoughts, and feelings to determine some of your eating triggers, such as stress or fatigue. It may be helpful to note your energy levels and recovery during and after various types of training sessions.

Assess your intake. Make sure that you are following the principles of post-exercise recovery nutrition. Monitor your hunger and fullness patterns. Do you often wait until you are ravenous before eating? Do you get overfull at meals? Do you eat for comfort or in reaction to stress fairly often? Do you have significant drops in your energy levels during the day?

You may be surprised at how much you actually consume during the day. Writing down your food can help you stay on track while you are trying to lose weight and, more important, can help you improve the quality of your diet and nutritional strategies, as it makes you accountable and conscious of your food choices.

Have a healthy strategy or plan for reducing your caloric intake and improving your diet. There are a number of effective ways to reduce your caloric intake and improve your diet. It is important that you do eat well after exercising, practicing the recovery nutrition guidelines supplied in Chapters 1 to 5, and that you time your meals and snacks appropriately before training. If you eat out frequently or consume too much fast food, you may have a large amount of hidden fat in your diet.

Other techniques for reducing fat intake include choosing leaner meats, switching to low-fat dairy products, minimizing added fats and those used in cooking, and decreasing the frequency of sweets. You can also cut back on high-calorie fluids. Alcohol is an obvious choice, as are sodas and perhaps juices. Pay attention to portions when you eat out or grab items on the run. A bagel or muffin can easily provide more than 300 calories.

Plan ahead. Preparing meals ahead of time can help you avoid fatty restaurant foods. Learning how to shop for quick, low-fat, nutritious foods can be extremely helpful in improving your diet and changing your body composition. You can also pack healthy snacks such as fresh fruits and vegetables. Programming your food environment for success or learning how to manage the environment in which you make your food choices will go a long way toward supporting you in reaching your weight-loss goals.

Eat balanced meals at the right times. Having real meals will leave you feeling satisfied. Make sure that you consume meals throughout the day, and don't set yourself up for periods of intense hunger. Have a complete breakfast and a full lunch, and don't consume all your calories in the evening. Your body works best on a steady supply of fuel throughout the day. As you can see from the nutrition guidelines outlined for pre-training eating, recovery nutrition, and nutrition strategies designed to optimize muscle building, eating small, frequent meals is ideal and effective.

Have some protein and fat with your meals and snacks. These foods will keep you feeling full longer and help prevent the hunger that leads to an unplanned trip to the vending machine. Choose lean proteins and small amounts of healthy fats. Look at your food journal to determine what times of day you get too hungry. Add a bit more protein or fat to the preceding meal or snack if hunger sets in quickly at specific times.

Tune in to hunger and fullness. Paying attention to your body's physiological signals is one of the best ways to gauge when to start eating and when to stop. Of course, you must plan your eating around your training and your schedule for work or school, but becoming aware of hunger and fullness can also provide valuable direction regarding your food intake and portions. You can also use the 20-minute rule: Stop eating before you are completely satisfied, then wait for 20 minutes to see whether you feel full. Usually, this amount of time allows your body to stop giving you hunger cues.

Enjoy the meal and have some treats. Food is not only fuel but also a source of enjoyment. This means sitting down and enjoying your meals whenever possible, eating slowly and savoring the food, and making sure that favorites are regularly included in your diet.

THE SPECTRUM OF DISORDERED EATING

When you train and compete, being able to move your body quickly over a given distance for a set amount of time offers a performance advantage. So having a lower level of body fat is considered to be a mechanical advantage. However, athletes can become overly focused on their weight and body-fat levels. Because athletes may be driven, goal oriented, perfectionistic, and highly competitive, some of the qualities that promote athletic success may manifest in unrealistic weight and body-fat goals. Placing undue emphasis on losing a few pounds is the result. Pressure to lose this weight may come from a number of outside sources, including trainers, coaches, athletic peers, and the media. Female athletes seem especially at risk of becoming dissatisfied with their bodies and distorting their body image, though males are also susceptible.

NUTRITION FOR PREGNANCY AND EXERCISE

Many pregnant female athletes desire to maintain a high degree of fitness during pregnancy and often return to training and competition as quickly as possible. It is no longer unusual for Olympic or professional athletes to have a child and resume training at a high level soon after the baby's birth. Although these athletes may be most concerned about consuming an adequate number of calories for a healthy and appropriate weight gain, the nutrients consumed while planning a pregnancy are also very important.

It is a good idea to see your physician before trying to conceive to discuss how to get the best nutrition during this time. He or she may recommend taking a prenatal multivitamin and mineral supplement in order to obtain folic acid and other important nutrients. Folate (found from food sources) and folic acid (from supplement sources) deserve serious attention from women athletes even contemplating pregnancy. An adequate intake of folate, both prior to conception and during the first several weeks of pregnancy, can help prevent birth defects such as spina bifida. Folate is used for the synthesis of DNA, the building block of all cells. During the first twenty-eight days of pregnancy, cells divide rapidly and form the neural tubes that become the baby's brain and spine. Many Americans fall short of the recommended 400 micrograms of folate.

Good food sources of folate include asparagus, lentils, spinach and other leafy green vegetables, dried beans such as kidney beans, and orange juice. Grain products such as bread, pasta, rice, and enriched flour have been fortified with folic acid for several years, and a decrease in these types of birth defects has been the result. Many health experts also recommend that any woman who may become pregnant take a multivitamin providing 400 micrograms of folate.

During the first three months of pregnancy, it is normal to have no weight gain or perhaps a small gain of up to 5 pounds. After the first trimester, a weight gain of up to 1 pound weekly is normal. Generally a total weight gain of 25 to 35 pounds is recommended. Underweight or lean women may be advised to gain more weight for a total of about 28 to 40 pounds. Adequate weight gain comes down to finding the right balance of calories to build your own tissue during pregnancy, to support the growth of the baby, and to meet your energy needs from exercise in order to prevent having a low-birthweight baby or a premature delivery. Starting in the second trimester, pregnancy requires only an additional 300 calories daily above your usual energy needs and another 10 to 12 grams of protein. These additional amounts are easily met with an increased food intake—for example, 8 ounces of milk and a small turkey sandwich.

CONTINUES

NUTRITION FOR PREGNANCY AND EXERCISE continued

The expectant mother's weight gain comes from growth in her own body tissues, the baby's body weight, and tissues that support the baby's growth. It includes an increased blood volume, body fluid, and breast tissue as well as the placenta, umbilical cord, and amniotic fluid. Body-fat stores increase in anticipation of lactation, which requires at least an additional 500 calories or more daily above normal nonpregnancy requirements. Your physician will monitor not only your total weight gain but also your pattern of weight gain to make sure that it is appropriate.

Fluid requirements also increase during pregnancy, and it is critical to maintain proper hydration during exercise and training. You need about 2.5 to 3 quarts of fluids daily plus whatever is needed to account for sweat losses during exercise. It is essential that you begin your training sessions well hydrated if you are pregnant. Overheating could have serious negative effects on the unborn baby. Plenty of fluids should be consumed several hours before exercise, and at least 4 to 8 additional ounces should be consumed every 15 to 20 minutes during exercise. Carbohydrates can be consumed several hours before exercise to prevent hypoglycemia. Sports drinks, carbohydrate gels, and energy bars can be consumed during exercise to maintain blood glucose levels, but make sure they do not contain extra vitamins, minerals, or herbal additives. Your training diet and your prenatal vitamin and mineral supplement should be more than adequate to meet your nutrient requirements; do not take more vitamins and minerals than your doctor recommends. Herbal products and teas have not been tested in pregnancy and should be avoided.

Do discuss your intake of iron and calcium with your doctor to make sure you are getting enough of these important minerals during your pregnancy. Iron requirements double during pregnancy owing to a pregnant woman's expanded blood volume. Most pregnant women receive adequate iron in their prenatal vitamin and mineral supplement, but some require an additional iron supplement in order to prevent anemia. Anemia can result in fatigue, shortness of breath, and increased delivery risks. The baby also runs the risk of developing anemia if iron stores run too low, and athletes may already have low iron stores. Your doctor should check your iron levels early in your pregnancy and again at regular intervals until the birth. Be sure to include plenty of high-iron foods in your diet (see Table 3.6).

Calcium plays an important role in every woman's health and deserves extra attention during pregnancy. Calcium requirements increase to 1,200 milligrams daily during pregnancy. As the baby builds bone, the mother's bones serve as a calcium source. If her diet is inadequate to

CONTINUES

supply the baby's needs and maintain this calcium reservoir, the risk of developing osteoporosis later in life increases. High-calcium food sources are listed in Table 3.5. You can also consider taking a separate calcium supplement during pregnancy to meet your elevated requirements. But do consult with your doctor first.

Certain nutrients and foods should be limited during pregnancy. Excess vitamin A intake from oversupplementation can increase the risk of birth defects. Intake from a supplement should not exceed 5,000 IU of vitamin A daily. There is also no room for alcohol in the diet, as it can produce severe negative effects for the baby such as fetal alcohol syndrome. Caffeine should be restricted to no more than 300 milligrams daily or avoided altogether. Avoid saccharin, and limit other artificial sweeteners as much as possible. Limit soft cheeses such as Brie, Camembert, blue cheese, and feta cheese because they can increase the risk of bacterial contamination. In general, pregnant women should be careful with food safety, never eat raw fish, and make sure that all meats are well cooked. Avoid any unpasteurized milk products and raw eggs.

Fish can also be contaminated with mercury, which can have adverse effects for the developing baby. Fatty fish such as swordfish, mackerel, shark, bluefish, tilefish, and striped bass should be avoided completely. Other high-mercury fish to avoid include marlin, red snapper, trout, fresh tuna, and white canned albacore tuna. Lobster can also be high in mercury and should be avoided. Limit your consumption of canned light tuna to less than 6 ounces weekly, and your total fish intake to 9 to 12 ounces weekly. Sole, tilapia, scallops, shrimp, canned salmon (wild Alaskan), and catfish are relatively low in mercury. Eat low-fat fish, and trim excess fat as much as possible.

After the birth, lactation and breast-feeding will increase your daily energy requirements 500 calories or more above your nonpregnancy requirements. Fat stores accumulated during pregnancy serve as an important energy source for lactation, but your diet should be rich in nutrients during the breast-feeding period. Your fluid needs will also be high during this time. Weight loss can occur gradually with lactation, but it is best to try not to lose more than 1 pound weekly, as an overly restrictive diet will decrease the quantity of milk that you produce. Maintain the high calcium and iron intakes that you established during your pregnancy, and ask your doctor about whether you should continue taking your prenatal multivitamin and mineral supplement. Limit alcohol and caffeine intake, as they can enter breast milk. It may be best to nurse before exercise due to transient changes that occur in breast milk with exercise. When women train at very high intensities or complete interval training, higher levels of lactic acid in the breast milk may result.

The estimated prevalence of eating disorders in athletes varies greatly depending on the screening technique employed, the athletes studied, and the definitions used. Estimates in female athletes range from a low of 1 percent to a high of 62 percent, and in male athletes from 0 to 57 percent. Despite this wide range, most experts agree that eating disorders pose a significant health risk to too many athletes, especially when eating disorders are defined broadly. Under the broad definition, disordered eating encompasses a full spectrum of eating behaviors, with misguided and unhealthy strategies for weight loss and occasional bingeing and purging at one end and full-blown anorexia nervosa, bulimia nervosa, and EDNOS (Eating Disorders Not Otherwise Specified) at the other end. There are many gray areas in disordered eating, and it can often be difficult to differentiate when a minor difficulty ends and a true eating disorder begins. Often behavior that begins as an attempt to lose weight takes on a life of its own and develops into an unhealthy group of behaviors that qualifies as disordered eating.

Although the incidence of full-blown eating disorders is not exceptionally high in most sports, studies indicate a high incidence of disordered eating behavior and distorted concerns regarding body weight, body fat, and body shape among athletes. Common disordered eating behaviors include skipping meals, constantly weighing oneself, eating very little fat, and fearing that specific foods may promote unwanted weight gain. Binge eating, as characterized by consuming large amounts of food while feeling out of control, can be part of disordered eating.

Another term, *anorexia athletica*, describes a syndrome characterized by disordered eating and compulsive exercising. It is associated with an intense fear of gaining weight, despite being at normal or below-normal weight, and is marked by food restriction, often to fewer than 1,200 calories per day, and excessive exercise. Bingeing, self-induced vomiting, and use of laxatives and diuretics may also occur. Some athletes are able to stop these behaviors when their participation in a sport stops. But for other athletes, the behavior continues to develop into a full-blown clinical eating disorder.

Eating disorders are complicated and multifactorial. Psychological and emotional issues such as anxiety and depression, an inability to cope with family and personal problems, life stresses, and the pressure to be thin or lean from both the athletic subculture and the society may be involved. Biochemical imbalances may also play a role. Triggers associated with eating disorders in athletes include traumatic life events such as relationship and family problems, recommendations to lose weight, prolonged periods of dieting, and a large discrepancy between actual weight and a self-defined ideal weight. It is possible that individuals at high risk for eating disorders will gravitate toward certain sports, but being involved in a sport may also trigger the eating disorder in a susceptible athlete. Risk factors that are more common among athletes than among the general population include prolonged periods of dieting or weight cycling; an increase in training

EATING DISORDERS

Anorexia Nervosa

- Resistance to maintaining body weight at or above a minimally normal weight
- Intense fear of gaining weight or becoming fat even though underweight
- Distortion in the way in which one's body weight or shape is experienced
- Denial of the seriousness of the current low body weight
- Infrequent or absent menstrual periods in females who have reached puberty

Physical Characteristics of Anorexia Nervosa

- Hair loss and growth of fine body hair
- Low pulse rate
- Sensitivity to cold
- Stress fractures, osteopenia, or osteoporosis
- Overuse injuries
- Abnormal fatigue
- Gastrointestinal problems

Bulimia Nervosa

- Recurrent episodes of binge eating characterized by a sense of lack of control and an excessive amount of food within a short period of time
- Purging behavior such as self-induced vomiting and misuse of laxatives, diuretics, enemas, or other medications
- Binge-eating and purging behavior that occurs on average at least twice weekly for 3 months
- Self-esteem inappropriately influenced by body shape and weight

Physical Characteristics of Bulimia Nervosa

- Frequent weight fluctuations
- Difficulty swallowing and throat damage
- Swollen glands
- Damaged tooth enamel from gastric acid
- Electrolyte imbalances and dehydration
- Menstrual irregularities
- Diarrhea or constipation

CONTINUES

EATING DISORDERS   continued

Eating Disorder Not Otherwise Specified (EDNOS)

This category includes disorders of eating that do not meet the criteria for a specific eating disorder.

- Episodes of binge eating without the use of compensatory behavior as seen in bulimia nervosa
- Repeatedly chewing and spitting out, but not swallowing, large amounts of food
- Anorexia nervosa–like symptoms in conjunction with regular menstrual periods
- Bulimia nervosa–like symptoms, but with the behavior occurring less frequently or for less than 3 months
- Regular purging behaviors after consuming only a small amount of food

Muscle Dysmorphia

This term describes a form of body-image disturbance described primarily in male bodybuilders and weightlifters.

- Preoccupation with not being sufficiently lean and muscular
- Preoccupation with muscularity that causes significant social impairment
- Excessive exercise, preoccupation with food, abuse of steroids, and/or abuse of dietary supplements aimed at increasing body size or decreasing body fat

CONTINUES

volume; stress related to sports and training, such as the loss of a coach; weight-loss pressures from coaches and trainers; and lack of guidance on appropriate weight and body-composition goals and healthy weight-management strategies.

Although eating disorders among men in the general population and male athletes specifically are not as prevalent as among females in both realms, they are still a concern. The figures currently available may underestimate the true prevalence of eating disorders in men. Males who develop disordered eating are more likely to previously have been overweight or even obese, and the fear of gaining weight may relate to this past experience. Male athletes may also diet in an attempt to improve performance or in response to an injury that limits training. Male athletes are in fact more susceptible to *muscle dysmorphia,* a body-image disorder characterized by an intense preoccupation with body size and degree of muscularity. Individuals with this disorder attempt to increase body size and may abuse performance-enhancing drugs or dietary supplements that

EATING DISORDERS   continued

Anorexia Athletica

This term has been used to describe a condition that is not a full-blown eating disorder.

- Disordered eating in conjunction with compulsive exercise
- Intense fear of weight gain despite weighing below the expected weight for age and height
- Weight loss achieved by food restriction and extensive compulsive exercise
- Self-induced vomiting and use of laxatives and diuretics

Binge Eating Disorder

This disorder is currently a subset of EDNOS but is expected to be classified as a separate diagnostic entity.

- Recurrent episodes of binge eating during a discrete period of time and characterized by a large amount of food and a sense of lack of control
- Binge episodes that are characterized by eating more rapidly than normal; eating until uncomfortably full; eating large amounts when not physically hungry; eating alone because of embarrassment of the volume of food; feeling disgusted, depressed, or guilty after eating; experiencing marked distress regarding the binge eating
- Bingeing at least twice weekly for 6 months

promise to increase muscle mass or decrease body fat. This disorder is more common in weight-lifting and bodybuilding than in other sports but can affect athletes in any sport.

There are several common warning signs for eating disorders. Someone suffering from a disorder may repeatedly express concerns about body weight, refuse to maintain even a minimal weight, enforce periods of severe calorie restriction, and/or engage in excessive physical activity that is not part of a balanced training program. Other warning signs are carrying out food rituals, engaging in self-induced vomiting, and abusing laxatives and diet pills. Some of these behaviors by themselves do not prove the presence of a full-blown eating disorder, but these signs do justify further attention to the possible presence of a problem. The sidebar "Eating Disorders" describes some of the characteristics of full-blown eating disorders.

Disordered eating and true eating disorders can lead to poor performance related to glycogen and electrolyte depletion, dehydration, and loss of lean body mass. Nutrient deficiencies can result, as can increased risk of infection, illness, and injuries. Other health-related effects are decreased metabolism, gastrointestinal complications, menstrual dysfunction in females, and decreased bone mineral density. To avoid these harmful effects, an athlete with an eating disorder requires the help of a team of skilled professionals trained in treating the condition, including a physician, dietitian, and psychologist or therapist.

7

ERGOGENIC
AIDS

Separating Fact from Fiction

THE TERM ERGOGENIC LITERALLY MEANS "work producing," etymologically speaking, but in modern parlance it refers to the numerous supplements and other substances said to enhance athletic performance. Nutritional ergogenic aids can be nutrients, metabolic by-products of nutrients, or other substances commonly found in foods. When put into supplement form they exist in concentrated amounts. Advertisers for these products claim they can provide performance benefits by increasing muscle size and strength, promoting fat burning, or improving speed. Several ergogenic aids, such as carnitine, for example, are touted as aids to "enhance fat burning," and creatine is reputed to enhance muscle building when taken during a strength training program.

Apparently many consumers have believed the promises behind the ads, as sales of these products have become a serious and lucrative business. When creatine first appeared on the market, sales skyrocketed to $30 million in 1995, $180 million in 1998, and $220 million in 2005. With all sports nutrition product sales, including sports nutrition supplements such as creatine, nutrition bars, and sports and energy drinks, reaching more than $11 billion in 2005 and projected to reach $14 billion in 2007, according to the *Nutrition Business Journal,* athletes have clearly embraced a wide selection of substances as an important component of their training programs.

Chapters 4 and 5 outlined practical uses for sports nutrition products such as sports drinks, gels, bars, and high-carbohydrate and meal-replacement supplements that are backed by both research and the practical experience of athletes. Using these products knowledgeably and appropriately carries minimal risk and provides some clear performance benefits that support your training and competition goals. However, some sports drinks and recovery drinks may also contain ingredients that are not necessary or even proven to be safe for athletes to consume, especially young and developing athletes.

The marketing surrounding ergogenic aids is effective, but it is important for you to verify that any product you ingest in the quest for top performance is legal, effective, and safe. Unfortunately, many of these products are backed solely by strong and enticing claims, anecdotal hearsay, high-profile athlete and coach testimonials, and referenced "research" that has not been published in full in a reputable scientific journal. In reality, many of these supplements have not been thoroughly and appropriately tested. Moreover, many of the supplements that have been tested independently of the manufacturers who supply them don't live up to their performance claims. Despite this lack of evidence that ergogenic aids can do what their manufacturers claim they can, or even that they are safe to take, it can be tempting to top off all your hard work with an easily ingested supplement that promises a quick and effective performance boost.

With new products coming out monthly, athletes need to be discerning when evaluating nutritional ergogenic aids or performance enhancers. It is important that you learn to make knowledgeable choices about these products. Keep these tips in mind before you use them:

- Understand how the ergogenic aid purportedly functions.
- Know both sides of the story of current research supporting or opposing the supplement.
- Be aware of any safety concerns surrounding the product.
- Know whether the product is a legal supplement for athletes to take.

Chances are you may try a supplement because it is widely talked about among other athletes you train with or compete against, or because it is surrounded by enticing marketing claims for building muscle, burning fat, or increasing energy output. But these supplements are never going to be an effective substitute for a solid training program and an optimal performance diet.

Another important consideration when evaluating the safety of these supplements is the age of an athlete. The American Academy of Pediatrics does not recommend high-performance supplements in the diet of child athletes. These supplements are also routinely tested on adults (if at all) and not on young and growing bodies or athletes of high-school age. Studies of collegiate athletes are limited, as are long-term safety data. What safety information is available does not usually address safety issues in high-school athletes. Some supplements are also banned by the National Collegiate Athletic Association (NCAA).

REGULATION OF ERGOGENIC AIDS

Athletes are bombarded with claims of the magical effects of nutritional ergogenic aids on performance. Advertising and claims surrounding these products have increased exponentially since the Dietary Supplement Health and Education Act (DSHEA) was passed in 1994. DSHEA significantly changed how all dietary supplements, such as vitamins, minerals, herbs, amino acids, metabolites, and even hormones, are tested, marketed, labeled, and manufactured.

Unlike regulation of makers of a drug or food additive, supplement manufacturers are not required to prove that a dietary supplement works. Under DSHEA, manufacturers are merely responsible for making sure that their products are safe. The government does not review these products before they are put on the market, but the Food and Drug Administration (FDA) can take action against any unsafe dietary supplement products. The FDA cannot evaluate the thousands of products on the market, and it makes selective use of its time and resources. It usually responds only to products that have caused significant adverse health effects on a large scale.

The labels on these products often include a somewhat loosely defined "nutrition support claim." These claims may relate to the "structure and function" of the body and "general well-being." Although a certain set of conditions must be met to make these claims, they do not require prior FDA approval. Manufacturers must be able to substantiate that the claim is "truthful and not misleading," but they cannot promise to prevent or cure a disease. Some nutrition support claims may include, for example, "maintains a healthy circulatory system," or "helps maintain a healthy intestinal flora." Note that supplements providing these types of claims must also state, "This product is not intended to diagnose, treat, cure, or prevent any disease."

The FDA assumes that the discerning consumer realizes that it is up to each company to decide how to prepare and package their supplements and that these manufacturing practices may affect the products' purity, safety, potency, and overall quality. According to the FDA, consumers can contact the manufacturer and request product safety information and research support, which would preferably not be only in-house data. They can also question whether the firm has a quality-control system in place and whether any adverse event reports have resulted from use of a particular product.

In 2003, the FDA began developing Good Manufacturing Processes (GMPs) in coordination with the supplement industry. Two Web sites, www.nsf.org and www.consumerlab.com, currently list products that have been evaluated for appropriate quality control. Both of these sites also test products for banned substances and can certify that products do not contain substances banned for athletes. Some supplement companies have their own GMPs in place and may be regulated under the National Nutritional Foods Association (see www.nnfa.org).

Consumers should also review the "Supplement Facts" labels on the packages of dietary supplements. Unlike serving sizes for conventional foods, the dosage on labels is not standardized. So remember that the amounts that are recommended may be higher than needed or safe. The label will provide the following information:

- Statement of identity
- Net quantity of ingredients
- A structure and function claim statement
- Directions for use
- Supplement facts
- Other ingredients, listed in descending order of predominance by common name or proprietary blend
- Name and address of packer, manufacturer, or distributor

Unfortunately, even if companies are accused and fined regarding false claims on dietary supplements, they may not be deterred from promoting new products. Often fines may be rendered insignificant by a large volume of sales generated while claims are investigated.

EVALUATING EROGENIC AIDS: SAFETY, EFFECTIVENESS, AND LEGAL ISSUES

When deciding whether to take an ergogenic aid, it is essential to understand how to evaluate a product's safety and effectiveness objectively and to take the trouble to make sure it is even legal in sports training and competition. The first question should be, Is this product effective? Does solid research back up the company's claims? After all, if a so-called aid is not effective, why bother taking it in the first place? Valid scientific testing of a nutritional ergogenic aid costs time, money, and resources. Tests of a supplement's effect on athletic performance should be conducted with well-trained athletes and can be specific to the type of sport, such as cycling or running. For these and other reasons, much of the supplement industry forgoes testing and relies heavily on testimonials, anecdotes, and untested scientific theories rather than valid research to promote their products. But a theory is not proof. A theory is a hypothesis or intriguing idea that requires testing. What the manufacturer calls a "scientific breakthrough" may be a new and interesting idea with little or no basis in fact.

Conducting a scientific trial remains the best way to examine the effectiveness of ergogenic aids on performance. Here, athletes' experiences can be helpful to researchers who desire to focus on potentially effective substances. Scientists can use reports of these experiences to determine what products are worth testing and what dosages are appropriate for test protocols. Testing should mimic real athletic performance conditions as much as possible. Researchers should also control for age, level of training, and nutritional status. Various dosages, supplementation periods, types of exercise, and performance testing may need to be incorporated.

Studies should control for the placebo effect as much as possible by incorporating a double-blind design. In this approach, different groups of subjects receive the substance being tested or a placebo. To minimize bias, the test subjects, and the researchers in direct contact with the subjects, do not know which product is being administered when and to whom. In addition to a placebo trial, there may be a control group who receives no treatment. These are only some of the features needed in a well-designed testing strategy. But even with a well-designed study, a large change in performance is required for the outcome to be considered statistically significant. In many cases, the changes produced by nutritional supplementation are small. Although a 1 to 3 percent change may not be statistically significant from the scientist's perspective, it may be useful in elite competition. In addition, researchers report only the overall performance effect within a group. The positive results of individuals within the group may be diluted by the negative or neutral responses of other subjects. Not all subjects respond in the same way to a particular substance.

Companies may state that they are in the process of conducting research, or that their research is "in-house" or has simply never been published in reputable peer-reviewed journals. The value of this research is difficult to assess. Unfortunately, even well-designed studies can be quoted out of context. Research findings are extrapolated to produce inappropriate conclusions. And good preliminary studies require verification through additional sound research. Studies published in reputable journals can provoke criticism when placed under close scrutiny. Furthermore, consumers may be impressed by an ergogenic aid because the company has patented its product. Yet patents are not granted based on the effectiveness of the product, but rather on its distinguishable differences. Patents can be obtained with a theoretical model rather than objective double-blind research.

False claims aside, the next question to consider in determining whether you should use an ergogenic aid is, Is this product safe? As previously mentioned, supplement manufacturers are not required to prove a product's safety. Negative effects from a product may be acute, mild, or temporary, but they can also be serious and chronic. Some dietary supplements may be toxic or decrease the absorption of other nutrients, especially in high doses. Surprisingly, independent testing has found that many supplements do not even contain the ingredients marked on the label. Often products are watered down or contain other unlisted ingredients that may be harmful or illegal. It is hoped that this concern will be resolved when all companies comply with adopted GMPs.

Finally, as a competitive athlete, particularly if you may be drug-tested both in and out of competition, you do not want to inadvertently take a dietary supplement that contains a banned substance. Therefore, the third question to ask is, Is this product legal for my sport? The past decade has seen a significant increase in the number of positive test results for illegal substances at the elite and professional levels that are claimed to be the result of contaminated or mislabeled dietary supplements. All athletic governing bodies have some regulation regarding the use of ergogenic aids. (Products banned by the NCAA, for example, are listed at www.ncaa.org.) Even if you avoid illegal products such as ephedra or androstenodione, checking labels does not guarantee 100 percent that you will avoid banned products. Cross-contamination can occur in the manufacturing process, and the purity of these supplements is often questioned. The World Anti-Doping Agency provides a complete list of banned substances at www.wada-ama.org/en/.

COMMON ERGOGENIC AIDS

Specific nutritional ergogenic aids can benefit athletes under certain conditions. However, the supplement industry is an extremely profitable business that relies on unsupported theories and testimonials to market products. Ergogenic aid theories may even be extrapolated from clinical research on disease states or nutrient deficiencies. To say that this product will then produce a performance improvement is not a scientific breakthrough but a leap of faith. Even with proven ergogenic aids, it is important to keep their role in perspective. Although they may produce small performance improvements, ergogenic aids are no substitute for proper training, nutrition, and psychological preparation.

This section will review some popular nutritional ergogenic aids for scientific validity as determined by quality research. It will also look at some of the safety concerns and practical issues regarding the use of these supplements. Not surprisingly, sports physiologists and sports nutritionists do not overwhelmingly support the majority of these supplements. They would prefer that athletes train and eat properly, two strategies that very effectively improve performance! Many professionals are especially concerned about young athletes taking supplements that have not been proven safe for them, as supplement testing is usually done on adults.

Ergogenic aids marketed to endurance athletes are often designed to increase muscle mass and strength and decrease body fat. Some are also reported to improve performance by increasing power output during exercise. Table 7.1 summarizes several ergogenic aids that are discussed in more detail here.

TABLE **7.1**	SUMMARY OF ERGOGENIC AIDS		
SUPPLEMENT	**CLAIMS**	**SCIENTIFIC DATA**	**SAFETY**
Creatine	Supports training for increased muscle mass	Well supported by scientific data	Can be used safely by adults when following scientific protocols
HMB	Builds muscle strength; inhibits breakdown of muscle and protein	Limited human data supporting claims; several studies found no benefits	Doses at 3 g taken for 6–8 weeks appear safe
Protein supplements	Facilitate muscle building	When consumed before and after resistance training in the proper dose and with the proper timing, can facilitate building of muscle tissue	Can consume 10–15 g high-quality protein in conjunction with carbohydrates before and after weight training Can consume protein from real foods; supplements not required Exceeding recommended dose provides no additional benefits
Amino acids	Facilitate muscle building and exercise recovery	Not supported by well-designed research	Can upset balance of amino acid metabolism when taken in large doses
Ribose	Improves muscle recovery, energy, and endurance; rebuilds ATP	Published research is limited; current data far from conclusive	Not enough safety data
Glutamine	Supports the immune system; promotes protein synthesis	May benefit athletes with a true glutamine deficiency; more data required	Often incorporated in sports nutrition supplements; too much could upset amino acid balance
Carnitine	Metabolic fat burner	Not supported by well-designed research	L-carnitine form only may be consumed in doses of 1–2 g daily for 6 months
Chromium	Builds muscle and burns fat	Not supported by well-designed research	Do not exceed 200 mcg daily
Pyruvate	Improves endurance; promotes muscle building and fat loss	Not tested on athletes; not supported by research	Not much safety data
Prohormones	Promotes muscle building	Increases muscle mass and strength	Banned by the USADA and IOC; long-term safety concerns and possible adverse health effects

CONTINUES

TABLE **7.1**	**SUMMARY OF ERGOGENIC AIDS** continued

SUPPLEMENT	CLAIMS	SCIENTIFIC DATA	SAFETY
Weight-loss supplements	Promote body-fat loss and weight loss	Many ingredients not supported by well-designed research; risks may outweigh benefits	Risks of supplements may be serious; some ingredients may be banned
Caffeine	Promotes endurance; may improve power output for shorter distances	Good data support claims for endurance exercise; limited data on power sports indicate need for more research	Can be used safely in moderate doses; high doses are not required for ergogenic effect
MCT oil	Provides fuel during training and spares muscle glycogen; enhances fat burning	Tested mainly for endurance exercise; not supported by well-designed research	May cause mild gastrointestinal symptoms

ERGOGENIC AIDS THAT AFFECT BODY COMPOSITION

Creatine

With sales in the United States at $400 million in 2001, creatine is clearly a supplement that shifted into high gear just out of the starting block. Fortunately, it is one of the best-researched ergogenic aids on the market, making it possible for sports nutritionists to provide clear and confident recommendations regarding this sports nutrition supplement.

Creatine is often advertised as a steroid alternative, but its use is really more comparable to glycogen loading. Just as carbohydrate ingestion maximizes the glycogen content of the muscle, "creatine loading" can increase muscle creatine stores. Your normal intake of creatine is about 2 grams daily (perhaps less for vegetarians), and it is also synthesized in the liver and kidneys. Creatine is an essential fuel of the adenosine triphosphate–creatine phosphate (ATP-CP) system. Loading the muscle with creatine is designed to increase ATP resynthesis. This power system typically stores enough fuel to last 6 to 8 seconds. Creatine can also buffer lactic acid and transport ATP to be utilized for muscle contraction.

Muscle biopsies have confirmed that rapid loading can be achieved with 25 to 30 grams of creatine daily, taken in five or six 5-gram doses per day for 5 or 6 days. A more gentle loading protocol is 3 grams daily over 28 days. Unlike carbohydrates, creatine appears to remain trapped in the muscle for 4 to 5 weeks after a loading phase without ongoing supplementation. About 30 percent of individuals who creatine load appear to be "nonresponders"—that is, they do not adequately load creatine into the muscle. To counter this problem, experts recommend consuming creatine with carbohydrates. Ingesting 75 to 100 grams of carbohydrates along with the creatine has been demonstrated to enhance creatine accumulation in the muscle. In addition, a 2- to 5-pound (1–2 kg) weight gain is associated with creatine loading. Scientists believe this to be water gain, however, as urine output decreases during the loading phase.

Though not documented in the scientific literature, anecdotal reports abound that creatine loading is associated with muscle cramping and GI upset. If you decide to load with creatine, make sure that you consume plenty of water to help prevent any side effects. Taking more than 30 grams of creatine daily over a 5-day period offers no additional benefits for loading. As is often the case with nutritional supplements, more is not better. In fact, there are some concerns that taking creatine in high doses or taking it over a long period of time can lead to liver and kidney damage. People with kidney disease should not take creatine.

We know that creatine ingestion can load the muscle, but how does it affect performance? Creatine loading appears to increase the rate of creatine resynthesis during recovery (20 seconds–5 minutes) from bouts of high-intensity exercise (6–30 seconds). Creatine loading delays fatigue during activity that includes repeated, all-out surges of energy interspersed with rest periods.

Creatine could potentially assist team sport players such as hockey players or soccer players, but it is unlikely to provide any performance benefit for most endurance training sessions and competitions. Of course, many endurance athletes incorporate resistance training into their programs, and creatine loading does appear to allow more repetitions to be performed and consequently to increase one's strength.

After completion of one loading phase of creatine, you can maintain these higher creatine levels with a low daily dose of 3 grams for at least 60 days. Creatine loading may actually only be necessary once or twice yearly due to the cyclical nature of your training and the muscles' ability to hold creatine for several weeks.

Creatine is currently legal. However, there have been concerns about cross-contamination of creatine products in recent years, as athletes ingesting this supplement have tested positive for banned prohormone products. No creatine studies have been done with high-school athletes or athletes who are still growing and developing. Many high schools and colleges likely have their own policy regarding creatine supplementation in their athletes. The NCAA does not allow use of creatine (see the sidebar "The NCAA and Nutritional Supplements").

Beta-Hydroxy-Beta-Methylbutarate (HMB)

Beta-hydroxy-beta-methylbutarate, or HMB, is primarily marketed to strength and power athletes and is one of the fastest-selling supplements on the market. Endurance athletes who weight-train and want to facilitate muscle recovery may be interested in this supplement because it is promoted to decrease protein breakdown, and in doing so to enhance muscle size and development, decrease exercise-induced muscle damage, and promote fat loss. HMB is not actually a nutrient but a metabolic by-product made naturally by the human body in small amounts when the amino acid leucine is metabolized. You produce only about 0.2 to 0.4 gram of HMB daily. The form used in supplements was first developed by scientists and then patented in the early 1990s by the company that produces HMB, which has sponsored much of the research on its effects.

The initial HMB research was conducted mainly with animals, but its effects on humans have also been studied. Some researchers found greater muscle mass gains and fewer markers of muscle damage in subjects taking the supplement; however, these studies have not always controlled for diet and training load, both of which can have a significant impact on muscle gain in conjunction with weight training. Several studies found no ergogenic benefit from HMB supplementation in regard to muscle mass and both anaerobic and aerobic exercise performance.

In one study of HMB use among collegiate football players, for example, no improvements in muscle strength and body composition were seen with HMB supplementation. Another study, which looked at the effects of HMB in elite male rugby players, found that both aerobic and anaerobic capacity were unaffected by supplementation with either HMB by itself or HMB in combination with creatine. Although a study on HMB use in runners did find that the supplement helped to prevent exercise-induced muscle damage, other studies have not produced similar findings. A recent review of existing studies on HMB supplementation suggested that this supplement may provide a small improvement in muscle size and strength when combined with resistance training. Further research is needed, however, particularly on trained athletes.

Further published data on this supplement are needed. A daily dose of 3 grams divided into three 1-gram doses appears to be safe when taken for a 6- to 8-week period. Higher doses have not resulted in greater effectiveness.

Amino Acids

The marketing of amino acid supplements is heavily targeted to athletes who benefit from building muscle mass. Supporters of amino acid supplementation claim that the protein used in these products is more readily digested and absorbed than the protein found in foods. This statement simply is false. Your body is well equipped to handle protein from whole foods by secreting a number of enzymes that help you to absorb amino acids. This absorption process occurs at a high level of effectiveness.

As explained in Chapter 6, timing your consumption of a high-quality protein source before and after weight training can facilitate muscle building and recovery. However, full muscle recovery entails following specific nutritional guidelines to obtain enough calories and protein in your daily training diet. Protein metabolism is very complex. It is affected by a variety of factors, including amino acid concentration in the blood, competition with other available amino acids, and the presence of other nutrients. Amino acid mixtures could potentially lead to nutritional imbalances, as an excess of one amino acid may negatively affect the absorption of another. Amino acid supplement dosing may also be misleading. A bottle listing up to 500 milligrams in a capsule actually contains less than 1 gram of amino acids, whereas only 1 ounce of chicken contains 7,000 milligrams, or 7 grams, of amino acids in the form of whole protein. Clearly, amino acid supplements cannot meet the dosing found in a compact source of natural protein. Purchasing expensive amino acid supplements simply is not necessary and could actually be harmful.

The amino acids arginine, lysine, and ornithine are often sold individually or in combination as "legal anabolic compounds" and "recovery agents." The advertisements claim that these products can promote the release of growth hormone and thus increase lean body mass and decrease body fat. These claims surfaced after two studies found that infusing these amino acids directly into the bloodstream stimulated the release of human growth hormone, which is involved in building muscle tissue. The effects of oral supplementation of amino acids on human growth hormone are very questionable, however. Several well-controlled studies have verified that oral supplementation does not have the same effect as intravenous infusion. Other studies have been criticized for their design. One study that provided a large oral dose of arginine and ornithine found a slight increase in growth hormone release. However, this increase was most likely stimulated by the resistance training itself rather than the amino acid intake. High oral dosages of these supplements are also associated with gastrointestinal problems.

Arginine, lysine, and ornithine are available individually or in mixtures in powder or tablet form. Several research studies have used 2- to 3-gram dosages; a dosage of 6 grams may cause gastrointestinal distress. High doses of certain amino acids may also inhibit absorption of other amino acids. Moreover, the dosages used in several studies can easily be obtained by consuming high-protein foods. The use of any amino acid supplement, either alone or in combination with others, is unlikely to be beneficial and is not recommended.

Ribose

Ribose is hyped as a supplement that can improve muscle recovery, boost energy, enhance endurance, support cardiovascular fitness, and rebuild ATP. A sugar formed from the conversion of glucose, it is considered the starting substance for ATP production and is part of the metabolic pathway that results in ATP resynthesis.

However, published research on the effect of ribose in athletic performance is relatively limited. Ribose did benefit one group of men who suffered from cardiac ischemia, but study results on these subjects are not applicable to athletes. Three other published studies measured its effects on repeated high-intensity exercise in trained male athletes. Ribose supplementation did not affect power output. Another study that combined the ribose supplements with creatine and glutamine found no improvement in muscular strength and endurance or in body composition. Many studies looking at the ergogenic effects of ribose have been presented at conferences, but not published in full for further evaluation.

Ribose is for sale, so its safety must be considered. Ribose has not been used for long periods of time, though doses of up to 20 grams appear to be tolerated. Higher doses may result in gastrointestinal side effects. Manufacturer labels often recommend taking 3 grams prior to and 3 grams after exercise. The patent holder recommends that ribose be consumed with carbohydrates on an empty stomach. Current data are far too limited to safely recommend a cycling or maintenance dose. In fact, much more data and solid proof are required before this supplement can be recommended.

Glutamine

Glutamine is an amino acid synthesized in the muscle tissue. It is the most abundant amino acid in the body and is used as a fuel source by the cells of the immune system. Impaired glutamine status has been associated with the overtrained state in athletes, and overtrained athletes are thought to be more susceptible to upper respiratory tract infections as well as other kinds of infections. Blood glutamine levels fall during endurance exercise and remain lowered during the recovery phase for several hours after exercise. Glutamine depletion is thought to become cumulative if recovery between sessions is inadequate, and overtrained athletes do sometimes have low blood glutamine levels. However, adequate daily carbohydrate consumption may be the most effective means of preventing glutamine depletion.

The theory behind glutamine supplementation is that it could help prevent the immune system problems suffered by overtrained athletes. Research data do not consistently support this theory. What is more likely is that glutamine supplementation benefits those athletes with a true deficiency and that it is not a general cure for immune system problems.

Another theory regarding glutamine supplementation is that it promotes protein synthesis and helps maintain a positive protein balance in the muscle by preventing protein breakdown during periods of heavy training. Glutamine may also stimulate the synthesis of muscle glycogen. Obviously, glutamine performs some very important functions in the body. However, more research on glutamine supplementation in athletes is needed.

A dose of less than 0.1 gram of glutamine per pound (0.3 g/kg) of body weight is safely absorbed and does not appear to cause any harm when taken for several weeks. Higher doses for up to 5 days also seem safe.

Chromium

Chromium is a trace mineral that is often marketed as a legal alternative to anabolic steroids and human growth hormone. Scientists have long known that chromium enhances the effects of insulin, which regulates glucose metabolism. Adults with impaired glucose regulation have been measured to have positive responses with chromium supplementation. Insulin also promotes the uptake of amino acids into muscle cells and regulates protein metabolism. Because of this protein-building function, some have theorized that chromium intake should lead to an increase in muscle mass.

Proponents of chromium supplementation for athletes maintain that many are chromium-deficient and that a supplement would improve their protein synthesis. Other proponents believe that high chromium doses could stimulate muscle building. It has not been firmly established that athletes are in fact chromium-deficient; however, the North American diet is high in refined grains, which may trigger a higher release of insulin and require more chromium in the diet than is normally consumed.

Studies on chromium supplementation have produced mixed, but mostly negative, results. The more recent and better-designed studies monitored and controlled for exercise training and carefully measured body composition. These studies found no significant gains in muscle mass with chromium supplementation. Earlier studies, which showed some positive results, were not as carefully controlled. Several studies have shown that even higher doses do not lead to significant gains in muscle mass.

Nevertheless, manufacturers recommend large doses, and sales of chromium are high. More information is needed about the safety of chromium supplementation, especially at these dosages. There is little long-term data on chromium doses beyond 200 micrograms. Because chromium is a mineral, large chronic doses are unwise. Minerals often compete with one another for absorption, and one study found that iron status was compromised with chromium supplementation.

Clearly, adequate chromium intake from whole foods is important. Especially good sources are whole-grain breads and cereals, mushrooms, asparagus, apples, raisins, cocoa, peanuts, peanut butter, and prunes. Various sports nutrition supplements such as recovery drinks and bars often include chromium as well, as do many regular multivitamin and mineral supplements. Try not to exceed 200 micrograms daily from supplemental sources. Most diets likely do not exceed 50 micrograms of chromium daily.

Overall, chromium's ability to build muscle mass in athletes appears highly doubtful. Supplementation in safe doses is only appropriate to correct a deficiency and compensate for an inadequate diet.

Prohormones

Prohormones are widely sold in dietary supplements and are currently banned by the World Anti-Doping Agency (WADA), an international, independent organization created in 1999. WADA developed and implements the World Anti-Doping Code, which harmonizes anti-doping policies in all sports and countries (www.wada-ama.org). The U.S. Anti-Doping Agency (USADA) was created in 2000 and is the independent anti-doping agency for Olympic-related sports in the United States (www.usantidoping.org). Like WADA, USADA bans prohormones. These products include the "andro" and the "nor" prohormones. Andro products, namely androstenedione, are testosterone precursors that transform to this hormone in the body. Other androgenic products include androstenediol and dehydroepiandrosterone (DHEA). Nor products are precursors to the steroid nortestosterone (nandrolone), which is similar in structure to testosterone. Available nor prohormones are 19-norandrostenediol and 19-norandrostenedione. These nor products break down to the same metabolites used to detect nandrolone usage. Andro prohormones may lead to an elevated testosterone-to-epitestosterone ratio. All of these substances carry the risk of a positive drug test and potential negative side effects.

Prohormones are easily purchased in the United States and over the Internet because they are classified as dietary supplements. Often these supplements are geared toward building muscle, enhancing recovery, and "maintaining hormone levels." Since the late 1990s, a rash of elite athletes have tested positive for the steroid nandrolone. Many of these athletes have claimed that it occurred through the inadvertent ingestion of the dietary supplements that contained nor hormones. Although athletes can read labels carefully to avoid these banned products, it is becoming clear that this may not be enough. A study conducted at the Olympic Laboratory at the University of California at Los Angeles checked urine tests after supplementation with androstenedione and 19-norandrostenedione. As expected, the 19-nor produced nandrolone metabolites exceeding IOC limits. But the results of the andro supplementation were especially of concern. This test actually produced nandrolone metabolites in the urine! Twenty of twenty-four positive urine samples exceeded doping limits. Based on these findings, researchers tested several andro supplements. Seven of eight tested capsules contained varying amounts of 19-nor. Researchers speculated that the supplements had been contaminated with 19-nor in the manufacturing process. Many supplement companies use the same equipment to blend, encapsulate, and bottle both prohormone and nonprohormone products.

Some of these prohormones may carry unwanted side effects as well. One study that supplemented with andro did not find higher testosterone levels or increased muscle strength but a rise in blood estrogen and a reduction in the good HDL cholesterol in male subjects. These side effects could result in potentially serious health effects. A second study tested andro combined with an herbal product designed to decrease estrogen production. The estrogenic profile was not reduced from the herbal supplements despite claims to the contrary from the manufacturer.

Of course, no athlete engaging in competition should take prohormones, because they are illegal. Read labels carefully to ensure that they are not contained in any of the products you purchase, and be aware that cross-contamination is a real concern. Banned substances may turn up in supplements even if they are not listed as ingredients.

Weight-Loss Supplements

Weight-loss supplements are typically marketed via strong claims purporting that they can speed up metabolism, burn fat, and decrease appetite. Although the ingredients found in some weight-loss supplements are legal (and ineffective), other weight-loss supplements contain banned substances and may be dangerous to use.

Until 2004, the most widely purchased weight-loss supplement was ephedra. Because it had a high incidence of reported side effects, the FDA banned it, and it is not currently available in the United States. Ephedra, also called ephedrine or Ma Huang, stimulates the central nervous system and improves appetite control. However, because it is a stimulant, reported side effects included nervousness, headache, heart palpitations, dizziness, insomnia, and anxiety. Ephedra was banned in sports before it was banned by the FDA and its use is easily detected in drug tests.

Another weight-loss supplement on the WADA monitoring list, which has products not on the prohibited list for patterns of misuse, is phenylpropanolamine (PPA), also known as norephedrine. This product claims to suppress appetite and stimulate metabolism. However, it can also increase the risk of a bleeding stroke, and its safety risks far outweigh its effectiveness. The FDA warned consumers to stop use of a product containing PPA, caffeine, an herb called yohimbine, and diiodothyronine, a form of thyroid hormone. The FDA received multiple reports of liver injury or liver failure with use of the product over a 2-week to 3-month period.

Many weight-loss supplements are currently marketed as being "ephedra-free." However, these supplements may also contain banned products that are sources of synephrine or pseudoephedrine, including citrus aurantium, or bitter orange. Synephrine is banned by the NCAA and is on the WADA monitoring list, and pseudoephedrine is banned by WADA. Many other ingredients in weight-loss supplements lack solid research backing. Other weight-loss supplement ingredients to avoid are caffeine, cola nut, ginseng, and willow bark. Many of these supplements contain high amounts of caffeine, and they are often strong stimulants. Like ephedra, they can produce potentially dangerous side effects.

ERGOGENIC AIDS THAT AFFECT EXERCISE PERFORMANCE

Carnitine

Often promoted as a "metabolic fat burner," carnitine is a nonessential nutrient formed in the liver from two amino acids. Your skeletal muscles contain at least 90 percent of the carnitine in your body. Carnitine is of interest to athletes because it carries fat into the cells to be burned for energy during exercise. If carnitine supplementation did increase fat burning and decrease your body's reliance on glycogen and blood glucose, it could enhance performance. Carnitine is found in large quantities in meat and dairy products, however, so a carnitine deficiency is unlikely.

Carnitine is unlikely to be an effective ergogenic aid, as carnitine supplementation does not appear to increase muscle carnitine levels (as measured by muscle biopsies). Glycogen sparing with carnitine supplementation was also not found in the studies conducted on its use. Only one study found a slight increase in muscle carnitine content after supplementation with 2 grams daily. Other studies found no improvements in exercise performance with carnitine supplementation. Two studies that did find a positive performance effect have been criticized for their methodology and design.

Carnitine supplementation appears to be safe if you consume the L-carnitine form of the nutrient only. DL-carnitine can be toxic, as it depletes L-carnitine and may lead to a deficiency. Two to 4 grams daily can be consumed for 1 month, though 1- to 2-gram doses have been taken for 6 months.

Pyruvate

Pyruvate is commonly sold as DHAP, which is a combination of pyruvate and dihydroxyacetone. Manufacturers claim that it can improve endurance exercise, promote fat loss, and increase muscle mass.

Studies that have tested pyruvate on endurance performance need to be put in perspective. These studies, using a small number of untrained subjects exercising at moderate intensity, may not have much relevance to endurance athletes. In addition, several of the study protocols used 25 grams of pyruvate combined with 75 grams of dihydroxyacetone. Many commercial preparations contain much smaller doses. However, these studies did measure an increase in endurance with the supplement.

Pyruvate does not appear to have much validity as a fat burner. One often-quoted study restricted participants to a 1,000-calorie diet daily and no activity—a result not applicable to an athlete participating in endurance sports.

Several more recent studies have evaluated aerobic exercise performance, mainly in cycling, with pyruvate supplementation. No positive effects were found.

Caffeine

One of the oldest known drugs, caffeine belongs to a group of compounds called *methyl-xanthines*. Caffeine is found naturally in coffee beans, tea leaves, cocoa beans, and cola nuts, and caffeine-containing foods are a normal part of the North American diet, from coffee, tea, and chocolate to soft drinks. Many of these products provide 30 to 100 milligrams per serving.

But does it enhance performance for endurance athletes? Although it appears that caffeine does provide some muscle glycogen–sparing effects, this appears to be limited to the first 15 to 20 minutes of exercise. Researchers are not certain exactly how caffeine produces this effect. The classic explanation is that caffeine elevates free fatty acids in the blood, which exercising muscles use for energy while conserving muscle glycogen. Caffeine may also impact the enzyme that breaks down glycogen. Besides sparing glycogen, caffeine stimulates the central nervous system (increasing alertness), stimulates blood circulation and heart function, and releases epinephrine, all of which could enhance a variety of performance-related functions. Caffeine also stimulates calcium release from the muscle, which stimulates muscular contraction, and could have other direct performance effects on the muscle.

Starting January 1, 2004, caffeine was removed from the WADA prohibited-drug list and was placed on the monitoring list. Previously caffeine intake was not to exceed a threshold dose checked with a urine test. Many recent, well-designed studies with elite athletes have found that caffeine can effectively enhance performance when consumed in relatively low amounts. Doses as low as 1.5 to 2 milligrams per pound (3–5 mg/kg) of weight are effective. The optimal dose appears to be 2.25 to 2.7 milligrams per pound (5–6 mg/kg). Consuming higher amounts provides no additional performance benefits and may result in rapid heart rate, nervousness, and gastrointestinal discomfort. Most studies have had subjects ingest caffeine 1 hour prior to exercise.

Caffeine can enhance performance over a wide range of exercise protocols. These include not only endurance events lasting 90 minutes or longer and ultraendurance events lasting over 4 hours but also high-intensity exercise lasting 1 to 5 minutes and prolonged high-intensity exercise lasting 20 to 60 minutes. There is also evidence that small doses of caffeine of 0.5 to 1.4 milligrams per pound (1–3 mg/kg) can aid performance if taken before competition, at various times during competition, or toward the end of an exercise session or race when an endurance athlete can become fatigued.

Not all athletes react to caffeine in the same way, however. Some individuals may have a performance response to caffeine, while others may not. Caffeine's diuretic effect has long been debated, but it appears that it is essentially insignificant. Studies indicate that caffeine does not increase urine output during exercise. Athletes who wish to use caffeine as an ergogenic aid in competition should experiment during training to determine their personal tolerance to caffeine during exercise and their own performance response.

Medium Chain Triglycerides

Medium chain triglycerides, or MCT oils, have been promoted to athletes for several years. Because of their shorter molecular chain size (compared to long-chain triglycerides), MCTs empty from the stomach more quickly and are more easily absorbed into the bloodstream. In fact, they are absorbed as quickly as glucose and transported to the liver, where they are metabolized and rapidly burned for energy. Their ergogenic benefit supposedly results from their ability to provide quick fuel during exercise and spare muscle glycogen during extended training.

Of the several studies conducted with MCT oil, one found a performance improvement, while the others did not. One study determined that the amount of MCT oil that can be tolerated within the gastrointestinal tract might be limited. GI symptoms ranging from mild to severe can result. Consuming carbohydrates prior to exercise (as recommended in this book) could also negate the effects of MCT supplementation. MCT oil is promoted as a metabolism enhancer and fat burner. However, these claims are not supported by research. Overall, this supplement is not recommended to athletes.

Glycerol

Glycerol is a colorless liquid alcohol found naturally in fats and is produced from the breakdown of fat. It is available as a glycerine solution or as part of hyperhydration supplements for athletes. Its use is thought to facilitate hyperhydration before training and competition because it holds and attracts water like a sponge. If taken properly and with the correct amount of fluid, glycerol can hold about 36 ounces of fluid in the body. It may be useful for offsetting sweat loss in environments where the possibility of dehydration is extreme.

Study results are still mixed on glycerol hyperhydration. Several studies have suggested that hyperhydration derived from glycerol ingestion can help an athlete maintain a low heart rate and body core temperature during exercise in the heat. Other studies, however, found that it exerted no beneficial physiological effect during endurance exercise.

When diluted and mixed properly, glycerol appears to be relatively safe to use. Dosages used in research have been limited to about 0.45 to 0.7 gram per pound (1–1.5 g/kg) of body weight, with each gram of solution diluted with 0.75 to 1 ounce (25–35 ml) of water. Glycerol solutions should be consumed 1 to 2.5 hours before exercise, but athletes experimenting with glycerol must be very careful. Some physiologists recommend that it only be used under medical supervision. Some athletes taking glycerol have reported headaches, bloating, nausea, vomiting, or dizziness. Pregnant women or individuals with high blood pressure, diabetes, or kidney disease should not use glycerol because of its potential negative side effects.

Glycerol hyperhydration supplements have been targeted toward endurance athletes because of their fluid needs in long-distance events. It may be appropriate for situations in which dehydration and excessive heat conditions are likely to occur. It may also be useful for rehydration in situations where quick recovery from fluid losses is required. But do not exceed the recommended amounts of glycerol, and experiment first with this product in training before attempting to use it in competition. You will experience some weight gain with glycerol use, and you will still need to consume adequate amounts of fluid while competing.

Bicarbonate

Sodium bicarbonate, commonly known as baking soda, is an alkaline salt thought to buffer the acid buildup in the muscle cells caused by training that stresses the anaerobic glycolysis (or lactic acid) energy system. During exercise that stresses the lactic acid system, acid accumulation inhibits muscle contraction and is associated with fatigue. The majority of both laboratory and field studies show that bicarbonate supplementation, or "soda loading," improves performance in high-intensity tasks, both continuous and intermittent, that last from 1 to 7 minutes. This effect appears to be moderate. Only two studies, however, have found that bicarbonate enhances endurance exercise lasting 1 hour. Overall, this supplement should not be of great benefit to an endurance athlete because its effect is more applicable to short, high-intensity tasks.

Sodium bicarbonate appears to be safe when taken in the recommended dose of 140 milligrams per pound (0.3 g/kg) of body weight. For a 150-pound (68 kg) athlete this translates to a dose of 5 teaspoons of baking soda, which provides 21,000 milligrams, or 21 grams, of bicarbonate. Baking soda should be consumed with plenty of water, about 1 to 2 quarts (1–2 L), when taken 1 to 2 hours prior to exercise. This fluid may or may not mitigate reported side effects in some individuals, which include nausea, bloating, abdominal pain, and diarrhea. Experimenting with this supplement in training can help you determine whether you are prone to these unwanted side effects and whether it seems to provide any benefit for you.

Ginseng

Ginseng is a popular substance that has been used for thousands of years in Chinese medicine. Its extracts contain several chemicals, the most important being glycosides or ginsenosides. There are various plant species and forms of ginseng. Ginseng is considered to be an adaptogen, that is, a substance that aids the body's response to stress and increases energy levels. This includes physical stress such as intense exercise. Numerous theories regarding how ginseng exerts this effect have been proposed, though the actual underlying mechanism has not been determined.

THE NCAA AND NUTRITIONAL SUPPLEMENTS

Collegiate athletes competing in the sports of swimming, cycling, cross-country track, rowing, and triathlon need to be aware of the National Collegiate Athletic Association's (NCAA) policy on supplements. The NCAA's current policy regarding sports nutrition supplements states that it is not permissible for an institution to provide any substance to student athletes unless it is a non-muscle-building product and is included in one of the four classes of permissible supplements. Permissible supplements include vitamins and minerals, energy bars, calorie-replacement drinks, and electrolyte-replacement drinks. A listing of nonpermissible supplements includes amino acids, chrysin, chondroitin, creatine and creatine-containing compounds, ginseng, glucosamine, glycerol, HMB, L-carnitine, melatonin, Pos-2, protein powders, and tribulus. However, a supplement that contains protein is permissible if it does not obtain more than 30 percent of its calories from protein and falls under one of the four permissible categories.

The NCAA is concerned with the lack of quality control in the production and manufacture of nutritional supplements. Supplements geared toward muscle building have been found to be contaminated with substances currently on the NCAA banned-drug list. In one study funded by the International Olympic Committee, approximately 15 percent of 600 over-the-counter supplements were found to contain nonlabeled ingredients that could result in a positive doping test. The NCAA promotes the superiority of a well-balanced diet over nutritional supplements and is concerned about the long-term safety of some of these products.

Currently, student athletes wishing to take muscle-building supplements must obtain them on their own. Athletes still need to seek out sound nutrition advice from qualified sports nutritionists and information on the scientific data behind these products, rather than depending on advertising claims and professional athlete endorsements. It is not worth risking eligibility to take products that may offer no real benefit. It is much safer—and more effective—to follow healthy nutritional strategies. Be sure to consume adequate calories and protein, take care to eat a variety of nutritious foods, and strive for optimal nutrient timing to reach your performance goals.

The NCAA encourages students to refer to the Resource Exchange Center (REC), which is sponsored by the National Center for Drug Free Sport, at www.drugfreesport.com/rec, for more information.

Many of the heavily marketed claims surrounding ginseng were from studies conducted in the 1960s and 1970s. Few of these studies were well controlled, and most had many research design flaws. Seven more recent, well-controlled studies have reported no significant effects on performance measures. Overall, the effects of ginseng have not been thoroughly researched.

Ginseng appears to be relatively safe when taken in doses recommended by the manufacturer. However, excessive use may result in high blood pressure, nervousness, and sleeplessness in some individuals. Ginseng is legal. Be wary of ginseng-containing products that may contain other substances, however, such as ephedrine, which is banned. The ginseng content of commercial products is likely to be highly variable, and some preparations have been found not to contain detectable levels of ginsenosides.

SPORT-SPECIFIC NUTRITIONAL GUIDELINES

Putting Your Sports Nutrition Plan into Action

Though all endurance sports are similar, they are not all exactly alike. Each one presents a unique set of challenges and demands. Triathletes, cyclists, runners, swimmers, rowers, and adventure racers all must function differently to achieve the top levels of their sport. Nutritional considerations must take this into account. The principles presented in Part II apply to all endurance sports, but they can use some fine-tuning for each specific type of sport. Part III shows endurance athletes how to do just that. Triathletes can adjust their nutrition race plan specifically for short-course and long-course racing. Cyclists can modify their nutrition plan for road, criterium, or mountain-bike racing. Runners can adapt their training, taper, and competition nutrition plans for 10K races or longer distances, such as the marathon. Endurance sports such as swimming and rowing, which impose large training demands for races measured in minutes, also have their own unique nutritional considerations. Finally, the sport of adventure racing, which has welcomed new participants in increasing numbers to its shorter events, has its own very specific nutrition training and racing techniques and strategies.

Although each chapter in Part III focuses on a different sport, many of the sidebars throughout this part of the book are applicable to all endurance athletes. Please refer to these sidebars for valuable information on, for example, keeping your immune system strong, training and/or competing in high-altitude environments, and preventing muscle cramping.

8

NUTRITION FOR
TRIATHLON

SINCE BEING INTRODUCED AS A MEDAL SPORT at the Sydney Olympic Games in 2000, triathlon competition has received a great boost in exposure. In the past several years there has been a rapid increase in both amateur and professional race participation. Membership in the sport's governing body, USA Triathlon (USAT), increased to 72,500 in 2006, up from 21,000 in 2000. USAT sanctioned 2,070 races in 2006, and there were approximately 500 other events across the country not sanctioned by USAT.

Many triathlon fans "discovered" the sport while flipping through television channels when they first came across weekend coverage of the inspiring and grueling Hawaiian Ironman Triathlon World Championship. While triathletes can participate in Ironman and half-ironman races around the world, and USAT sanctioned 111 long-distance events and 19 ultradistance events in 2006, race events designed to attract first-timers wanting to participate in the sport at a recreational level have increased exponentially. These new events, particularly the sprint-distance and the women-only races, have greatly fueled the sport's growth. Triathletes can now also take their act off-road with events such as the XTERRA® series. These events draw endurance athletes who have participated in one of the three triathlon disciplines and who are looking for some crosstraining, variety, and new challenges in their exercise and competition programs. Some single-sport endurance athletes participate in events as part of a relay team.

Triathlons also have a broad age appeal. The World Triathlon Corporation, which has branded the Ironman name, and USAT statistics show that most triathlon participants are between the ages of thirty and forty-four, but there are many younger athletes competing at the shorter distances as well as older competitors embracing the triathlon lifestyle beyond their middle years. Although triathlon competition is essentially an individual sport where competitors attempt to set their own best time, triathletes often train together and there is a real sense of community within the sport.

And although certain physiological characteristics seem essential for competitors at the elite level, people of all shapes and sizes are embracing the sport at the recreational level. Elite competitors have a high VO_2max, low body fat, high anaerobic threshold, and economy of movement. Of course, many other factors influence competitive success, but at the age-group level, anyone who is willing to train in all three events can participate. Multisport athletes can choose from a variety of races and distances, and special nutritional considerations are appropriate to each.

TYPES OF EVENTS

TRIATHLON

Sprint Distance (short): 0.5-mile swim, 12.4-mile cycle, 3.1-mile run

Distances for the shorter races can vary slightly, with even a few "super-sprint" options available for the newbies or super-speedsters in the sport. Sprint race distances may also vary slightly to fit the course. In 2006, USAT sanctioned more than 834 sprint or short races.

Olympic Distance (intermediate): 0.93-mile swim, 24.8-mile cycle, 6.2-mile run

Olympic hopefuls compete at this distance, but plenty of race options are available to the amateur triathlete. USAT sanctioned more than 286 races of this distance in 2006. At the elite level competitors can compete on the International Triathlon Union (ITU) circuit around the world. XTERRA races are often held at this intermediate distance or at shorter distances.

Half-Ironman (long): 1.2-mile swim, 56-mile cycle, 13.1-mile run

The new Ironman 70.3 race series (70.3 designating the sum of the course miles completed) offers eighteen races around the world. Long-course triathletes can choose from this race series or take part in independent races at or near this distance. The half-ironman race attracts participants who prefer the long-course events but cannot carve out the time for full Ironman training each season. In addition, full Ironman competitors may race this distance in advance of their final race of the season as part of their race preparation.

Ironman (ultra): 2.4-mile swim, 112-mile cycle, 26.2-mile run

With more than twenty races to choose from around the world, triathlon competitors craving the ultradistance in triathlon events have more options than ever. Despite the challenge of this race distance, it is not unusual for the full Ironman races to fill up within 24 hours after registration opens.

DUATHLON

Duathlon races combine the sports of cycling and running, typically in a run-bike-run sequence. Distances can vary and include:

- 2-mile run, 10-mile cycle, 2-mile run (Formula One® race)
- 5K run, 30K cycle, 5K run
- 10K run, 40K cycle, 5K run (international or short-course race)
- 10K run, 60K cycle, 10K run (Powerman® or long-course race)

Duathlon events are popular with athletes who do not have a swimming background, and the number of duathlon races has increased in recent years. USAT sanctioned 261 duathlon races in 2006, and athletes can also compete in the worldwide Powerman Duathlon Series.

AQUATHLON

Aquathlons combine the sports of running and swimming, and races are generally completed in less than 45 minutes. The races follow the run-swim-run format and distances generally include a 1.5K run and a 1,000-meter swim followed by another 1.5K run. The 2006 ITU Aquathlon World Championships were held in Lausanne, Switzerland, in conjunction with the ITU Triathlon World Championships.

WINTER TRIATHLON

Winter triathlons are not just regular triathlons held between the months of November and March; rather, the winter triathlon is a separate sport that combines running, mountain biking, and cross-country skiing. The ITU has been holding winter triathlon championship races since 1997. Much of the winter triathlon activity in the United States is based in the Rocky Mountain region, and the number of such races is increasing.

TRAINING NUTRITION

Whatever the distance a multisport athlete is racing, the proper training diet is essential to a successful and enjoyable racing experience. Because of the diverse nature of their sport, many triathletes complete training for two disciplines daily. Though some schedule two training sessions back to back, others schedule two separate training sessions with a recovery period in between—training, for example, for one sport in the morning and for another in the afternoon or evening. For those who schedule two workouts, weekends are often reserved for long back-to-back training sessions.

Depending on the race distance, triathletes may train anywhere from 8 hours weekly (for the sprint distance) to 25 hours weekly (for the ultradistance). Clearly, the nutritional demands of multisport training are varied depending on the type and distance of the course. Race nutrition demands can also vary depending on the level of the competitor. Racing itself can last over 1 hour for a sprint first-timer, from 2 to 4 hours for Olympic-distance competitors, from 4 to 8 hours for a half-ironman, and from 8 hours to just under the 17-hour cutoff for the Ironman distance. Despite spreading the work out among various muscle groups, any race distance can challenge muscle fuel stores and blood glucose levels. Multisport athletes are also often challenged by the environmental conditions in which they compete. Their races often take place in hot and humid conditions, challenging fluid and electrolyte stores. Long-course racing presents its own unique set of challenges as competitors must fuel and hydrate for several hours within the constraints of their own stomach and intestinal tolerances.

Because of the nature of their training, multisport athletes need to match energy intake, and particularly their intake of carbohydrates, to their training sessions and training cycles. They must also know how to adjust their protein and fat intake levels for optimal training. It is important for the multisport athlete to understand sensible meal and snack timing as well in order to ensure a steady cycle of fueling before training and refueling afterward, particularly when there is a short recovery period between training sessions.

Optimal daily hydration remains essential for multisport athletes, but with multisport training and competition it is more important than ever for an athlete to become familiar with his or her own sweat rate for each training discipline and to develop techniques for rehydrating and refueling during training. And although it is important for any multisport athlete to meet his or her fueling needs during training, this aspect of nutrition can make or break the efforts of the long-course triathlete.

NUTRIENT REQUIREMENTS

Triathletes often plan their race season well in advance. This type of planning should allow triathletes plenty of time to map out their training program and look at weight and body-composition goals.

Multisport athletes, particularly long-course triathletes, have training days that demand a very high energy intake. Energy needs can vary throughout the week depending on the level of training for the day. For example, say an intermediate-course male triathlete who weighs 165 pounds (75 kg) completes an easy 45-minute swim one morning followed by an easy 45-minute evening spin on the bike. His energy needs for the day would amount to approximately 3,000 to 3,300 calories. For this same athlete, a weekend endurance ride lasting 3 to 4 hours would require an intake ranging from 3,800 to 4,450 calories. The same athlete would require more calories if he were training for a long-course distance. Two hours of moderate training would require him to take in 3,600 calories, while a long bike ride of 5 hours or more would demand an intake of more than 5,000 calories for the day.

Refer to Table 4.4 to appreciate the peaks and valleys of an athlete's carbohydrate requirements as training builds and progresses and then decreases during recovery weeks. Carbohydrates are an important fuel for the triathlete during any period of training. Although fuel demands can be low during the preparation phase of training, long-course triathletes often require hefty doses of carbohydrates even early in the season owing to the volume of their training. Fat intake may need to be higher for long-course competitors on high-volume days that include more than 4 hours of training. Protein requirements build steadily as training increases in both duration and intensity; both long workouts and shorter speed workouts have high carbohydrate demands.

CHANGING BODY COMPOSITION

Without exception, elite competitors in triathlon events exhibit low levels of body fat. Although this is not the case with competitors at the recreational level, some age-groupers may also want to improve body composition over the course of the season. (Refer to the weight-management guidelines outlined in Chapter 6.) Triathletes wanting to lose weight should start as early in the season as possible, since weight loss is more easily tolerated during the preparation cycle. As you approach the build phase of your training, the rate of weight loss should slow down because the fuel demands of your training program will increase and adequate recovery is essential. It is important to have realistic weight and body-composition goals and to monitor your changes in body composition throughout the season. Weight-loss efforts are not advised during the last build to an important race or during a race taper.

Regardless of your competition focus, meeting your energy needs is essential for recovery. Attempts to lose weight quickly may result in fatigue and lackluster training. Keep in mind that optimal body-fat levels are not the same for all individuals—an "ideal" weight that results in hormonal imbalance, loss of muscle and power, and compromised immune function will not make you a better triathlete. Lean triathletes who are also successful competitors achieve their low body-fat levels through an intense training program and proper fueling.

TIMING YOUR MEALS AND SNACKS

As a triathlete, you may faithfully keep up a vigorous schedule of training twice a day all year-round. Although multiple training sessions are essential for refining your swimming, cycling, and running skills and accelerating your conditioning, they also present a nutritional timing challenge. It may sometimes seem that your life is one continuous cycle of training, eating, and recovery.

It can be a challenge to determine how to time your meals and snacks around multisport training schedules. You don't want to train with an empty or even half-empty tank, or one that is too full prior to exercise. But figuring out just the right amount of fuel to consume for training more than once daily—and when to consume it—can be tricky. Depending on when you have swimming, cycling, running, or resistance training planned in your training schedule, you may find that it is difficult or even impossible to eat several hours prior to exercising.

Even if you find that your gastrointestinal (GI) system can adapt fairly well to eating close to exercise, as many triathletes do, clearly you must think ahead to the day's schedule in planning your food choices. Three factors will most likely affect those choices: whether you are going for a swim, bike ride, or run; how hard you expect to train; and the timing of your training sessions. Generally, the higher the intensity, the lighter the pre-exercise meal. Running will likely present the greatest digestive challenge, with swimming next in line and cycling the most gentle on your GI system. And although large meals before exercise could make you drowsy and lethargic and possibly cause digestive distress, your real challenge lies in determining the size of the meal and the meal choices that work best for you before particular types of exercise sessions.

In general, a moderate snack providing 1 gram of carbohydrates per pound (2 g/kg) of body weight can be consumed 2 hours prior to training. This snack can include some easily digested solid food, such as a granola bar and yogurt, along with fluids. If you need to eat within an hour of exercise, try an easily digested energy bar, piece of fruit, carbohydrate gel, 24 ounces (720 ml) of a sports drink, or another high-carbohydrate sports nutrition supplement to boost energy levels. Your training schedule may dictate that you have a full meal during the recovery part of your day. Plan ahead, and be sure to include enough meals and snacks to supply the energy you need to train at your best.

Early-Morning Sessions

Early-morning training sessions are not uncommon for the serious triathlete. Often this early session is a swim, but it could easily include a run or bike ride. If your early-morning schedule does not leave much time for digestion before exercising, make sure that you consume a high-carbohydrate dinner, or perhaps even a high-carb evening snack, the night before. You want to start the training session with full muscle glycogen stores and minimize as much as possible the effects of the liver glycogen breakdown that occurs overnight. You can also experiment with small, low-fiber snacks beforehand to determine tolerances. Well-tolerated early-morning noshes may include an energy bar, half a bagel or English muffin, a small yogurt, a glass of juice, or a piece of fruit. These carbohydrate choices can boost your early-morning blood glucose levels and help keep them nice and steady during training. Aim for about 50 to 75 grams of carbohydrates before exercise. Of course, you should also drink plenty of water in the morning. If your early-morning training session is a long workout, you may also want to consider consuming a sports drink while you train. This strategy is easy on your GI system and ensures a steady supply of blood glucose. It can also help you compensate for eating just a small amount of food before the exercise session and can be a useful fueling strategy even during a short workout.

During Training

Anytime that your schedule or personal food tolerances preclude adequate food intake prior to training, think about what you can consume while exercising. Sports drinks, bars, and gels provide glucose for your exercising muscles and can offset muscle glycogen losses that occur later during exercise. Proper refueling during exercise prevents your body from entering a greatly depleted state and will ultimately speed your recovery. Try to consume 30 to 75 grams of carbohydrates, or 0.5 gram of carbohydrates per pound of body weight (1 g/kg) per hour for workouts lasting longer than 75 minutes or during high-intensity interval sessions. If you decide to consume only water during very low-intensity workouts, keep in mind that muscle glycogen and blood glucose stores will eventually drop to low levels as training time progresses. Keep in mind your training goals for that day and that week. Consuming carbohydrates during training sessions is especially important if another training session will quickly follow with limited recovery time in between. If your training schedule is not as demanding, then you may have more recovery time. But consecutive training sessions are not uncommon for multisport training. Hydration is important during any workout and during any part of your training cycle, and sports drinks provide the right balance of carbohydrates and fluid, as well as electrolytes, to stave off the depletion that can occur during heavy training.

RECOVERY NUTRITION

Because you are in a constant cycle of training and recovery, it is very important that you pay close attention to recovery nutrition. If you go into your second workout dehydrated or low on energy, you may not have a high-quality training session. In fact, you may end up digging yourself into an even bigger hole of energy depletion that will affect your training for the next day. Improper refueling can start a downward spiral of poor training and low energy. Follow the recovery nutrition guidelines provided in Chapter 5. Make sure that you plan to have foods on hand that will provide anywhere from 50 to 100 grams of carbohydrates, or at least 0.5 gram of carbohydrates per pound (1 g/kg) of body weight, and up to 20 grams of protein. Check your weight loss from the training session to see how much fluid you lost in sweat, and drink to rehydrate. You should drink about 16 to 20 ounces for every pound of body weight. Consume foods and fluids containing sodium after training in hot, humid weather to replace sodium losses and to enhance rehydration efforts.

The food choices that suit you best after exercise depend to a large extent upon your training schedule for the day. If your next training session is within 2 hours, a between-workouts snack is likely your best option. Aim for easily digested choices. You can try real-food options such as a banana smoothie and toast with jam after a hard session, knowing these foods will sit well until the next training session. At other times, a recovery drink that can be mixed quickly after training or ahead of time may be the most convenient choice. However, if your next training session is several hours away, you should consider having an actual meal. This will allow you to fill up not only on carbohydrates, but provide you with the opportunity to round out your protein and fat intake. Some triathletes practice both nutrition strategies after an arduous training block. They make certain that a good recovery snack is readily available immediately after training and follow this snack shortly afterward with a well-balanced meal.

FOOD AND YOUR TRAINING SCHEDULE

As a triathlete you need to plan ahead to have the proper meals and snacks available. Pack recovery foods and sports drinks the night before. Know what deli carries your favorite healthy lunch that provides just the right balance of protein, carbohydrates, and fat. And make sure that you have just the right afternoon snack available when hunger strikes—and to prevent hunger during an early-evening workout.

The meal plan in the "Meal Plan Outline" sidebar reflects the food and training schedule of a half-ironman competitor. It provides about 3,400 calories, including 530 grams of carbohydrates, 170 grams of protein, and 77 grams of fat. This plan is for a full day of training with 2 to 3 hours of total training time. Short-course athletes could pare down the portions at meals, as they likely would train less and have lower energy, carbohydrate, protein, and fat requirements, but the meal timing and types of food choices would remain the same.

If you train both in the morning and over the lunch hour, the timing will be a bit tighter. After a strenuous morning workout, have recovery foods available in the form of a quick snack, followed by a large breakfast. If it is feasible, your recovery meal can be a nice-sized breakfast. You may want to follow with a mid-morning snack so that hunger does not set in during your lunchtime training session. If needed, consume a sports drink during the lunchtime training session. Lunch should follow as your recovery meal. Depending on the intensity of your training, you may be hungry for an afternoon snack or an early dinner. The meals and snacks following

MEAL PLAN OUTLINE

Early-morning snack
12 oz. (360 ml) apple juice
16 oz. (480 ml) water

Morning workout: 60-90 minutes
32–40 oz. (960–1200 ml) sports drink

Recovery breakfast
8 oz. (240 ml) yogurt with fruit
½ c. (120 ml) granola
1 banana

Lunch
5 oz. (150 g) turkey
1 oz. (30 g) low-fat cheese
2 slices bread
1 pear
1 c. (240 ml) pasta salad with vegetables
3 tsp. (20 ml) olive oil

Pre-exercise snack
1 energy bar
8 oz. (240 ml) cranberry juice
1 apple
2 tbsp. (40 ml) peanut butter

Afternoon workout: 60-90 minutes
32–40 oz. (960–1200 ml) sports drink

Dinner
5 oz. (150 g) fish
1.5 c. (360 ml) cooked brown rice
1 c. (240 ml) broccoli
3 tsp. (20 ml) sesame seed oil

Evening snack
1 c. (240 ml) frozen yogurt
1 c. (240 ml) strawberries

your last training session of the day are your opportunity to refuel for the next day. Make sure that you continue to recover for the next 12 to 24 hours or up until the time when your next training session presents itself.

Evening training could definitely receive a good fuel boost from an afternoon snack. Later training sessions often take place 5 hours or more after your last good meal. Dinner can follow an evening training session as a recovery meal, and depending on the intensity of your training, you may even be hungry for an evening snack.

SPORT-SPECIFIC GUIDELINES

SWIM WORKOUTS

Triathletes frequently experiment with nutritional strategies specifically around their cycling and running workouts and during these workout sessions, but you should view your swim workouts in the same way. Even though you will not rehydrate and refuel during the swim in an actual race, the proper nutritional strategies for any workout enhance the quality of your training and recovery. What you eat and drink, and how much you eat and drink, before, during, and after swimming depend on the timing of your swim workout and other details of that day's training schedule.

Before an early-morning swim, aim for some liquid carbohydrate sources such as juice or a sports drink. A light solid food such as toast or a banana could also be tolerated. Experiment with easily digested foods and fluids to give your early-morning blood glucose levels a needed boost. For afternoon and evening swims, experiment with a light afternoon snack providing at least 50 grams of carbohydrates. Swims late in the evening present a logistical challenge. Some triathletes do well with a small dinner 3 hours beforehand and a sizable recovery snack after swimming. Another option is a very late afternoon snack and a moderately sized post-swim dinner for refueling. You can aim for both solid and liquid carbohydrate choices, with moderate portions of lean proteins.

When your swim training is greater than 60 minutes, or is scheduled back to back with another workout, consider refueling during the swim session. Although sweat rates in the pool can be significantly lower than during land training, hydration is still a focus. And even a relatively short swim of 45 minutes can start the fuel-depletion process. These problems are only compounded by another workout in quick succession. Hydrating with a sports drink can offset glycogen depletion from the swim and help prepare you for the workout directly following your swim. Keep a sports drink at the end of your lane to rehydrate and refuel. Check your weight before and after training to gauge your fluid loss during a swim workout.

Very long swim workouts completed by long-course triathletes may even require a gel shot for a needed carbohydrate boost. Most sports drinks provide 13 to 19 grams of carbohydrates per 8-ounce (240 ml) serving. Sixteen ounces (480 ml) of a sports drink should provide 26 to 38 grams of carbohydrates, and a gel shot can provide another 25 to 30 grams and may be appropriate during harder workouts and for large athletes. Experiment to determine the mix that works best for you. You can replenish after the swim with a sports drink and/or gel if your next workout is in 15 minutes; otherwise, just refuel with a good meal or snack.

BIKE WORKOUTS

Regardless of the distance for which you train, your cycling sessions are likely to be the longest workouts of your training program. The cycling leg of a race also presents the most opportune and convenient time to rehydrate and refuel. So practicing your on-bike nutrition is essential for race preparation. The longer the ride, the more important this key skill becomes, as fuel, fluid, and electrolyte stores can easily become depleted if you neglect this part of your nutrition plan.

Your GI system is relatively stable during a cycling workout, allowing you to consume a greater volume of fluid during the bike ride than during the run. In addition, your water bottle is more accessible on the bike. Check your sweat rate while cycling. If it is reasonable and gastrically possible to do so, aim to match this sweat rate with your fluid intake. It can be difficult at first to consume more than 1.5 quarts (about 1.5 L) per hour on the bike, but it does become easier with practice. At the very least, minimize dehydration on the bike, and of course, avoid drinking in excess of your sweat rate. This is only likely to occur in athletes with low sweat rates, however. Optimizing your fluid intake on the bike with your favorite sports drink results in a higher carbohydrate intake, which allows you to better meet your fueling needs, and a higher sodium intake, which better replaces sodium sweat losses.

Some practice tips may be helpful. First, use a larger water bottle if necessary, especially if your sweat rate indicates that you need at least 40 ounces (1,200 ml) of fluid per hour to prevent or minimize dehydration. Second, practice drinking while on the bike to increase your ability to handle the water bottle easily during the race. Third, you can set a watch alarm to remind you to gulp every 15 minutes. Sports drinks work on the bike for any triathlon distance. Short-course athletes can pack their own fluids for the race, whereas long-course athletes should anticipate taking advantage of the drinks offered on the course. In fact, they should train with this product to be fully prepared for race day. Depending on the volume of fluid that you consume, sports drinks can nicely meet your fueling needs, particularly for the shorter events. But you may need to add in gels and other carbohydrate sources for long-course racing. More information on race nutrition strategies is provided later in this chapter.

RUNNING

Hydrating and fueling during runs can be challenging for several reasons. First, running jostles your stomach, and drinking may not always be comfortable. Second, it is not as convenient to carry fluids with you on a run as it is during a bike ride. Just as you can train your stomach to take in greater volumes of fluid during bike workouts, however, you can also practice during the run. The racecourse does offer fluid stations. To mimic this setup, you can run a loop with a safe place to stash your fluids. Track workouts allow you to hydrate conveniently, though high-intensity training runs can still pose an intake challenge. At the very least, train with a hydration belt.

RACECOURSE-SPECIFIC GUIDELINES

Many of the hydration and fueling strategies that you practice in training are an all-important rehearsal for race day. Still, there are some nutritional considerations unique to each race distance in the days leading up to the race, on race morning, and during the race.

TABLE **8.1**	RACE NUTRITION FOR SPRINT- AND OLYMPIC-DISTANCE TRIATHLONS

SPRINT DISTANCE	**OLYMPIC DISTANCE**
Consume adequate carbohydrates during the race taper.	Taper and consume adequate carbohydrates in the 48 hours before the race.
Consume carbohydrates in excess of requirements 24 hours before the race.	Hydrate optimally in the 48 hours before the race. Monitor the color of your urine.
Consume a high-carbohydrate pre-race meal 2–3 hours before the race.	Increase salt intake 48 hours prior to the race if you are a salty sweater and if the race is likely to take place in hot and humid conditions.
Hydrate with a sports drink in the hours leading up to the race.	Consume a high-carbohydrate meal providing 1 g of carbohydrates per pound (about 2 g/kg) of body weight for 2–3 hours before the start of the race.
Drink 20–32 oz. of fluid, preferably a sports drink, during the bike leg.	Consume fluids from a sports drink in the hours leading up to the race. Top off your pre-race meal with a carbohydrate gel, if tolerated.
Stop at aid stations for fluid during the run to prevent further dehydration.	Drink a sports drink on the bike to minimize sweat losses. Amounts needed can range from 24–40 oz. per hour.
	Stop at aid stations on the run and consume the sports drink provided to prevent further dehydration.

SPRINT DISTANCE

This race distance may be short, but arriving at the starting line fully prepared still requires some savvy nutritional planning. Focus on a diet ample in carbohydrates 24 to 48 hours prior to the race, and make sure your intake matches the energy needs of your training taper. Drink plenty of fluids to hydrate well, and have an early high-carbohydrate dinner the night before the race. Stick with easily tolerated foods and fluids for a couple of days before the race. Time your pre-race meal on race morning according to your personal preferences and tolerances, with plenty of fluids and easily digested foods. Though race starts are likely early, pre-race eating 2 to 3 hours before the start time seems to work best. In the 48 hours leading up to the race, make sure that you stay optimally hydrated. Drink fluids to stay hydrated before the race start—a sports drink is an excellent choice—and time bathroom breaks appropriately. (See Table 8.1 for a summary of nutrition guidelines for sprint- and Olympic-distance triathlons.)

Enjoy the swim, have a good transition, and consume a sports drink on the bike leg of the competition. With typical race times ranging from under 1 hour to just under 2 hours, it will be important for some sprint-distance triathletes to play it right nutritionally on the bike. Cycling presents the opportune time to drink and maintain blood glucose levels. By race day you should be a pro at on-bike drinking due to plenty of practice. Pack two bottles of your favorite sports drink on the bike and drink as you are able for the quick run to the finish. Make sure that you have practiced drinking the sports drink available on the course during your runs.

OLYMPIC DISTANCE

Although top competitors may complete this race around the 2-hour mark, for many age-groupers an Olympic-distance triathlon is a test of both technique and endurance, with 4-hour finishes commonly listed in race results.

Again, eat according to your energy needs as determined by your taper for 24 to 48 hours and emphasize high-carbohydrate foods. Consume 3 to 4 grams of carbohydrates for every pound (6.5–9 g/kg) of body weight 2 days before the race, and close to the same amount the day before the race. Be aware that you may gain a bit of weight when carb loading over 2 days.

Try to time and size your meals appropriately for your start time, consuming 1 to 2 grams of carbohydrates per pound (2.5–4 g/kg) of body weight 3 to 4 hours prior to the race (see Table 5.1). You may wish to time your pre-race meal closer to the start time and decrease your carbohydrate intake accordingly. Practice the pre-race fluid tips outlined in Chapter 5 so that you start the race well hydrated. Hydrate to maintain fluid balance during the taper, and take care not to overhydrate. Large volumes of very clear urine may indicate that you are overhydrating. Include some sodium in your pre-race foods, especially if you are a salty sweater and susceptible to muscle cramping.

When you complete the swim and start the bike portion of the race, begin fueling up with a sports drink. Some competitors may also prefer gels and water for their carbohydrate and fluid combination. If you are racing in hot and humid conditions, make sure that the sports nutrition products you use contain adequate amounts of sodium. Sports drinks are more likely to contain adequate sodium than gels and other products. You can also increase your regular sodium intake for 48 hours before the race to prevent sodium depletion. Age-groupers who have longer finish times are at greater risk of sodium depletion than elite athletes who complete the course quickly. Ingesting low-sodium fluids such as plain water over several hours can dilute the blood and reduce your sodium to below-normal levels. Pack a relatively high-sodium sports drink for the bike leg of the race if needed.

You should still focus on maintaining an adequate fluid intake during the run. Chances are that your efforts on the bike have not replaced 100 percent of your fluid, carbohydrate, and electrolyte losses. Drinking during the run is not as easy as during cycling, but you can practice and acquire this technique in training. The sports drink available on the racecourse should provide better hydration than a gel- and water-combination.

OFF-ROAD

Most off-road races are similar to the Olympic-distance event in terms of length, but finish times are longer owing to the necessity of having to navigate the terrain on the mountain bike and while running on trails. Both present unique nutritional challenges. Carb load in the 48 hours before the race, and have a good pre-race meal as you would for an intermediate-course race. Start the race well hydrated, and consume adequate sodium in the days leading up to the race. By the time race day arrives, you should have had plenty of miles of practice fueling on the bike. A sports drink is essential for completing an off-road race, and both fueling and hydration are essential if you plan to be on the course for more than 3 hours. During the race, a back-mounted hydration pack is a good off-road race option because it leaves your hands free to navigate the off-road bike terrain. But packing water bottles is also helpful, and with relatively long bike times, a gel shot can provide a handy carbohydrate boost. A gel flask mounted on your bike presents yet another practical fueling option.

LONG-COURSE

The impact of optimal nutrition when competing in a half-ironman or Ironman triathlon cannot be overestimated. Having a good fluid-and-food day can make or break your race. Long-course triathletes often search diligently for the perfect food and fluid choices, and many top competitors have developed their own distinct rehydration and refueling choices and strategies. Half-ironman competition is challenging, and Ironman competition is grueling, so it is imperative that you begin the race with glycogen-loaded muscles, adequate liver glycogen stores, optimal hydration and topped-up fluid levels, and a placid and satisfied GI system. One recent study indicated that male Ironman competitors burned more than 10,000 calories of fuel during the race, and female competitors more than 8,000 calories. Energy intakes during the race, however, were less than half the amount of calories burned. It is not expected that fuel intake match fuel burned. The logistical constraints of the race make it difficult to refuel, and the GI system does not always tolerate adequate refueling during the race.

EATING FOR THE TAPER

Regular Ironman training can take up to 25 hours weekly and necessitates a high calorie intake with the proper balance of carbohydrates, fats, and proteins. However, Ironman competitors also have a welcome training taper prior to competition. The taper allows the body to fully recover before the race and gives the athlete an opportunity to refuel and carbohydrate load. Ironman triathletes may actually cut their training down by a full 50 percent during the taper, and this reduction decreases their calorie and carbohydrate requirements.

Even with carbohydrate loading, your calorie and carbohydrate requirements may dip below training levels during the taper. When you load carbohydrates, you rest your muscles and burn minimal amounts of glycogen. You then eat to exceed your carbohydrate requirements in order to bring your glycogen levels to above normal. Your typical training diet should be more than adequate to accomplish this pre-race loading. In fact, continuing your normal caloric intake can lead to unwanted weight gain, as you may be training for only 1 to 2 hours daily.

During the carbohydrate-loading phase of your program, your portions may be smaller than on training days. But do maintain a high percentage of your calories from carbohydrates. Of course, it is the total grams of carbohydrates that matter most, rather than percentages. If you are training for up to 2 hours daily, consume anywhere from 3 to 4.5 grams of carbohydrates for every pound (6.5–10 g/kg) that you weigh. For a 165-pound (75 kg) triathlete this translates into at least 500 grams daily, a significant amount that requires knowledge and planning. Gauge your hunger and fullness carefully. If you are too hungry or become hungry quickly, you are not eating enough to fuel up your body. However, feelings of uncomfortable fullness are not appropriate either. High levels of carb loading may be better tolerated 2 days before the race than the day before—you do not want to wake up race morning feeling bloated and too full.

At the very least, your normal diet will fill up your muscle glycogen stores during a taper; at worst, you will gain some weight. But do keep in mind that a bit of weight gain may be inevitable, as the glycogen you store in your body will hold water in your muscles. This fluid gain does not have any detrimental effect upon performance and can be valuable during competition.

Carbohydrates clearly matter the week prior to competition, but another important focus of your pre-race nutrition plan should be staying optimally hydrated. Fluid intake is especially important if you are racing in a location where heat and humidity can reach extreme levels. You need several quarts or liters of fluids daily regardless of the training level for the day. During training, average sweat losses can range from 1 to 3 quarts (about 1–3 L) per hour. If possible, weigh yourself before and after training during your taper phase and consume 24 ounces (720 ml) of hydrating fluid for every pound of weight lost. A large volume of pale urine should be an adequate indicator of hydration. Pay close attention to your sodium requirements during this time as well. Have recovery drinks containing sodium, add sodium to the foods you eat for several hours after training, and include plenty of sodium in your carb-loading diet.

Chances are you will be traveling to compete in an Ironman. Pack some of your favorite foods, such as sports nutrition supplements and other portable items, including cereals, dried fruit, and granola bars, to take with you. You can also call ahead to your destination or surf the Internet to determine what types of restaurants and menus are offered near where you are staying.

Well-trained triathletes are already glycogen-storage machines, but the 48-hour period before a race is a critical time for true carbohydrate loading to ensure optimal fuel stores. Even if you simply eat "normally" during the bulk of the taper, increase your carbohydrate intake 2 days before the race. Aim for 4 to 5 grams of carbohydrates per pound of body weight. Keep in mind that during this 48-hour carb-loading phase, the types of carbohydrates you choose are just as important as the amounts you consume. Placing less emphasis on high-fiber foods can keep your GI system settled and help you "race light." You should try to rely on carbohydrate-containing fluids and low-fiber foods. Concentrated low-fiber carbohydrate sources include jam, honey, soft drinks, energy bars, refined pastas, breads, cereals, sports drinks, and concentrated sports nutrition supplements. You don't want to encounter any digestive surprises in the 48 hours prior to Ironman competition. Be sure to limit hard-to-digest foods, excess fat and spices, and any unusual or new items. Stick with bland, simple, plain foods, and request special preparation as needed. Your meals may not be a culinary delight in the 48 hours prior to racing, but at least they won't talk back to you during the race. During this period, you may also need to streamline your protein and fat intake to make room for the carbohydrates.

Hyponatremia, or low blood sodium levels, whether mild, moderate, or severe, has been an increasingly serious problem at Ironman competitions, and some cases have received a generous portion of media attention. As a result, many Ironman competitors have become very sodium conscious in recent years. Certain individuals may be more susceptible to excess sodium losses than others, but what you consume before an Ironman can make a difference. Before the race, you may want to consume some high-sodium foods and salt your food at mealtime. Levels of sodium loss due to sweating and regulation of blood sodium levels are unique to each individual, but it would be prudent to start an Ironman, or any long-course race, with blood sodium levels at the high end of normal. Although you need to drink fluids steadily during the pre-race period, don't overdrink, since overhydration can dilute the sodium levels of your blood.

THE NIGHT BEFORE

The night before an Ironman, your favorite easily digested, tried-and-true foods low in fiber are your best option. Many athletes like potatoes, rice, refined breads, and pasta choices with a mild sauce. You may want to limit salads and other raw vegetables, which are harder to digest. You can also have a reasonable amount of easily digested protein with the night-before meal. A late-evening snack can provide a little carbohydrate insurance, but it is probably best to consume a larger meal by early evening. Remember, you do want to wake up hungry the morning of the race so that you can enjoy and easily down your pre-race meal despite any race-day nerves.

RACE MORNING

Race morning is another time for following sensible strategies regarding your food and fluid intake, so plan your breakfast in advance. This pre-race meal should allow your body to refill its liver glycogen stores after the overnight fast that occurs when you sleep. Be sure to top off your fluid

TABLE **8.2**	IRONMAN RACE NUTRITION STRATEGIES

TIMING	NUTRITION STRATEGIES
3–7 days prior to race	Consume a high-carbohydrate training diet. Decrease protein and fat portions slightly during taper in training.
	Maintain a carbohydrate intake of 3–3.5 g/lb. (6.5–8 g/kg) of body weight.
	Increase sodium intake. Hydrate optimally during training and rehydrate after training. Monitor the color of your urine to assess hydration status.
48 hours prior to race	Carbohydrate load with 4–5 g/lb. (9–11 g/kg) of body weight.
	Emphasize concentrated sources of carbohydrate low in fiber.
	Consume salt and salty foods. Optimally hydrate.
Night before	Finish the pre-race meal early, by 5:00–6:00 p.m.
	Keep the pre-race meal simple and somewhat bland.
	Keep fat intake low and choose very low-fat protein foods in small amounts.
Race morning	Consume breakfast containing easily digested carbohydrates in the amount of 1–1.5 g/lb. (2–3 g/kg) of body weight 2–3 hours before race start.
	Hydrate with a sports drink.
	Top off carbohydrate intake with a gel or energy bar.
T1 and bike	Have a predetermined fueling plan for the bike and practice on your long rides.
	Consume a sports drink for fluid, sodium, and carbohydrates in amounts required to minimize dehydration. Work within gastric tolerances regarding volume.
	Add a gel, banana, energy bar, or concentrated carbohydrate drink to your sports drink intake per hour as needed for fuel.
T2 and run	Have a pre-determined fueling plan for the run and practice in training.
	Vary fluid intake with a sports drink and cola. Add a gel to intake as tolerated and needed.
	Maintain adequate sodium intake with a high-sodium sports drink and electrolyte tablets, if needed.
Post-race	Consume easily digested carbohydrates and small amounts of protein, if tolerated.
	Consume sodium-containing foods and fluids for several hours after the race. Eat and drink at regular intervals.

levels enough to carry you through the swim and the first transition (T1) leading to the biking portion of the race. Some competitors find that small amounts of easily digested protein can also be tolerated the morning of the race. Experiment with some of your favorite choices on training days that mimic the timing of the race, and don't try anything new on race day. Table 8.2 summarizes some pre-race nutrition strategies for the Ironman.

DURING THE RACE

Despite all your heroic efforts to prepare nutritionally prior to an Ironman, consuming adequate calories and carbohydrates during the Ironman itself is essential to completing the race and performing at your best. Optimal eating and drinking fuel you to the finish after months of preparation, whereas inadequate nutritional intake can leave you feeling depleted and disappointed. When preparing for your Ironman competition, it certainly can't hurt to visualize a "good stomach day." As an Ironman competitor, you need to translate the nutrition guidelines for eating and drinking during exercise into combinations and amounts of sports drinks, sodium sources, gels, bars, and other foods that work for your individual preferences and tolerances and that maintain your energy levels toward the finish.

As in your pre-race preparation, the most important nutrients during a race remain fluids, carbohydrates, and sodium. The basic sweat rate of 1 to 3 quarts (about 1–3 L) per hour can vary with heat, humidity, exercise intensity, acclimatization, and fitness levels. The more pronounced the factors, the greater your fluid losses. Studies indicate that the rate at which fluid empties from the stomach exhibits a great deal of individual variability, but in general, it ranges from 24 to 40 ounces per hour. Aim to consume this amount of fluid during your race, and practice maintaining this intake during training. Seasoned competitors have learned to tolerate greater volumes.

Estimated sodium losses from sweating range from 115 to 700 milligrams per hour, but they can reach as high as 2,000 milligrams per hour in nonacclimated athletes or salty sweaters. Check the labels of your favorite sports drinks to determine their sodium content, and choose those that seem to match your typical level of sodium loss. If you are prone to muscle cramps, it may be because you have very salty sweat. You can also add small amounts of salt to a sports drink if needed. One-quarter of a teaspoon of salt contains 550 milligrams of sodium. Salt tablets generally contain several hundred milligrams of sodium per tablet. All salt or electrolyte tablets should be consumed with at least 8 ounces of water.

Of course, you need carbohydrates to maintain blood glucose levels and provide fuel for your muscles as glycogen stores are burned for energy. Try to replace carbohydrates at a rate of 0.5 gram or 2 calories per pound of body weight per hour. This translates to about 60 to 100 grams of carbohydrates, or 250 to 400 calories per hour. This may sound like a lot of calories, but Ironman competitors expend several thousand calories in a race. Generally, 32 ounces of a sports drink provides 55 to 75 grams of carbohydrates. Check the labels of any items you may consume during a race, such as energy bars or gels, to determine their carbohydrate content.

TRANSITION 1 (T1) AND ON-THE-BIKE NUTRITION

After a swim in choppy waters or saltwater, your stomach may feel a bit unsettled. You may swallow some water during the swim and even feel a bit nauseated. But the bike leg is your opportunity to consume adequate fuel and set yourself up for the run. It is also the longest leg of the long-course triathlon. Try not to wait more than 30 minutes on the bike before you start consuming fluids.

Once you and your stomach are settled on the bike leg, it is time to get down to business. Start consuming fluids as soon as you can tolerate them. Fuller stomachs empty faster to quickly replace sweat losses, so drink enough to produce that effect. Sports drinks can provide a perfect balance of fluid and carbohydrates and varying amounts of sodium. Plain water can wash down the taste of sweet gels and beverages in hot and humid conditions. Try out your favorite sports drinks and gels (and the brand available on the racecourse) during long training sessions on your bike that are near race pace. The more efficient you become at drinking on the bike, the less energy you expend doing it. You may want to slow down slightly when you refuel, but the more you practice, the better you can maintain your pace.

Despite the fact that biking keeps your GI system relatively stable, most triathletes prefer to consume the majority of their calories from fluids. Gels are also well tolerated. Many top competitors have come up with their own fluid-replacement formulas so that they can have something a bit more concentrated than a sports drink while on the bike, perhaps even adding a bit of protein at times as well. Of course, anyone who consumes these personalized products has experimented with them in training. As far as solids are concerned, they are generally kept to a minimum, but they can provide a nice chew in the middle of all that drinking. Make sure that you limit solids to well-proven, tolerable foods. Some good options are fruit bars, cut-up sports bars, and bananas. But only your stomach knows for sure what works best. You can also take along some items that you may possibly crave during the long day.

Pack more gels, bars, and other treats than you think you will need. This allows you to have some choices and satisfy cravings. You can tape gel packets to your bike for easy handling or plant them ahead of time in a pack or the pockets of a cycling jersey. Experiment with various carrying systems. You may want to try a bladder hydration system or seat-mounted and/or aerobar-mounted bottle carriers in addition to the traditional frame-mounted water bottles. Pack your turnaround bag with fluids and foods, and allow yourself enough choices that you can select an item that appeals to you at the time.

MUSCLE CRAMS

Any endurance athlete who has suffered a muscle cramp probably remembers it well. These rapidly ignited and long-sustained muscle spasms can be painful and inconvenient, particularly when they occur during competition. The exact cause of muscle cramps remains a mystery, however, and research data on cramping are limited. What is known is that muscle cramping generally occurs during relatively long exercise sessions in the heat and that it is often associated with overexertion. Some cases of muscle cramping may be due to simple muscular exhaustion or low fuel stores; others may result from biomechanical problems or mineral and fluid deficiencies. Whatever the cause, there are some methodical nutritional steps that you can take to help prevent muscle cramps. You may need to experiment with these possible solutions: Prevention in recurrent sufferers is often a matter of trial and error.

Although scientists have not yet figured out a way to look directly at the muscle cell to see precisely what is causing a heat cramp as it is occurring, research suggests that muscle cramps are related to salt and fluid imbalances. Muscle cramps during exercise have been linked to low levels of sodium in the blood. If there are large amounts of sodium chloride in an athlete's sweat, or an athlete replaces his or her sweat losses with low-sodium drinks or plain water, diluting the sodium in the blood, or both, the chance of getting a muscle cramp increases. Dehydration and other mineral deficiencies, such as shortages of calcium and magnesium, may also be predisposing factors.

Some age-groupers experience severe muscle cramps during races, especially when they do not yet have much experience in competition, and even if they have not been prone to cramps in training. Increasing salt intake when training in hot, humid weather prior to competition can help. Maintaining hydration levels before, during, and after exercise can also help. During exercise, try to consume the amount of fluid necessary to match or minimize your sweat losses. Recheck your sweat rate for different training disciplines in varying weather conditions, and monitor the color of your urine. Sports drinks with some sodium content are better than plain water for making sure you do not dilute your blood sodium levels.

It is also prudent to obtain plenty of sodium in your diet while training in hot weather. Foods that contain sodium include canned soups, pretzels, cereals, various cheeses, crackers, and yogurt. You can salt your food prior to training in the heat or on competition days. If you find yourself craving salt, your body may be telling you that it needs more. Sodium losses in 1 quart (960 ml) of

CONTINUES

MUSCLE CRAMPS continued

sweat can range from 400 to 1,800 milligrams, or even more in some endurance athletes. Having a high sweat rate only compounds the level of sodium losses each hour during training and competition. Cramp-prone endurance athletes can use high-sodium sports drinks during training to replace sodium losses. Electrolyte tablets that contain sodium are also available for very salty sweaters. However, they should be taken with plenty of fluids and not overconsumed.

Other reasons for muscle cramping are sometimes cited, and if you are prone to cramping you may receive advice based on these theories. There has been some speculation that potassium losses can lead to muscle cramping, for example. Your diet can easily supply ample amounts of potassium. Excellent sources include all fruit juices, fruits, and vegetables, with some of the best sources being grapefruit, orange, and pineapple juice; apricots, bananas, papayas; greens, carrots, potatoes, and tomatoes. Milk, yogurt, and dried peas and beans are also good sources of potassium. Although sodium losses are a more likely culprit, you may want to eat generous portions of these high-potassium foods anyway, as they provide carbohydrates. A lack of calcium is also sometimes blamed for muscle cramps, though its involvement has not been conclusively proven. Although blood calcium levels do not typically fall below normal during long-distance training, low levels may play a role in cramping for some individuals competing in ultraevents. Calcium is the most abundant mineral in your body and plays many functional roles, including a role in muscle contraction. To be on the safe side, athletes suffering from muscle cramps should at least correct inadequate calcium intake. Being sure to consume enough calcium won't hurt, and it will help to preserve bone mass, if nothing else. Good sources of calcium, including milk, yogurt, and leafy green vegetables, are listed in Chapter 3. A calcium supplement can also compensate for a low dietary intake of this important mineral. Yet another theory is that a lack of magnesium, a mineral that plays an important role in muscle relaxation, may be related to muscle cramping. Good sources of magnesium include nuts, seeds, legumes, green leafy vegetables, and unrefined grains.

Make sure that you test strategies for preventing heat cramps carefully in training. Any nutritional plan for preventing heat cramps will depend on your medical history, usual diet, and usual sweat and sodium losses. If following these nutritional strategies does not help you in solving the mystery of heat cramps, look to resources that can help you determine whether there is a biomechanical cause or problems with your stretching or training techniques.

Practice keeping up with your fluid requirements. Once you become dehydrated, it can become difficult to empty fluids adequately from your stomach. As you attempt to catch up with your fluid losses and drink more, your stomach will become uncomfortable and bloated. Despite your intake of fluids, you may experience the symptoms of fluid and carbohydrate depletion. It can be hard to differentiate among the symptoms to know whether you require more fluid or more carbohydrates. If you don't need to urinate, then you are not drinking enough or emptying your stomach adequately.

TRANSITION 2 (T2) AND THE RUN

Maintaining proper hydration and carbohydrate intake can be a challenge during the run portion of a triathlon. Running is harder on your GI system than cycling and more likely to result in nausea and bloating. Moreover, by the time the running leg rolls around, you have been exercising for several hours and your fluids and glycogen stores may already be running low. If you do try to drink, you may feel fluid jostling around in your stomach. Nevertheless, it is important that you stop or slow down at aid stations and make a point of drinking fluids. Most competitors choose to stay away from solids and stick with water, sports drinks, gels, and cola during the run. Because the risks of hyponatremia can increase as the race progresses, many competitors also bring along salt or electrolyte tablets or continue to hydrate with a high-sodium sports drink.

There are a variety of steps you can take to set yourself up for good GI tolerance during the run. The plan that is best for you depends upon your own individual tolerances. Some competitors find that it is best not to consume anything for the last 15 to 30 minutes on the bike and to keep their intake very light for the first few miles of the run. Other competitors successfully down a whole bottle of sports drink in T2. Knowing how you will fare best during this transition takes practice and experimentation in training.

Alternating among gels, sports drinks, water, and cola can support your carbohydrate and fluid needs during the run. Alternating cola with water can help dilute the higher carbohydrate concentration of the former. The caffeine in the cola may also stimulate your central nervous system and improve your focus and concentration during the race. Slow down when you approach aid stations. If you try to gulp fluid from the cups provided while keeping up your running pace, you may not actually get much of it down—most of the drink will spill out. Taking the time to drink should improve your overall performance.

If you consume gels during the run, make sure that you take them with plenty of fluid. Also, look for some flavor variety in your gels and drinks to relieve the taste boredom that can occur during a long race. Switching to a different flavor may be just the change you need to increase your intake. Keep in mind that some gels—and cola—are not as high in sodium as sports drinks. Often competitors make a point of consuming salt tablets during the run, but make sure that you do not take excessive amounts of them and that you have no medical contraindication to taking these tablets. Also, like gels, salt tablets should be consumed with plenty of fluid. When a race is held in a hot climate, triathletes who arrive from cooler environments and have not had time to acclimatize are at greater risk for hyponatremia. Slower triathletes are also at risk for developing this condition, as longer race times provide more opportunity for sodium losses that are not adequately replaced.

Unfortunately, it can be difficult to discern whether your stomach is emptying properly. The symptoms of inadequate emptying of fluids from the stomach and of inadequate carbohydrate consumption and absorption are similar. If you are not producing adequate amounts of urine, however, the chances are greater that the fluids are not emptying properly. Once you become dehydrated, your risk of GI upset increases significantly. Dehydration will delay emptying, and attempts to rehydrate at that point will upset your stomach further. It is best not to stop drinking altogether, so try sipping fluids a little at a time. If you overfill and vomit, regroup and slowly continue to sip fluids. Your body needs the fluids, but try not to give it more than it can handle at this point.

It can be equally difficult to discern whether you are suffering from low blood sugar during a race. If you feel mentally sharp, you probably have adequate glucose available to fuel your brain; if you feel irritable or spacy, however, you may be experiencing low blood glucose levels. If symptoms of hypoglycemia occur, try a gel or soda and see if symptoms improve. Experienced triathletes know that every Ironman is different and that one key to success is learning how to listen to your body and how to provide what it needs during the race.

HALF-IRONMAN RACING

The nutritional strategies for the Ironman need to be slightly modified for the half-ironman distance. Although many age-group competitors can expect to be on the course for more than 5 hours, most athletes tackle this race at a slightly higher intensity than the rate at which they would approach an Ironman, at the upper end of their aerobic zone. You may compete at more of a "tempo" speed, or at a higher heart rate, during some sections of the race, particularly if the race is the most important one of the season for you.

Because of the higher intensity sustained during this type of race, you may wish to temper your nutritional strategies. You should continue to hydrate with a sports drink, choosing one high in sodium if you have high salt needs. Gels can also be added to the mix. But when you exercise at higher intensities, the more concentrated carbohydrate sources do not empty from your stomach as quickly as they do during less intense exercise. Be very careful with any solid items, if you use them at all. Drink to match or minimize sweat losses on both the biking portion of the race and the running portion. You may not start the run with the same level of dehydration as in an Ironman, but the higher running speed can affect your stomach tolerances.

9

NUTRITION FOR ROAD CYCLING, MOUNTAIN BIKING,
TRACK CYCLING, AND CYCLO-CROSS

CYCLING IS UNDOUBTEDLY ONE OF THE MOST physically challenging sports that an athlete can pursue. It requires muscular strength, power, and endurance. Cyclists complete long aerobic training rides to prepare for competition, but they also incorporate a significant amount of anaerobic exercise into a program that includes intervals, sprints, and weight training. It is important that cyclists develop both the aerobic and anaerobic systems in order to compete at their best. Tactical savvy is also essential to success in cycling.

USA Cycling (USAC), the official cycling organization recognized by the U.S. Olympic Committee, now has a membership of over 60,000 and sanctions more than 2,500 events across the country annually in a variety of formats from early spring to late fall. These competitions include road races varying in length from 15 to 80 miles, criterium racing, and time trialing. The sport of mountain biking is also popular, and in some areas of the country, track cycling is available. Cyclo-cross is a traditional off-season option, and many cyclists choose to participate in strength training during this time of year. Thousands of other cyclists participate in recreational long-distance rides, some at a serious and focused level.

Road racing requires muscular endurance, the power to undertake surges in speed, and the ability to sprint at the end of a race. Depending on the level at which you compete, road races may last from 45 minutes to several hours. The ultimate in road racing is professional stage racing, particularly the 21-day Tour de France. Mountain bike racing requires mainly muscular endurance, but it also requires power for climbing steep hills and for sprinting at the finish. Cyclo-cross events are shorter but very intense and require superb bike-handling skills, the ability to ride well on varying terrain, and excellent technique in such skills as dismounting and mounting the bike. Although track racing demands mostly power from the cyclist, a good training program for this event incorporates long endurance rides. Of course, many recreational riders also complete long bike rides, especially in the warmer months, thus altering their nutritional requirements.

Cyclists typically train once daily but incorporate longer rides lasting several hours weekly, particularly on the weekends. Training can also include high-intensity rides as well as anaerobic threshold training, interval training, and sprint workouts, with the training becoming more specialized as the cyclist builds to his or her event during race season. It is not unusual for cyclists to train for 10 to 20 hours weekly during heavy training cycles. The training programs are unique to each discipline within cycling, but no matter which discipline a cyclist chooses to specialize in, meeting specific fuel demands for the type of training program and the period of training allows the cyclist to have optimal energy for both training and daily recovery.

TRAINING NUTRITION

TRANSITION PHASE (OFF-SEASON)

In the transition phase of a periodization training schedule, cyclists may train on the road, indoors on a wind trainer or rollers, or in an indoor cycling class or clinic. This off-season period is also a time to concentrate on strength training. Cyclists who live in parts of North America with friendly climates may put in some steady miles, but overall the volume and intensity of their training on the bike decrease at this time. Some choose to take a short break from cycling during this time and participate in other sports in order to crosstrain.

If you strength train, proper nutrition can make the most of your program. Strength training can help you maintain lean body mass that is normally lost with the aging process. It can also improve your aerobic performance and help prevent injury. Depending on your level of aerobic exercise, however, your overall calorie and carbohydrate requirements may be lower than at the height of the season. Training in the off-season simply does not usually require as much energy as training more than 15 hours weekly and completing rides lasting several hours.

You do need to consume enough calories to build muscle (see specific guidelines in Chapter 6). It takes 350 to 400 additional calories daily to build 1 pound of muscle. If you are trying to shed a few pounds during the off-season, strict dieting can hamper your muscle-building efforts. Your protein intake should not increase significantly while weight training and may even be a bit lower than during the build cycle of the regular training season, though novice weight trainers may have slightly higher protein requirements. Protein requirements of 0.5 to 0.8 gram per pound of body weight are easily met with a well-balanced diet and nutritious food choices.

Muscle glycogen is an important energy source during weight training, so arrive for training sessions in a well-fueled state. To support your muscle-building efforts, aim for 10 to 20 grams of high-quality protein combined with 35 grams of carbohydrates within the hour before weight training. You can consider consuming a sports drink during training to maintain blood glucose levels, supply your muscles with fuel, and maintain adequate hydration. You should also practice recovery nutrition after a hard weight-training session, combining both protein and carbohydrates to support muscle repair and rebuilding and to stimulate muscle glycogen resynthesis.

If you train outside during the colder months, you still need to replace fluid losses from sweating, though these losses may not be as significant as in hot and humid weather. If you are dressed warmly, you can lose up to 2 quarts (about 2 L) of fluid per hour through sweating. During cold-weather exercise, try to drink at least one full 20-ounce water bottle per hour. If the thought of a cold sports drink makes your teeth chatter, prepare your drink with warm or hot water. Hot decaffeinated tea mixed with plenty of honey can provide a carbohydrate boost. You can even dilute sweet drinks such as hot chocolate or hot apple cider for a warming treat while training. These warm liquids provide several advantages. They are easier to drink when it is cold outside, they provide a feeling of warmth, and they increase blood flow to the extremities by dilating blood vessels. And better yet, your body does not need to expend extra energy to warm them as it does with cold liquids. For the same reasons, keep any food you bring with you as warm as possible. Cold weather does create a greater demand for calories. Be sure to consume some carbohydrates while training, as shivering uses up fuel. So do your muscles during these winter sessions. In fact, long, low-intensity "fat-burning" rides slowly drain carbohydrate stores at a steady rate. It may be a good idea to eat close to your exercise session as this can have a warming effect. Make this meal or snack predominately carbohydrates.

PREPARATORY PHASE (EARLY SEASON)

As spring draws near, most cyclists begin looking ahead to the racing calendar. The great outdoors begins to beckon to you for more miles, greater intensity, and perhaps even an early-season race or two. It is now time to carefully match the calories you burn on the bike with those you consume both on and off the bike. You may come into early-season training a bit on the heavier side of your ideal racing weight and may be tempted to diet to shed a few pounds. Try to resist the temptation to reduce calories too severely, however, or to refrain from eating altogether during longer rides. Although these techniques may produce quick weight-loss results, they can also produce negative results, such as poor recovery, hypoglycemia during training, and intense hunger and subsequent overeating. Ultimately, restricting calories too much can hold you back in training. You don't want to end up feeling tired and overtrained just at the time when you were hoping to whip yourself into shape. After long rides, pay attention to the immediate post-exercise recovery nutrition guidelines outlined in Chapter 4. Refer to Table 4.4 for guidelines in matching your nutritional intake to your training volume and intensity.

BUILD PHASE

When training and racing season are in full gear, the number of calories your body burns—and its carbohydrate expenditure—become significant. Review Chapter 4 on daily recovery nutrition to ensure that you match your training with your carbohydrate intake and round out your meals with adequate protein and fat. It can be difficult for cyclists to meet their energy and carbohydrate needs by consuming only three meals daily. Plan on having snacks and possibly even incorporating high-calorie sports nutrition supplements into your diet. Some cyclists need more than 4,000 to 6,000 calories on heavy training days, an impossible food-consumption task without careful planning. Most successful cyclists are constantly grazing during the day. Large meals may make you feel heavy and sleepy, whereas several steady meals and snacks keep the recovery process going throughout the day.

Recovery nutrition is essential after long or intense training rides. You need 0.5 gram of carbohydrates per pound of body weight and smaller amounts of protein within 30 minutes after exercise to recover. When you train in hot and humid weather, make sure that you also consume some sodium afterward to replace electrolyte losses and optimize fluid replacement. Have these recovery snacks readily available after rides. Fluids are an important part of your daily training diet. Carry or have fluid with you everywhere you go, on public transportation, in the car, and at your desk. Keep drinking, and make sure that you produce several full bladders of light-colored urine daily. Follow the daily hydration guidelines presented in Chapter 1. Check your weight before and after hard training to determine your sweat rate, and consume 24 ounces of fluid for every pound lost. If you are losing greater than 1 to 2 pounds of fluid weight during training, you are not keeping up with your fluid requirements as well as you should during your training sessions. You may have a high sweat rate, or you may need to refine your drinking skills on the bike. You should also recheck your sweat rate at different points throughout the season, as it may increase as your fitness level improves, as the weather heats up, and as you become acclimated to the warmer weather.

Cyclists should also pay close attention to their iron intake. They can lose large amounts of iron through sweating and may have elevated iron requirements from their heavy training. Female cyclists should be especially careful to include good iron sources in their diet because of higher iron losses, though male cyclists are susceptible to being deficient in this nutrient as well. Have a physician monitor your iron stores, and supplement safely if necessary.

Cycling is not considered a weight-bearing sport, though it does put some pressure on your spine. Cyclists therefore need to pay close attention to maintaining good bone health and preventing osteoporosis. This includes both men and women. While the causes of osteoporosis are multiple, consistent weight-bearing exercise and adequate calcium intake are two of the cornerstone recommendations for preventing this debilitating condition. Cyclists should incorporate weight-bearing exercise into their training year-round and consume at least 1,000 milligrams of calcium daily. If your diet does not provide this amount of calcium, a calcium supplement can make up the difference.

Body-fat levels are also a big concern for cyclists. Many successful elite and professional competitors are extremely lean, but they also put in long hours of training, which is the most effective way to safely reach low levels of body fat. Severe dieting or attempts to become too lean too fast can result in fatigue, loss of muscle mass and power, and possibly overtraining. Some cyclists may have unrealistic body-fat goals, and though losing excess body fat may improve climbing, it likely will have little impact on time trialing and sprinting. Striving for too low a level of body fat can compromise energy levels and even your health. Follow the guidelines for sensible weight loss presented in Chapter 6, and remember that a good cycling program requires quite a bit of energy to be successfully maintained. Be patient, and let the weight take care of itself with good training and proper eating.

HYDRATING AND FUELING

Cycling is a unique endurance sport in that refueling while you train is a relatively simple task in contrast to swimming or running, which present challenges in this regard. No other sport keeps your gastrointestinal system so stable or so conveniently allows you to carry your food and fluids. This is fortunate, as the fluid and carbohydrate demands during training are high. Cyclists experience significant fluid losses, though they may be unaware of this as their sweat can evaporate quickly in the wind. This wind effect can also keep you from overheating and hide your need for fluid. Start training with a moderate volume of fluid to distend your stomach and enhance emptying, and start drinking as soon as you settle into the rhythm of your training ride. Aim for 4 to 8 ounces every 15 to 20 minutes, or the amount appropriate for matching or minimizing your sweat losses. Set your watch or heart-rate monitor to remind yourself to drink on schedule. Once you become dehydrated, it will be difficult to catch up with your fluid requirements. Remember that riding in the heat, wind, or humidity also increases your fluid losses and therefore your fluid requirements.

You will dip significantly into your muscle glycogen stores during aerobic endurance rides lasting longer than 90 minutes, which steadily deplete your muscle glycogen stores. Muscle glycogen is also rapidly used for fuel when you complete interval and sprint training sessions, and it can reach low levels within even 1 hour of this type of training.

To obtain both fluid and carbohydrates, it makes sense for you to consume a sports drink during almost any type of training ride. Cyclists seem to be more susceptible than other endurance athletes to "bonking," or reaching low blood glucose levels. Consuming a sports drink will maintain blood glucose and provide your muscles with a fuel source when they run low on glycogen. If you anticipate a longer training ride, consume a sports drink from the start. You can also bring along gels, bars, or bananas, which can be consumed with some water if you need an occasional change from liquid carbohydrates. Just as it is difficult to catch up with your fluid needs when you are already dehydrated, it can be challenging to consume carbohydrates when your blood sugar is already low, so hypoglycemia is best prevented.

Because food and fluid can be carried on your bike, you can pack large fluid bottles filled with a sports drink. For longer rides, pack powdered drinks and reconstitute them in your emptied bottles along the way. You can plan out a route where water fountains are available or where water or sports drinks can be purchased. Bladder systems work well during more technical, off-road rides because they allow you to drink without taking your hands off the handlebars. You can also pack gels and bars in your jersey pockets or tuck them conveniently in the leg of your cycling shorts. If you find the taste of sports drinks too sweet in hot weather, look for milder or unflavored drinks. You can also alternate a good full swig of a sweet sports drink with a gulp of water on occasion.

Some cyclists may believe that consuming plain water during long rides early in the season encourages more fat burning during the ride. This practice likely can only be tolerated for a limited time at very low intensities, however. Moreover, it takes more time to recover from a carbohydrate-free ride than it does to recover from a ride that includes refueling, so if you do try to lose body fat this way, plan accordingly. You may need more time between training sessions, or you may decide that this strategy is not worth the stress that it places on your body. Don't plan on having good energy levels during the end of such a ride. You should never skip carbohydrate consumption on a ride when your primary goal is a good solid training experience designed to prepare you for a race.

Another technique for preparing yourself nutritionally is to eat and drink adequate amounts of fluid before a long training ride. Start with a good breakfast 2 hours beforehand, and consume plenty of carbohydrates according to the guidelines presented in Chapter 5. If you train in the evening, make sure you have a substantial afternoon snack providing 50 to 100 grams of carbohydrates 1 to 2 hours beforehand. Before very early morning rides, you may not have time for a good breakfast. But at least take a few minutes to down something simple, such as juice and toast. A small dose of pre-training carbohydrates is better than none at all, but make sure you consume carbohydrates during the ride to offset low morning liver glycogen stores.

DISCIPLINE-SPECIFIC GUIDELINES

A proper nutritional program matched specifically to your training helps you to progress faster and reach your training goals, but what you eat in the days and hours before an important race can have a positive performance impact. Smart pre-race eating provides several performance benefits. In particular, cyclists can lower their chances of developing hypoglycemia, or low blood sugar ("bonking"), along with the accompanying feelings of fatigue, poor concentration, and light-headedness. Eating right for the race can also top off your muscle glycogen stores and provide your exercising muscles with fuel during the race. Eating before racing will help to settle your stomach and prevent hunger pains during long races. Following the proper pre-hydration strategies before competition decreases your risk of developing dehydration during the race. You will also benefit psychologically from knowing that your body has been properly fed and you are as race-ready as you can be.

Cyclists should arrive at any race lasting longer than 60 minutes with adequate body stores of carbohydrates. Depending on your racing schedule, rest or taper for 24 to 48 hours and consume a diet adequate in carbohydrates. You can load up on carbohydrates before longer criteriums, time trials, road races, and a full race schedule of track cycling. It is especially important to rest and replenish your stores before a series of races that will take more than several days to complete. (See Chapter 5 for tips on carb loading.)

The foods you choose, the amounts you consume, and how you time your pre-race meal will largely be determined by your race start time, the type of race in which you are competing, and your personal tolerances. For races lasting longer than 60 minutes, consume 30 to 60 grams of carbohydrates per hour during the race to prevent hypoglycemia and provide muscles with fuel later in the race. However, fluid consumption during a race is not as simple as fluid consumption during training. Depending on the type of race, bike racing often requires that you respond to sudden changes in speed, race tactics, and varying terrain.

ROAD CYCLING
Training Nutrition

Because of the nature of road cycling and the distance of the races, high training volumes are not uncommon in the sport, even for cyclists new to the racing scene. Early in the season, cyclists constrained by cold weather may participate in indoor wind-trainer sessions, indoor cycle classes, and weight-training sessions.

Serious cyclists need to consume adequate carbohydrates for daily recovery, as well as protein to prevent muscle tissue breakdown during the long race season. Calorie requirements may be best met with three meals and several snacks daily. Adequate nutritional intake is also essential to maintaining a strong immune system during the season. Cyclists often attempt to achieve low body-fat levels to improve their power-to-weight ratio for climbing. Weight loss is best accomplished early in the season, and peak levels of leanness can be achieved through quality training.

Both male and female road cyclists should take care to have adequate intakes of iron and monitor iron status during the season.

Competition Nutrition

During a full season of racing, a cyclist may compete almost weekly and even participate in a stage race. Cyclists should start all road events with good fuel and fluid stores. Road race start times can be as early as 8:00 a.m. and as late as 4:00 p.m. on a full day of racing that includes the various racing categories. You may have to travel to the race and eat your pre-race meal in the early-morning hours on the road or even in the car. For road races that last longer than an hour, you should rest from training and consume adequate carbohydrates for 24 to 48 hours before the race. Most cyclists prefer to consume their pre-race meal 2.5 to 3 hours beforehand. As mentioned in Chapter 5, consume about 1 gram of carbohydrates per pound (2.5 g/kg) of body weight at this meal, more if tolerated. Small amounts of low-fat protein and tiny amounts of fat can also be included if your tolerances allow. Be sure to provide enough time for digestion to compensate for pre-race nerves.

If you have an early start time, it may still be worth eating 2 hours prior to exercise and then taking some time for a good warm-up. You can make this meal especially high in easy-to-digest carbohydrates such as liquid carbohydrates and sports nutrition supplements. If you need a smaller meal, consume ample amounts of a sports drink in the hour leading up to the race for both extra carbohydrates and hydration. Later morning starts may allow time for a large pre-race breakfast 3 or even 4 hours beforehand. You can top off this meal an hour before exercise with an easily digested item providing 50 to 75 grams of carbohydrates, and of course consume plenty of fluids. Late-afternoon start times may allow you to sleep later and have a large pre-race breakfast followed by a snack. You can also consider having an early breakfast and then a small lunch-type meal 2 hours prior to the start time. Experiment with various start times and meals in training. Try to mimic the start time scenario of the most important races of the season during training so that you feel comfortable with all your decisions on race day.

Make sure that you drink adequately during your warm-up. Aim to drink a sports drink in the hours leading up to the race. You can start the race with some fluid in your stomach to prime the stomach for gastric emptying during the race.

During road races you should make an effort to maintain good hydration levels as soon as you settle into the race. If the race lasts more than 60 to 75 minutes, a sports drink can maintain blood glucose levels and prevent glycogen depletion, ensuring adequate stores for your muscles later in the race. Make sure to drink gulps when the pace is relatively steady, as surges in the race may preclude drinking on the bike at key moments. Large volumes of fluid leave your stomach more rapidly than sips, and the pressures of racing are not conducive to steady sipping. Practice your

TRAINING AND RACING IN THE HEAT

In addition to causing greater fluid losses and increased body temperature, training in the heat imposes other stresses on your body. When you train in hot weather, your body experiences an increased rate of muscle glycogen use, which can result in premature fatigue. Lactic-acid production is also greater, and your heart rate increases to compensate for fluid losses. Consequently, training at a given intensity is harder than it would be in cooler weather.

The key to training in hot weather is to appreciate that your body must adapt to the heat. Although a few training sessions of 30 to 60 minutes each at 70 percent of VO_2max may be helpful, full adaptation to the heat may take from 7 to 14 days and is a highly individual response. After 10 days of training in the heat, the sweat response adapts in several ways—you start to sweat sooner, you sweat more, you sweat over more of your body, and your sweat contains fewer electrolytes, decreasing your sodium losses. Other adaptations include an increased blood volume and decreased sodium excretion in the urine. After 10 days of training in the heat, your sweating capacity during exercise can double.

Though these adaptations are all essential to cooling your body, they do result in greater fluid losses. Clearly, if these fluid losses are not replaced, you run the risk of becoming dehydrated and the benefits of heat acclimatization are lost. Because your sweat capacity is greatly enhanced after adapting to the heat, dehydration can occur quickly. And in addition to fluid replacement, you should emphasize glucose replacement to meet the accelerated fuel demands imposed by training in the heat.

Keeping up with fluid losses is often a matter of logistics. Make it a priority to bring fluids with you on your bike, and set your watch to remind you to drink at specific intervals. Sports drinks are a great choice. Besides providing carbohydrates, they provide the important electrolyte sodium. Sodium and chloride, which form salt, are the major electrolytes lost in sweat. When you go out for a very long training session or compete in races lasting several hours, you may be at risk for developing hyponatremia, or low blood sodium levels. Hyponatremia results from losing large amounts of salt from sweating or from replacing fluid losses with plain water, diluting the sodium concentration of your blood.

To prepare for these sodium losses, you can increase your intake of salty foods for a day or two before a long ride or race, unless this is medically contraindicated. Avoid drinking plain water

TRAINING AND RACING IN THE HEAT	continued

when a sports drink or sodium-containing gel plus water can be consumed to maintain blood sodium levels. If plain water tastes better in the heat, consider one of the sports drinks with little or no flavor. These products are often very appealing in hot weather.

Weigh yourself before and after training to determine the amount of fluid lost in a typical training session (see the sidebar "Estimating Your Sweat Losses" in Chapter 5). Try to consume 24 ounces of fluid for every pound of weight lost to replace both sweat and urine losses. Sweeter products or something a bit salty may stimulate your desire to drink. Cool drinks are usually more palatable. Sodium may stimulate your drive to drink and enhance the rehydration process. Sweating results in large fluid losses and relatively small sodium losses for most endurance athletes, but some athletes are salty sweaters. Consuming large amounts of plain water after exercise can dilute your blood before your full blood volume has been restored. This dilution effect shuts down the thirst mechanism, and you urinate to bring your blood concentration back to normal. The end result is that you will produce a large amount of diluted urine before you are fully rehydrated.

drinking technique in training as much as possible—trying to mimic race conditions—and follow the pre-hydration guidelines from Chapter 5, starting 36 to 48 hours before the race.

During longer road races you may wish to try more concentrated sources of carbohydrates such as gels and pieces of energy bars. Just be sure to consume them with at least 6 to 8 ounces of fluid. If you are racing in very hot weather, sports drinks are probably your best choice, but you may need some plain water as well. Some very disciplined elite racers have trained their stomachs to consume one full bottle every half hour. Practice will also improve your ability to drink at very high intensities. Aim for at least 30 to 60 grams of carbohydrates per hour from the various products you consume and tolerate while racing. Commit to a specific number of bottles for the entire race, and try to drink on schedule. Practice your technique for receiving additional food and fluid in the feed zone.

If you are competing over the weekend in several back-to-back daily races, make sure that you pay close attention to recovery nutrition. Stage races place plenty of stress upon your fuel and fluid reserves. Pack supplemental products to ensure that you meet your carbohydrate needs and replenish glycogen stores prior to the next start time. It is essential that your recovery nutrition begin immediately after the race with ample carbohydrate intake combined with some protein.

You should eat every 2 hours after completing a stage and even continue to fuel with a light snack before bedtime. When eating at restaurants, emphasize concentrated carbohydrate sources such as pasta, rice, potatoes, breads, and cereals. Pack some of your favorite high-carbohydrate snacks and supplements for the race, and try to stay away from unusual foods to avoid any gastric surprises during the event.

CRITERIUM RACING

Criteriums, or circuit races, are exciting to watch—they are often shorter in length than road races and higher in intensity, and are held on spectator-friendly courses. They require good bike-handling skills for cornering and surges in effort to keep up with breaks and maintain a good position during the race.

When preparing for a criterium, the pre-race meal and snack timing are especially precarious. You definitely want to allow enough time for digesting the pre-race meal, probably at least 3 hours to compensate for the very high-intensity pace of a criterium. Start the race optimally hydrated, as drinking during criterium racing can be difficult. To keep blood glucose levels nice and steady, you can even down a carbohydrate gel in the 30 to 60 minutes before the race starts.

Consider keeping a sports drink in your water bottle, even for shorter races. The flavor can stimulate your desire to drink, and the carbohydrates keep blood glucose levels nice and steady. Drink whenever the opportunity presents itself, and become accustomed to drinking at higher intensities. Practice recovery nutrition after criterium racing, and make sure that you consume sodium and fluid after racing in hot weather.

TIME TRIALS

Time trials also require rest and adequate consumption of carbohydrates. Your competition efforts will take mental concentration, focus, and steady-state exercise in the crouched position. A full stomach could interfere with being comfortable in this position. Allow yourself at least 2 to 3 hours of digestion time following your pre-race meal. Rest and consume adequate carbohydrates for at least 24 hours prior to the time trial. Pre-hydrate, and consume a sports drink leading up to your start time for both the 40K individual time trial and the 50K or 100K team time trials.

You may consider consuming only water for a 20K time trial, as maintaining blood glucose may not be as much of a challenge for this distance when a proper pre-race meal is safely digested in your system. Choose a drink that stimulates your drive to drink. A sports drink is not necessary for shorter time trials, but it will not be detrimental, either. Sports drinks should definitely be used for efforts lasting longer than 1 hour. Make sure that your stomach does not get too bloated, and consume your fluid in sips. Practice consuming fluids in the crouched position so that you can drink as efficiently as possible during your time trial. You may want to try a bladder hydration system that will allow you to hold a more steady position on the bike while drinking. After the time trial, rehydrate and practice recovery nutrition.

TRACK RACING

Track racing takes place indoors or outdoors on a velodrome. Cyclists compete on fixed-gear bikes without brakes, and they are forced to pedal even when slowing down. Track cyclists use large gears, which take enormous amounts of power, and athletes competing at the elite level hit high speeds. Competitive track cycling includes very short individual and team sprints that last for less than a minute as well as longer sprints, such as the 500- and 1,000-meter time trials and the Kieren (2,000 meters), which last for about two minutes. Middle-distance events, which last for several minutes, include individual races (3,000 meters for women and 4,000 meters for men) and the 4,000-meter team pursuit. "Track endurance" events range in time from over 15 minutes to over 45 minutes and include races such as the Scratch Race (10K for women, 15K for men), the Points Race (25K for women, 40K for men), and the Madison (50K for men).

Training programs are specific to the types of events being raced. Sprint track cyclists usually have high levels of muscle mass and low body-fat levels, and they strength train to build lean body mass. Their training rides generally consist of short, high-intensity repetitions with adequate periods of recovery. Training sessions are longer, with some endurance rides, when preparing for longer sprint events. Endurance road cyclists often compete in the longer track races, developing their sprint training for these events.

For training, sprint track cyclists need to maintain a caloric balance and a carbohydrate, protein, and fat mix that will optimize the power-to-weight ratio by maintaining muscle mass and keeping body-fat levels down. Too much calorie restriction can result in inadequate carbohydrate intake for the volume and intensity of training and can cause loss of lean body mass. Instead of undereating, these cyclists may need to engage in crosstraining sessions to decrease body-fat levels. Endurance track cyclists tend to have a lighter and leaner build than road cyclists.

Because of the highly intense nature of track racing and the number of races an athlete may complete in a day, meal and snack timing for race day is a complicated matter, and good planning is essential. Although inadequate body-fuel stores are not a performance-limiting factor for a single sprint event, the fuel demands of competing in successive multiple events can be high. Prior to the event, carb loading is not necessary, but the cyclist should eat adequately in the days leading up to competition and maintain adequate muscle glycogen stores for the start of a competitive day. Your pre-race meal should consist of comfortable and familiar carbohydrate foods. Endurance track cyclists should keep the carbohydrate amounts high to top off glycogen stores for their event. If you race in the evening, what you eat earlier in the day is essential for maintaining fuel stores for the later start. Make sure that your last meal is at least 3 hours before the start of your warm-up. You can consume easy-to-digest carbohydrate supplements such as gels and bars 1 or 2 hours before the start to keep your blood glucose levels steady, especially if you compete in longer track events.

Track bikes do not have bottle cages, and it is not practical to hydrate during these short, high-speed races anyway. But it is important to pre-hydrate leading up to the warm-up with water or a sports drink. Look at the timing of your race schedule. Hydrate between races with a sports drink to offset fluid losses and keep blood glucose levels elevated for each race. If your schedule allows for some digestion time, plan to consume some easy-to-digest carbohydrate foods between events. Gels can provide a quick carbohydrate hit between sessions when more solid items would not be tolerated. Energy bars can also be useful for fueling and refueling, providing protein as well as carbohydrates for longer time intervals between events. Liquid meal replacements can be consumed somewhere in a full day of track racing. Hydration throughout the day should be steady, particularly in hot environments.

OFF-ROAD RACING

Mountain bike racing is performed on varying terrain and includes climbs, descents, and challenging single-track sections. What started as a fun recreational sport is now included in the Olympic Games. Competitive races include a number of disciplines. Cross-country events can be point-to-point races, with distances ranging from 15 to 62 miles (25K–100K), or they can take place on a circuit course with a loop of at least 3 miles. In the circuit events, riders complete a predetermined number of loops based on their racing category, with races lasting from 1 to more than 2 hours. Short-course circuit events are also available. Mountain bike races can be timed, and they can be quite long. Some go as long as 12 to 24 hours. These longer races can be completed solo or in teams.

Besides a solid endurance base, cross-country mountain bikers develop a high level of skill, and their training combines road and off-road riding, with the mix changing throughout the season. Downhill mountain bikers complete the majority of their training on the trails, and they may include aerobic work and a strength component in their training to develop power.

Many recreational mountain bikers ride off-road regularly and include road riding only when they do not have access to trails. Others may have to travel some distance to spend a day training or competing off-road. Elite cross-country riders tend to be lean and strong, as an excellent power-to-weight ratio is optimal for hill climbing.

Training Nutrition

The volume and intensity of training required for cross-country mountain bike racing call for a diet matched to energy expended in calories, carbohydrates, and protein. These athletes should plan an optimal daily training diet when preparing for races and events. Recovery nutrition is essential after hard workouts and between two-a-day training sessions. High-intensity sessions deplete muscle glycogen stores quickly and should be followed by proper recovery nutrition and daily fueling. Nutritional guidelines should also be followed before and after weight-training sessions (see Chapter 6). Recreational riders can match their intake to training levels as well. Although they would be expected to have somewhat lower levels of energy expenditure than focused racers most of the time, they may have periods of high-volume exercise on the bike on some excursions.

Achieving an optimal level of body fat can improve performance when climbing, but body-composition goals are best achieved through a combination of quality fueling and training. Calorie restriction that would compromise recovery is not recommended and could ultimately hurt your performance if you attempt to lower body fat too much. Dieting could also result in the loss of power if there is loss in muscle mass and inadequate body-fuel stores for rides and races.

During rides lasting over 1 hour, plan to hydrate and fuel with a sports drink. Off-road fluid supplies can be carried in a back-mounted hydration system, and two water bottles can be mounted on the bike. Other portable sources of carbohydrate are gels, energy bars, and dried fruit.

Competition Nutrition

Race start times for men and women competing in the various off-road categories are generally staggered throughout the day, so it is very important that you time your pre-race meals and snacks carefully for your start. Your stomach can experience some jostling during a mountain bike race or when you ride over tricky terrain, and race-day nerves can also affect your digestion. Focus on consuming optimal amounts of carbohydrates, sodium, and fluids the day before, the night before, and the morning of the race.

You can carb load for long race events by consuming 3 to 5 grams of carbohydrates per pound of body weight. Keep protein portions moderate and fat intake low in the 24 hours prior to the event. Hydrate enough that your urine is pale yellow in color, and salt your food if you are a salty sweater and anticipate racing in hot and humid conditions. Consume your pre-race meal about 3 hours before the start time (see Chapter 5 for more on the pre-race meal size), and include tolerable amounts of low-fat protein. Although early-morning starts may necessitate that you simply get up early and consume the pre-race meal in the appropriate time frame, later start times can be a bit trickier. For example, for a noontime start you may need to consume a hearty breakfast 4 to 5 hours prior to the start, and then a small to moderate carbohydrate snack 2 hours before the start. Plan ahead for your race start and experiment with food choices, portions, and timing. You should also consume a sports drink to steadily hydrate in the hours leading up to the start. Many mountain bike racers like to down a gel in the 30 to 60 minutes before the start for one last carbohydrate boost.

It is more difficult to drink fluids during mountain bike races than during road races, so it is important to start the race well hydrated. Consume 8 to 20 ounces (240–600 ml) of fluid 2 hours before the start, and another 8 ounces (240 ml) in the hour before the start, to prime your stomach and improve stomach emptying during the race. In many sections of the race it may be impossible to let go of the handlebars. Make a conscious effort to drink during gradual climbs, dirt roads, paved sections of the course, and relatively comfortable descents. During tricky descents or when climbing over rough terrain, you will be less inclined to drink. If you have an opportunity to preview the course before the race, try to determine which sections are more conducive to refueling and rehydrating.

Many mountain bike racers use a bladder hydration system so that they will have access to at least one source of fluids without having to let go of the handlebars. These systems provide adequate fluid for the first one or two laps; after that, you can consume a sports drink from a water bottle or have a helpful friend pass you a bottle in the feed zone. Set a goal for yourself to consume a certain amount of fluid per lap as dictated by your sweat rate—a bottle per lap may work well. Sports drinks work best because of the carbohydrates they contain. Aim to consume 30 to 60 grams of carbohydrates per hour from your sports drink. For longer races you may want to consume a carbohydrate gel, but during hot races keeping up with your fluid needs is essential. Choose a sports drink or gel relatively high in sodium if you are a salty sweater.

24-HOUR RACES

Twenty-four-hour races require riders to complete as many laps of a cross-country circuit as possible within a 24-hour time frame. Riders may compete solo or in groups, with the groups ranging in size from two to ten. Each individual lap can be completed in anywhere from 45 to 90 minutes depending on the level of the rider and the distance of the lap. Obviously, solo riders have a daunting nutritional challenge ahead of them. Team members have time between laps to rehydrate, refuel, digest, and even nap. The larger the team, the more time individual riders have for recovery. Because they get a break to rest, riders in 24-hour races can monitor their weight for sweat loss to prevent becoming dehydrated and even to prevent overhydrating.

Solo Riders

Solo riders need to contend with the challenge of riding the entire race with only short stops or slowdowns through the transition zone to refuel and rehydrate. Keeping up with fluid, carbohydrate, and sodium requirements while working within gastrointestinal tolerances during an ultraendurance race can be challenging. Carb loading in the 2 to 3 days before the race is recommended to arrive at the start with full body-fuel stores. Sports drinks provide a good balance of fluid, carbohydrates, and sodium, and the relatively high-sodium options are recommended for a race of this duration. Depending on the course profile, riders can drink regularly every 15 minutes or on specific sections of the course that are conducive to drinking, such as fire roads and the start/ finish of the loop. Riders should be familiar with their rate of sweat loss at the planned race pace and in various weather conditions. Other sources of carbohydrates that work well are gels, energy bars, bananas, and high-sodium items such as salted crackers. It is important to bring a variety of foods to the race so that you can choose from a number of items as your tastes and cravings change throughout the long race. A variety of sports drink flavors that you have tested out in training can also prevent flavor fatigue. Choose more solid items carefully, as you are racing the entire time and your stomach can become more sensitive as the race progresses. Consume solid bites or more concentrated drinks as needed for a carbohydrate boost. Cola can provide a caffeine boost during the race to help with mental focus and concentration.

Pairs

Teams of two generally trade places every one to two laps, allowing one rider to rest and refuel while the other is on the course. Depending on the length of the lap and the speed of the rider, the resting rider may have 60 to 120 minutes or more to refuel in preparation for his or her next turn on the bike. A sports drink high in sodium should be consumed on the course. Riders can bring gels, bars, jam sandwiches, a variety of fruits, and dry cereals to eat between laps as tolerated. Experiment with various carbohydrate food items while simulating race conditions to see what works best for you.

Small Teams

Riders on small teams consisting of three or four members have longer recovery times between laps than pairs, often at least 2.5 hours, and sometimes even 3 to 4 hours. Although these team members should still focus on maintaining their fluid, carbohydrate, and sodium intake on the bike to some degree, there is less pressure to keep up with rehydration and refueling on the bike in this kind of race. To allow plenty of time for stomach emptying, digestion, and absorption of nutrients, however, riders should consume both food and fluids immediately after coming off the bike. Try solid items such as sandwiches, pasta, energy bars, and fruit. Keep taking fluids up to your next lap, but don't overhydrate, and be careful not to overeat. Consume protein foods wisely, keeping portions small, and avoid fat because it takes longer to digest. Include items that are high in sodium, such as broth and other soups, as well as a variety of flavors and choices over the 24-hour period.

Large Teams

Teams of six or more riders have ample time to digest between laps. They can keep their hunger under control and their blood glucose levels steady by eating a large carbohydrate snack 3 to 4 hours or more before their next lap start and a smaller snack of easily digested carbohydrates 1 to 1.5 hours before the lap start. Your consumption of solid foods should decrease the closer you get to the start time for your next turn. Riders should consume some fluid during the lap and hydrate as needed at the completion of each lap.

CYCLO-CROSS

Cyclo-cross takes place on a grassy loop, usually a few miles long, with a few short road or dirt road sections. There are numerous sections where riders must dismount to navigate man-made barriers. Muddy, wet, and snowy conditions are not uncommon for this race discipline, which is technically challenging and fast. Cyclo-cross training and competition are very high in intensity. Riders often train twice daily, and they need to take care to get enough calories and nutrients to support this training. But the most important nutritional considerations for cyclo-cross have to do with what takes place 24 hours before the race start time.

Though cyclo-cross race times may last only 45 to 60 minutes, it is prudent to optimize your muscle glycogen stores the day before a race. Because of the high intensity of cyclo-cross racing, muscle glycogen depletion can occur quickly. To boost muscle glycogen stores, allow yourself 24 hours of rest or light training, and focus on adequate carbohydrate consumption during this taper. Avoid scheduling training sessions close to race day that could result in muscle damage, as this would impair your muscle glycogen stores. If you are competing twice in one weekend, practice good recovery nutrition after the first race.

With pre-race meal timing it is best to err on the side of caution and allow plenty of time for digestion in order to avoid "cross-gut." Pre-race nerves may further accentuate gastrointestinal upset. Most cyclo-cross racers prefer to allow 3 to 4 hours of digestion time and to focus on easy-to-digest carbohydrate foods. If your race begins after noon, factor in two pre-race meals. Have a large breakfast, and then a small "lunch" 3 hours prior to your race consisting mainly of carbohydrate-based breakfast foods. Drink plenty of fluids several hours before the race for optimal hydration. Many seasoned cyclo-cross racers prefer to stop fluids 30 minutes before a race to avoid feeling bloated on the bike. Gels and sports bars can also be consumed in the 2 hours before race time if well tolerated.

Once you arrive at the starting line, your nutritional options are likely to remain limited, as cyclo-cross racing is done without a water bottle cage. Many racers try a carbohydrate gel at the starting line or halfway through the race for a carbohydrate boost, as the risk of bonking during cyclo-cross seems to be high. Even with a bottle hand-up once a lap you may be able to manage only a few gulps of fluid because of the course and race dynamics.

DOWNHILL RACING

Downhill races typically last from 2 to 5 minutes over a 1.5K to 3.5K course. Racers need to navigate a mix of rapid descents and technical sections over single tracks, rocky tracks, and forest roads. The "4 Cross" is a downhill event in which four riders compete against each other and pass through a series of gates, with riders typically taking 30 to 40 seconds to cover the course. In the "Dual Slalom," two riders race head to head down two parallel slalom courses, with runs lasting 20 to 45 seconds. And in the "Observed Trials," competitors navigate a series of obstacles, and points are deducted for mistakes.

When you are preparing for a downhill event, it is important to make sure you are well fueled, well hydrated, and physiologically and psychologically comfortable at the starting gate. Although each individual race takes only a matter of seconds or minutes to complete, you may do some practice runs that day, and you may have to make several runs during the full schedule of competition. Whatever your training regimen was the day before, make sure that you have matched your output with adequate carbohydrates and calories for your intake. In fact, consuming carbohydrate amounts slightly above your requirements will ensure that your glycogen stores are fully replenished for race day.

When planning your pre-race meal, allow ample time for digestion. Three hours is ideal, but if this is not practical for your start time, modify the timing and the meal accordingly. If this time interval is feasible, aim for 1 to 1.5 grams of carbohydrates per pound (2–3 g/kg) of body weight. Practice with food choices and portions before high-intensity training sessions similar to your expected competition efforts. In the hours leading up to the start time, you can maintain blood glucose and fluid levels by sipping a sports drink. Try consuming gels to maintain adequate blood glucose levels, which are imperative for adequate concentration, focus, quick decision making, and skillful bike handling.

You may need to consume a steady supply of easily digested carbohydrates throughout the day to maintain your energy levels through multiple runs. High-carbohydrate energy drinks, sports drinks, gels, and energy bars make good choices, so plan ahead and organize your nutrition supplies. Fluid losses may be exacerbated in downhill racers who wear heavy protection equipment and clothing that covers arms, legs, and hands, so steadily hydrate throughout the day of competition.

RECREATIONAL DISTANCE CYCLING

Recreational cyclists often ride a significant number of weekly miles, though they may exercise at lower intensities than cyclists preparing for competition. However, if your goal is to complete a century or another long ride in a specified period of time, there may be a sufficient amount of high-intensity training in your weekly program to make it worth your while to pay special attention to nutritional considerations. Overall, your diet should emphasize the carbohydrate amounts that match your training for both shorter weekday rides and longer rides. Especially with the longer rides, you need to focus on replenishing your muscle glycogen stores. After very long rides, recovery nutrition is helpful not only for replenishing these stores but also for minimizing your fatigue over the next several days.

If you ride after work or commute back and forth to work on your bike, make sure that you always carry adequate fluids and focus on hydration both on and off the bike. Pale urine indicates that you are well hydrated.

When preparing for longer weekend excursions, including centuries, you may want to rest for 24 to 48 hours before your ride and consume a diet rich in carbohydrates in order to fill up your muscle glycogen stores. Eat a meal high in carbohydrates several hours before the ride to replenish your liver glycogen. When you ride longer than 90 minutes, even at lower intensities, make an effort to consume 30 to 60 grams of carbohydrates per hour from sports drinks to maintain your hydration and blood glucose levels. Because you will likely be riding at a relatively low intensity in comparison with competitive cyclists, consuming solid foods and gels during the ride along with water may be simply a matter of taking an enjoyable and relaxing break.

One of the benefits of being part of an organized ride is the accessibility of the fuel stations that supply water, fresh fruit, sports drinks, treats, and a variety of easily digested carbohydrates. You can also pack some of your favorite on-bike foods and store them in your jersey pockets and in various bike bag options. Experimentation will teach you what foods work best for your stomach. It is best to start refueling early to prevent hypoglycemia. If you do start to manifest some of the symptoms of hypoglycemia, slow down and take in some carbohydrates.

Aim for a steady supply of fluid and fuel. Know your sweat rate for the conditions and intensity at which you plan to ride. One quart (960 ml) of a sports drink provides around 56 grams of carbohydrates. Add in semisolid and solid items carefully, and take in these products with at least 8 ounces of water. If you consume several hundred calories at a rest station, make sure that you give yourself a bit of digestion time at rest. Seasoned cyclists can learn to increase their tolerance for more solid items on the bike, but keep in mind that hydration with a sports drink is always your first priority.

NUTRITION AT HIGH ALTITUDE

Cyclists and other endurance athletes who live, train, or compete at altitude should be aware of how the elevation can affect their body and performance. Breathing at high elevations can be challenging, if you are not used to it, and exercising at high elevations places special demands on the respiratory and circulatory systems. The higher the elevation, the less dense the air that you breathe. Altitude "hypoxia," or a reduction of oxygen in your body tissues, can be the result. Fortunately, your body adjusts or "acclimatizes" to altitude, though this process can take up to three weeks. When you travel quickly to altitude, you may experience symptoms such as rapid heart rate, headache, shortness of breath, fatigue, nausea and vomiting, loss of appetite, decreased urine output, and insomnia, often referred to as acute mountain sickness (AMS). This complex of symptoms is most likely to occur in individuals who reside at sea level and ascend rapidly to a high altitude. Symptoms normally develop in 6 to 12 hours, peak at 24 to 48 hours, and subside in 3 to 7 days as your body acclimatizes to the new conditions.

Upon arriving at a high altitude, your body will experience an initial drop designed to concentrate the red blood cells that carry oxygen in your blood. During the adjustment period, your blood volume will return to normal. You will also develop more red blood cells if you stay at altitude for several weeks, and your muscles will begin to extract more oxygen from your blood. Altitude clearly causes metabolic adaptations that affect your nutritional needs. Even relatively moderate elevations of up to 5,000 feet can affect how you should eat and drink.

The air at high altitudes is extremely dry, and every breath you take results in fluid loss. "Insensible" fluid losses through your skin also increase. Normally these insensible fluid losses amount to only about half a quart daily; this amount can increase to 2 quarts daily at high altitudes. This is in addition, of course, to your urinary output and sweat losses during exercise, all of which implies that hydration should be your top concern when you are training or competing at a high elevation, especially if you are not yet acclimatized. Replacing your fluid losses at altitude takes a conscious effort. Always try to keep some source of fluid with you. You may require 4 to 8 quarts (3.8–7.6 L) of fluid daily depending on your training schedule. Light-colored urine indicates that you are matching your fluid losses.

When at altitude, you also have to consider your carbohydrate and calorie intake. Your basal metabolic rate can increase by as much as 40 percent the first few days at altitude; it then gradually drops off to about 15 percent above sea-level values. Overall, your energy needs at

CONTINUES

NUTRITION AT HIGH ALTITUDE   continued

altitude may increase by 200 to 300 calories daily. Although this may sound like a simple problem to cure, there is a real decrease in appetite that sets in at altitude, causing you to undereat by several hundred calories daily. Undereating and losing weight at altitude do not result in body-fat loss. What is more likely to occur is that your body will utilize valuable protein stores for fuel.

It is best if the extra calories that you take in at altitude come from carbohydrates. High-carbohydrate diets may reduce the effects of acute mountain sickness. They also delay the depletion of muscle glycogen, which will support endurance training at altitude. Another benefit is that carbohydrates are more easily digested and better tolerated than high-fat foods. Keep these foods handy, and have snacks to meet the additional caloric requirements. Small, frequent meals may be better tolerated with the decrease in appetite. "Bonking" can creep up on you at altitude, making adequate intake of glucose during exercise imperative. Sports drinks clearly provide both needed fluids and carbohydrates.

Although research on vitamin and mineral requirements at altitude is limited, enough is known about iron to suggest that it deserves your attention at higher elevations. Athletes training at altitude should have their iron status monitored regularly. Having adequate iron stores ensures that you will be able to produce needed red blood cells at altitude. Besides emphasizing good food sources of iron, you may want to take an iron supplement to boost and maintain your stores of this nutrient. Be careful not to supplement to excess, however, and only take supplements under a physician's supervision. Too much iron causes oxidation and free radical production. Adequate intakes of folate and vitamin B12 are also needed for red blood cell production.

Focusing on foods high in antioxidants like vitamins C and E may also be beneficial, as exercising at high altitude places "oxidative stress" upon your body. Exercising at altitude may also raise your vitamin E requirements. Food sources of vitamin E include fortified cereals, whole grains, wheat germ, nuts and seeds, green leafy vegetables, and vegetable oils. Recommendations for vitamin E supplementation are currently at 100 to 400 IU daily.

10

NUTRITION FOR
DISTANCE RUNNING

PARTICIPATION IN THE SPORT OF RUNNING currently stands at an all-time high. The number of marathon finishers in the United States exceeded 400,000 in 2005. In fact, the average running time for the marathon is getting longer, reflecting the extent to which participation in this race has expanded. The half-marathon distance also has a high level of participation, with more than 500,000 finishers in 2005. By March 2006, more than 500 marathon and 500 half-marathon courses had been certified by USA Track & Field (USATF). Running is no longer just for the lean and elite—people of all ages and fitness levels are joining in and becoming healthier in the process.

The shorter races remain the most popular, with more than 3 million 5K finishers and more than 1 million 10K finishers in 2005. Other race distances are 8K (4.8 miles), 5 miles, 10 miles, 15K (9.3 miles), and 20, 25, or 30K (12, 15, or 18 miles). More than 8 million participants completed races of all distances and more than 10,000 racecourses were certified in 2006. There are also ultradistance events, such as 50K (31 miles), 100K (62 miles), and 100-mile events. Although these do not attract as large a number of participants, they are nevertheless as popular as ever, with more than 90 certified ultrarunning events in 2006.

The largest age groups at the races are now men in their late thirties and early forties and women in their twenties. Runners are often club members, frequently train with a coach, and may prefer to enter events that raise money for charity. Fitness and fun runners are mainly females between the ages of eighteen and twenty-nine. Runners who prefer to compete in longer distances are often quite competitive and goal-oriented. Many of the runners in this group train year-round, and the majority are male participants averaging forty years old. Charity runners—primarily women—tend to enter just one event per year. Trail runners, primarily men, average twenty-nine years old.

Distance runners tend to improve their performance with age, and many run and train for more than a decade before they reach their best running times. Recreational runners are often satisfied to simply run for optimal fitness and health and enjoy the social aspects of running. Whatever a runner's level of training and competition, paying heed to nutritional considerations can enhance his or her participation in the sport. For recreational runners, that might mean simply feeling better and enjoying greater health benefits. For elite runners, however, proper nutrition can provide just the boost in performance that is needed to reach top goals.

TRAINING NUTRITION

Because there is such wide variation in running—with some runners just starting out at the 5K level and others running marathons or ultradistance events—training programs vary widely. Some runners may have just signed up for their first charity run, while others are planning to race in a dozen or more events during the year, perhaps at a variety of distances. Even an experienced marathoner may choose to compete in an early-season 10K race and a half-marathon as he or she builds up to the marathon of his or her choice for the season. Because of the broad range of competitive goals, training programs are somewhat specific to the athlete. Running sessions may include longer runs designed to develop aerobic endurance, on the one hand, and intense runs and interval work designed to improve the anaerobic system and speed, on the other. Training nutrition has to take all this into account and be flexible enough to be adapted to any level.

Weekly training sessions for a 10K may consist of 30 to 60 minutes of running, a longer run, and track sessions and tempo sessions. As a runner's competitive distance increases, the length of his or her base training runs and long run should also increase. When training for a marathon, many runners find it useful to incorporate a 5K or 10K race into their plan. And marathon training requires months of preparation, with carefully scheduled long runs and time for adequate recovery. Weekly marathon training can approach 30 to 45 miles weekly. Elite marathon runners may train twice daily and up to 90 miles weekly. Water running and/or weight training may also be included in a runner's program.

PRE-EXERCISE HYDRATION AND FUELING

Fueling for Training

Eating too much too close to training or competition for your own personal tolerances is probably the biggest nutritional mistake that you can make as a runner. Because running jostles your gastrointestinal system, GI disturbance is a more common problem in running than in other endurance sports. Timing your pre-exercise meals is important for feeling "light" during your run and avoiding unpleasant symptoms such as a sloshing stomach, bloating, cramping, and diarrhea.

Prior to a short, relatively easy run, what you eat before training may simply be a matter of comfort and fending off hunger or hypoglycemia. It is not uncommon for runners to train in the early-morning hours. Some experiment and find that having something light, such as juice and a plain piece of toast, works best at this time. Regardless of your tolerances, make sure that you drink water or even a sports drink to hydrate. On long morning runs, consider taking a fluid bottle or fluid belt with you. Consuming a sports drink maintains blood glucose levels in the latter part of a longer run, but even on shorter runs it is good practice. It prepares you for longer races, and it helps in any run that occurs after you have not eaten for several hours, whatever the time of day.

Consuming regular meals and snacks replenishes your fluctuating liver glycogen stores and consequently helps maintain steady blood glucose levels throughout the day and during training. For afternoon or evening runs, try to time your meals carefully and eat 3 or more hours before running. Leave enough space between meal or snack times and training times, especially for high-intensity runs and speed work. Emphasize carbohydrate sources that are easily digested. You may want to consider a liquid sports supplement, a meal-replacement product, or an easily digested gel before longer training sessions. Real food products also work well if you have experimented and determined your own tolerances.

The Long Run

Experiment with pre-race eating before your long weekend run. This practice sets the stage for race day—it is particularly important to know your tolerances and preferences when racing a distance of 10 miles (16K) or longer. Although it may be tempting to sleep as late as possible before a long early-morning run, the pre-exercise meal is necessary for filling both liver and muscle glycogen stores. Liquid meals may work best, but you can also experiment with carbohydrate foods that are low in fiber. Knowing what works for you in training will help lighten pre-race nerves and help you feel more comfortable about your nutritional choices on the big day.

Ideally, take in as much carbohydrate as you can tolerate up to 1 gram per pound (about 2 g/kg) of body weight 2 hours before the long training run. Although you may leave a longer time interval after eating before a race start, this is still essential practice for having a quality and well-fueled long run. If you decide to eat even closer to the long training run, lower your carbohydrate intake to half a gram per pound (about 1 g/kg) of body weight. Food choices should be kept simple. Two hours prior to a long run, a 160-pound (73 kg) runner could consume more than 100 grams of carbohydrates from 2 slices of toast covered with 2 tablespoons (40 ml) of jam, plus 12 ounces (360 ml) of orange juice. After this meal and leading up to the run, 24 ounces (960 ml) of a sports drink would provide another 40 grams of carbohydrate or more.

Some simple morning noshes that sit easy in your stomach and pick up your run include:

- ½ bagel with 1 tsp. (8 ml) peanut butter and 1 tbsp. (20 ml) jam with 8 oz. (240 ml) juice
- ½ cup instant oatmeal with 4 oz. soy milk and 1 tbsp. (20 ml) raisins
- 1 medium-sized high-carbohydrate energy bar and 1 banana
- Pretzels and hummus with a glass of juice
- Liquid meal replacement
- Crackers with a nut spread and banana
- Smoothie with milk, yogurt, and fruit
- Tortilla with peanut butter and raisins
- Chocolate milk and grapes
- Toasted waffle with syrup and fruit
- Bowl of rice and juice

Of course, coffee or tea, or a glass of water, can be included with all of these suggestions. Even with a good morning carbohydrate boost, longer or higher-intensity morning runs may call for use of sports drinks. Experiment with pre-run foods and fluids, as well as with water or sports drinks during your run, to determine what provides the best energy boost within your tolerances.

Hydration and Fluids

Runners should focus on consuming fluids throughout the day and maintaining adequate hydration. Light-colored urine indicates that you are well hydrated. Try to consume about 8 to 12 ounces every hour when not training, and practice the pre-hydration guidelines outlined in Chapter 5. Find the best timing to prevent sloshing in your stomach during training. It is helpful to hydrate well during the day, but step up your fluid intake within an hour of your run. Some of your early-morning carbohydrate food choices can also be hydrating fluid choices, such as a high-carbohydrate sports beverage, a sports drink, juice, soy milk, or dairy milk. Hydrating before a morning run, especially a run of more than 45 minutes, is important, so consume what you are able beforehand as your stomach and time allow.

RECOVERY NUTRITION

Hard training runs, and particularly twice-daily sessions, require that you pay attention to recovery nutrition. Running can cause some damage to muscle fibers, which can delay glycogen recovery. Carbohydrate intake immediately after training will start the process of muscle gly-cogen resynthesis and prevent the gradual process of muscle glycogen depletion that can occur over several days' time or longer. Consume half a gram of carbohydrates per pound (1 g/kg) of body weight immediately after exercise and plenty of fluids for recovery. You can also add 10 to 20 grams of protein, as this may aid in muscle repair. Monitor your weight before and after running to determine sweat losses, and consume 24 ounces of fluid for every pound lost. Consuming sodium after training, particularly in hot weather, can aid in the rehydration pro-cess. Make sure that you continue to rehydrate the rest of the day, and use your weight as a gauge of hydration.

After a morning run, you could consume a breakfast of cereal, milk, and fruit with a glass of juice. After an evening run, a recovery drink can hit the spot. Don't forget to consume the same amounts of carbohydrates and protein again in 2 hours to continue the recovery process. This could mean a mid-morning snack of yogurt and fruit, or a dinner containing carbohydrates from rice, pasta, potatoes, or some type of whole grain. Remember that thirst is not the most sensitive indicator of fluid needs. Continue to rehydrate in the hours after the run.

Runners training in hot weather may find that their appetite is limited immediately after training. Smoothies are a refreshing and hydrating choice that pack in plenty of carbohydrates and protein. Frozen fruit is also appealing, as is frozen yogurt and similar cold treats, including sorbet and sherbet.

Runners who incorporate high mileage for distance running need to pay close attention to re-covery nutrition. If you plan two training sessions in one day, be sure to refuel immediately after the first training session. Then, consume a meal or snack every 2 hours until the next workout, taking care to choose easily digested foods as the time for the next run approaches. If the second workout is a weight-training session, consume the recommended amounts of protein and carbo-hydrate beforehand as outlined in Chapter 6.

BODY COMPOSITION

Elite distance runners are typically lean and thin, most likely due to a combination of genetics and a high volume of training. Runners at any level, aware that carrying "dead weight" does not enhance performance, may develop weight-loss goals. An important first step when losing weight is to have your body composition assessed. If you are already lean, decreasing body-fat levels fur-ther may offer no performance improvement. If your body type just is not that of an elite runner, dieting offers no further benefit. It is better to focus on proper nutrition strategies to fuel and hydrate your body for optimal performance. Serious runners should aim for a target weight that is not unrealistically low and that can be maintained without excessive training or stringent dieting.

An overtrained or underfed runner does not produce his or her best performance. It is best to focus on sensible weight-loss strategies such as those outlined in Chapter 6.

Choose a body-composition assessment method that you can use at regular intervals throughout the season. Look at the big picture when setting your weight-loss and body-composition goals. Gradual weight loss is less likely to compromise your performance, energy levels, and recovery than rapid weight loss requiring a higher level of calorie restriction. If you have a modest amount of body fat to lose, lose it earlier in the season, well ahead of your important race dates. If you have only a small amount of body fat to lose, stick to quality eating, and let quality training take care of the body fat.

IMPORTANT NUTRIENTS
Iron

Distance runners, especially females, seem to be at higher risk for developing compromised iron status. Left untreated, iron deficiency can lead to anemia, which clearly impairs exercise performance. But even before it reaches the stage of anemia, iron deficiency appears to affect training and performance in some athletes. Clearly, iron deficiency needs to be corrected before it progresses.

Iron deficiency should be treated with a diet high in heme iron. Good sources are listed in Table 3.6 and include lean red meat, chicken, and fish. Nonheme iron can also be emphasized and consumed with a food rich in vitamin C to enhance absorption. For example, you can consume iron-fortified cereal with orange juice, mix beans and tomatoes in dishes such as chili, and include a baked potato and broccoli at the same meal. Iron-fortified breads and cereals are a major source of iron in the diet. If you purchase natural foods that are not iron fortified, you may be inadvertently reducing your iron intake. To maximize your iron absorption from foods, do not consume them with foods that inhibit iron absorption, such as coffee, tea, or an excessive amount of bran. Bran products contain phytates, which inhibit iron absorption. Phytates are also found in nuts, seeds, wheat cereals, peanut butter, and soy products. If you don't eat adequate amounts of heme iron, consider taking a low-dose iron supplement as part of a multivitamin providing 15 milligrams of iron daily.

It makes sense for runners, especially females, to screen for iron deficiency once yearly. Low levels of serum ferritin may warrant safe and monitored supplementation to bring levels back up into the middle range. Occasionally, increases in serum ferritin result in a slight increase in hemoglobin, reflecting that a mild anemia may have been present. Some athletes may benefit from a slightly higher level of hemoglobin.

An iron treatment dose is often more than 50 milligrams daily, and up to 300 milligrams daily for more severe anemia. But don't start taking therapeutic iron doses without first seeing a physician. Some individuals are susceptible to hemochromatosis, or iron overload, in which excess iron is deposited in the liver and other internal organs, causing serious damage. Too much iron when it is not really warranted can also decrease absorption of other important minerals like copper and zinc. Also, never self-diagnose an iron deficiency just because you are feeling run-down and tired. Fatigue can be related to a number of health, nutritional, and training factors.

When you have true anemia, a physician can prescribe a therapeutic dose of iron. Liquid ferrous sulfate is well absorbed. You can increase your dose slowly to minimize any gastrointestinal side effects of taking the supplement. Ferrous gluconate is often better tolerated than other forms of iron. Take your supplement on an empty stomach with a dose of vitamin C or a glass of orange juice. Iron supplements should be taken separately from calcium supplements to prevent a decrease in iron absorption. Your physician can monitor your serum ferritin and hemoglobin levels for several months afterward and continue, adjust, or discontinue supplementation as appropriate.

WOMEN, BODY WEIGHT, AMENORRHEA, AND BONE DENSITY

Bone health is an issue that has received heightened attention over the past two decades owing to the increasing rate of osteoporotic fractures and stress fractures. Exercise levels, hormone balance, genetics, and nutritional factors such as calcium intake all influence the maintenance of this important body tissue. Your calcium balance depends on the amount of calcium you consume and absorb as well as the amount you lose in your urine. The athlete at risk for development of compromised bone health must take all of this into account when making decisions about his or her diet and supplementation.

Bone is a dynamic tissue that is constantly being broken down and rebuilt under the regulation of your body's hormones. When the process of bone breakdown or bone resorption exceeds bone formation, bone loss occurs. If this bone loss is prolonged, osteoporosis, a condition in which low bone mass has developed and bone is fragile, can result, and there is greater risk for fracture.

The hormone estrogen plays a crucial role in maintaining bone tissue in women. When estrogen levels are low, bone serves as a source of calcium to maintain normal levels of calcium in the blood and perform important physiological functions in the body. Even if physical activity is high, low estrogen levels, as seen in amenorrhea and after menopause, can result in bone loss.

Female athletes seem to have a higher incidence of menstrual irregularities than women in the general population. *Athletic amenorrhea* has been used to describe menstrual imbalances

CONTINUES

in female athletes. A variety of factors have been implicated in the development of amenorrhea in athletes. It appears that the predominant factor is inadequate calorie intake. An excessive training load, or an increase in training that is not matched with proper food intake, creates a caloric deficiency that can result in amenorrhea. Of course, disordered eating or a full-blown eating disorder can also result in a chronically low intake of calories and amenorrhea. Amenorrhea may be more common in certain sports that emphasize small frames, such as running, gymnastics, and dance, but it can occur in any endurance sport under certain precipitating conditions.

Whatever the causes, one thing that is clear is that female athletes with amenorrhea have lower bone mass than athletes who menstruate regularly. A greater incidence of stress fractures has also been reported in athletes with current or past menstrual disturbances. Athletes with these health concerns should see a sports medicine physician for assessment of bone mass, hormonal status, and appropriate medical treatment. This may include hormone replacement, weight gain recommendations, nutritional guidelines, and modifications in training. These female athletes can benefit greatly from the guidance a sports nutritionist can offer regarding appropriate calorie intake and the balance of other nutrients in the diet.

Athletes being treated for amenorrhea should increase their calcium intake to 1,500 milligrams daily and their vitamin D intake to 400 to 600 IU daily. Refer to Table 3.5 for a list of foods high in calcium. If this amount cannot be achieved through diet, calcium supplements can make up the difference. Doses of 500 milligrams of calcium carbonate or calcium citrate combined with vitamin D can be taken once or twice daily. Excessive intake of protein, when combined with inadequate calcium intake, and high intakes of caffeine and sodium can also aggravate calcium absorption. Overall balance in the diet, especially adequate calorie intake, should also be restored. Weight-bearing exercise may be continued, though not at excessive levels.

COMPETITION NUTRITION

Competition in running is primarily an aerobic activity. Elite runners can complete a 10K in less than 30 minutes, and elite marathoners race for just over 2 hours, but recreational runners may take more than twice this long to complete the same runs. Many marathons also include walkers who enter for fundraising purposes and take even longer to complete the 26.2-mile event. Hydration is critical for all entrants in any running event, and fueling during the race is also essential for any race lasting longer than 90 minutes. The pre-race meal is also a key consideration, as races often have early-morning starts, race nerves can affect food tolerances, and early-morning liver glycogen stores are typically low. The perfect pre-race meal will prevent hunger before and during the race, be easily digested, and top off blood glucose levels before the start.

5K, 8K, 10K, and 10-Mile Races

Because of the typical times in which races ranging in distance from 5K to 10 miles will be completed, these races will not significantly challenge your muscle glycogen stores if you have eaten properly in the 24 to 48 hours before the race. You do need to arrive at the starting line not only with properly fueled muscles but also with replenished liver glycogen stores and a content and settled stomach. A pre-race meal can help keep blood glucose levels nice and steady throughout your warm-up and race and prevent feelings of hunger. Of course, you will want to be cautious when choosing your pre-race foods and timing your meal. Experiment in training with timing and portions, and consume easily digested carbohydrate foods and/or liquids that you know you can tolerate. Determine your best pre-race food and fluid tolerances through practice and experimentation prior to early-morning runs.

Once you address your fueling needs, your major nutritional risk during a race of this length will be dehydration. Faster runners competing in cool weather in the shorter distances are unlikely to waste time to stop and drink. But as race finish times increase and the temperature rises, optimal pre-race hydration becomes even more crucial. You need fluid when you wake up in the morning, and you can lose fluid in the hours prior to the race through sweating and urination. Gauge your fluid status by monitoring the color of your urine. Drink adequately to fill and empty your bladder before the race. Consider your warm-up time, travel time to the race, and waiting-around time, and use these moments to drink plenty of fluids, without overhydrating.

You may want to experiment with a sports drink for both fluid and a carbohydrate boost before racing, sipping it in the time before the race. Carbohydrate-sensitive athletes can experiment with this pre-race strategy in training. Fluid intake during the race should benefit racers running for more than an hour. Stick with about 16 to 32 ounces (480–960 ml) per hour. You may want to consume only water during a 5K or 10K, but a sports drink is fine if it appeals to you. Slower finishers in the 10-mile race should consider hydrating with the sports drink provided at aid stations.

Half-Marathon (21.1K) and 20K, 25K, and 30K Races

Races ranging in distance from 20 to 30K (or 12–18 miles) present their own set of nutritional challenges and definitely require an on-course fueling and hydration plan. For some top competitors, the half-marathon—a 13.1-mile race—does not present a significant fuel challenge, as the race is completed in less than 90 minutes. However, the vast majority of runners will complete the half-marathon in more than 90 minutes, and perhaps even in 2 to 3 hours. What matters for any of these race distances is that you are aware of your projected race time and plan your nutrition program leading up to the race accordingly.

For most competitors, all of these race distances require carbohydrate loading the day before the race, careful pre-race meal planning, and refueling with a sports drink to compensate for sweat losses. Taper your training up to 2 days before the race, and boost your carbohydrate intake to 3 to 4 grams per pound (6.5–9 g/kg) of body weight. Stick with low-fiber carbohydrate sources, keep protein portions low to moderate, and keep fat intake very low. Follow the same plan the day before the race, but have your large meal fairly early so that you wake up hungry and anticipate your pre-race meal.

In your pre-race meal, emphasize easily digested carbohydrate foods. Liquid sources low in fiber should be well tolerated. Aim to consume 30 to 60 grams of carbohydrates during any race lasting longer than 90 minutes. Sports drinks are generally the best-tolerated source of carbohydrates, but many runners have also experimented successfully with gels during longer races. Choose gels that contain sodium, and make sure that you take them with at least 8 ounces of water.

Marathon (42.2K)

Clearly, the marathon—a 26.2-mile race—requires careful nutritional planning on the part of even the most elite competitors. Lasting more than 2 hours for the world's top runners, the marathon is most challenging at about the 20-mile mark, when "hitting the wall," or running low on muscle glycogen, becomes a real possibility for any race participant. Having a nutrition strategy that puts your fuel gauge on full at the starting line is essential. This means knowing how to carry out a successful carbohydrate-loading plan during the pre-race taper.

Carbohydrate loading is synonymous with the marathon. The principles of carbohydrate loading, and the most current research-based guidelines, are provided in Chapter 5. After your last long run prior to the marathon, pay close attention to matching or even slightly exceeding your carbohydrate requirements for the remainder of your training during taper week. For maximum glycogen stores, an intake of 4 to 5 grams of carbohydrates per pound (9–11 g/kg) of body weight has been recommended, or about 500 to 700 grams daily. However, carbohydrate loading does not necessarily require enormous amounts of food and calories. On rest days, your calorie needs may not be especially high, and you simply need to eat enough carbohydrates to fill up your glycogen stores. This may only necessitate that a greater percentage of your calories be derived from carbohydrates, preferably those low in fiber.

During this critical time, make sure that noncarbohydrate foods do not crowd out the foods high in carbohydrates. Exceeding your protein and fat requirements serves little purpose during

FLUID AND SODIUM BALANCE FOR LONG-DISTANCE RUNNING

Hyponatremia, or low blood sodium levels, seems to be more prevalent in the marathon than in other long-distance events. Some hyponatremia-related fatalities have even occurred in marathons over the past several years, and other problems related to overhydration and dehydration during competition persist. There are a number of possible reasons for this trend, including the increased number of marathon participants who are racing recreationally and taking longer than 4 to 5 hours to complete the race—which translates into more sweating and sodium loss for these competitors. And the fitter a runner becomes, the more he or she sweats. So as runners new to distance racing increase their fitness and training levels, their sweat levels are increasing as well, causing greater sodium losses. Hyponatremia also seems to occur more often in women than in men, and women are signing up for marathons in increasing numbers.

But hyponatremia may also be caused by excessive consumption of fluid, which dilutes the concentration of sodium in the blood. Women generally have lower sweat rates than men and consequently lower fluid needs during a distance race, and women who do not realize this can drink too much, reducing their sodium levels. Women also have less blood volume than men, and when they overdrink, they overfill more rapidly. Drinking a sodium-free fluid does not adequately replace the sodium lost in sweat as the marathon progresses.

Part of the problem seems to be that marathoners often receive the message that they need to drink a lot of fluid. Rather than taking the time to determine their own personal sweat rate by weighing themselves before and after training (see the sidebar "Estimating Your Sweat Losses" in Chapter 5 for proper procedure), they may drink too much, often with a sodium-free fluid such as water. It is easier to drink when running at a recreational pace than when running at the elite level, and recreational runners often slow down to fill up at the water stops. It is ironic that most of the winners of any given marathon are probably the most dehydrated finishers on the course. At their fast pace, they not only have limited time for drinking, but also likely produce a higher amount of sweat. Even marathoners finishing in the 3- to 4-hour range are likely to sweat more than they replace. Finishers taking 4 to 6 or even more hours to complete a race are much more likely to overhydrate. To prevent overhydration and hyponatremia during a marathon, practice the following precautions:

- Determine your sweat rate during long training runs. Check your weight before and after training, and measure your fluid intake during the run with a graded water bottle. If you are gaining weight during long runs, you need to decrease your fluid intake.

CONTINUES

FLUID AND SODIUM BALANCE FOR LONG-DISTANCE RUNNING | continued

- Use a sports drink during all your long runs, and practice training with the sports drink offered on the course.
- Choose a relatively high-sodium sports drink if you are a salty sweater, as evidenced by salt marks on your clothing. Check the sodium content of the drink to be offered on the racecourse.
- Develop and practice a drinking plan for your long runs, based on the information you learn from monitoring your weight before and after training.
- Consume a sodium-containing fluid after long runs based on the weight-monitoring results. Aim for 20 ounces (600 ml) for each pound (about 0.5 kg) of weight loss.
- Don't drink obsessively in the days leading up to a marathon. Hydrate so that your urine is pale yellow in color, but don't overhydrate. Remember that your sweat losses decrease considerably during your pre-race taper. Just drink to maintain a good level of hydration.
- Don't rehydrate indiscriminately after a marathon. Your risk of hyponatremia can remain high for several hours. Have a variety of recovery foods and drinks that provide sodium.

---

the 48 hours preceding a marathon: Just keep reasonable amounts of protein and fat in your diet. Have a menu prepared ahead of time to ensure that you not only choose high-carbohydrate foods but also consume enough of them. Refer to the food lists providing 30-gram carbohydrate servings in Chapter 4, and draw out some sample meals. Beware of sweet foods that may provide some carbohydrates but also plenty of fat. They may fill you up and taste good, but they won't adequately fill your muscle glycogen stores. This may also be a good time in which to consume some extra sugar and high-carbohydrate fluids such as juices and smoothies, which have the added bonus of being low in fiber. You may wish to avoid high-fiber foods for 24 to 48 hours before the event to ensure that you can "race light" and reduce gastrointestinal difficulties.

It is important to be aware that your body stores a considerable amount of fluid when you carbohydrate load. Don't be alarmed if your muscles feel a bit stiff, or if the number on your scale increases, when you are carbohydrate loading. The additional stored water helps to delay dehydration during the race. Of course, you should also hydrate your body by drinking plenty of fluids in the 48 hours prior to the race. Keep a water bottle and hydrating fluids with you at all times. Monitor the color of your urine to ensure that it is light in color and that you are optimally hydrated, but not overhydrated. During your race taper, your sweat losses go down considerably. Just make sure you rehydrate sufficiently after any activity. At rest, try to stay in fluid balance. There is no need to hyperhydrate for the marathon, a practice that could actually increase your risk of developing dangerous fluid overload and hyponatremia. Several full bladders of light-colored urine should indicate that you are in fluid balance.

Plan to consume a high-carbohydrate breakfast the morning of the race. You can somewhat diminish your overnight liver glycogen losses by consuming a late-evening snack; however, eating the right pre-race meal, and timing it appropriately, can be much more effective in refilling your liver glycogen stores and helping you maintain blood glucose levels when racing. Eating properly is far superior to not eating the morning of the race. Eating breakfast also settles your stomach and prevents hunger during your warm-up and at the starting line. Some runners may prefer to have a liquid meal replacement or breakfast shake in order to avoid eating solid foods before starting several hours of hard running. Experiment during long training runs to determine your favorite and best-tolerated pre-race meal. If you are traveling to the race, you may want to pack some of your favorite race foods to supplement your restaurant diet. Avoid trying new foods in the days leading up to the race. If you will be running in hot weather, or for several hours, increase your salt intake prior to the race to prevent a decrease in blood sodium levels while racing.

What you consume during the marathon is just as important as what you had beforehand. Meeting your fluid needs while running in competition is also crucial. The faster you run, the more heat you produce and the greater your risk of dehydration. Even if your marathon starts in the early morning to avoid excess heat, be prepared for temperatures to rise in hot climates. Running longer than 90 minutes will also challenge your body's carbohydrate stores, no matter how careful your pre-race eating. Focus early in the race on consuming carbohydrates in order to delay depletion of your glycogen stores. Sports drinks are your best-tolerated option and provide both needed fluid and carbohydrates.

Aid stations are generally provided every mile in a marathon. Find out ahead of time what sports drink will be provided at the race and drink it during training to develop a taste and tolerance for the product. You need to average about 4 to 8 ounces every 15 to 20 minutes, or consume the amounts that most closely match your sweat rate or minimize your sweat losses. Depending on your sweat rate, which you should know beforehand from monitoring during training, you may only need to drink at every other aid station. Practice drinking and running in shorter early-season races. Even seasoned racers do not consume the full amount of liquid provided in the cup, but you can practice your technique. Pinch the cup to form a funnel, and take down two gulps. If you have to slow up in order to drink, you will still improve your race time by consuming adequate fluids and carbohydrates.

Many runners also consume carbohydrate gels during a marathon. Make sure that you consume a gel packet with 8 ounces of water. If you think that you will require several energy gels

RUNNING AND GASTROINTESTINAL DISTRESS

Runners seem to be more susceptible than other endurance athletes to gastrointestinal (GI) distress and diarrhea during training and racing. The causes of these problems are unknown, but they may be related to the constant jarring and repetitive motion of running. GI upset may also be related to the intensity of your running, decreased blood flow to the GI tract, and dehydration. Some runners may be able to identify specific foods that aggravate GI problems.

Drink plenty of fluids before and during exercise to prevent dehydration and maintain adequate blood flow to your intestinal system. Start drinking early to prevent dehydration. Some runners have benefited from lowering their fiber intake close to exercise. You may even want to reduce your fiber intake at dinner the night before an early-morning run. Caffeine, particularly from coffee, is known to have a laxative effect. Limit or avoid caffeine, as well as artificial sweeteners such as sorbitol and aspartame, which may aggravate symptoms, if they seem to cause problems for you. Make sure that you are not taking any medications or over-the-counter supplements that aggravate GI symptoms, and if you are experiencing chronic GI difficulties, see a physician to eliminate the possibility of intestinal parasites and other medical problems. Some runners may need to experiment with removing specific foods from their diet to determine which items may be aggravating their symptoms. You can also experiment with pre-run meal timing and food choices. Remember that although fueling before a run is important, plenty of time should be left for stomach emptying. Some runners may tolerate liquid choices, easily digested energy bars, and gels more easily than other foods before a run.

during the race, consider carrying them in a waistband or waist pack. Your goal is to consume at least 30 to 60 grams of carbohydrates every hour. Practice with gels during training. By race day, you should have mastered the best fluid- and fuel-replacement techniques to support your individual preferences and tolerances. You should also be flexible enough to consume the products offered on race day and adjust your plan as needed during the race.

Ultrarunning

Ultradistance races typically start at 31 miles but can also be 50, 62, or 100 miles. Other races are organized around a time frame, where you run as far as possible for 12, 24, or 48 hours. For races of these lengths, nutritional factors can determine whether you complete the race. Runners training for ultras extend the long weekly run that is the core of marathon training and put in high mileages on a regular basis. Besides building stamina and mental fortitude, these training runs give you the opportunity to develop your skills in fueling and hydrating for the long haul.

For competition, the taper presents the opportunity to carbohydrate load, as discussed earlier in this chapter (in the section "Marathon [42.2K]") and in Chapter 5. Eat a large snack the night before the race, and have your tried-and-true pre-race breakfast already planned out. Use liquid supplements as needed to be optimally fueled and hydrated before the race. Increase your salt intake to compensate for salt losses during the race, as the long running times and constant fluid intake can increase the risk of hyponatremia. Many ultrarunners do finish races with some weight gain, lower sodium levels, and even hyponatremia.

Dehydration can prevent an ultrarunner from completing a race. Drink at least 20 ounces of fluid per hour, or more or less depending on your sweat rate. Know your sweat rate for your race pace and various environmental conditions (for method, see the sidebar "Estimating Your Sweat Losses" in Chapter 5). Set your watch if you need to remind yourself to drink, and have a predetermined fluid schedule outlined. Carry a sports drink for both carbohydrates and fluids, and make sure a specific number of bottles will be available to you at each aid station. Because of the length of the race and the degree of hunger that can set in, ultrarunners often take in gooey carbohydrate gels or the more solid and chewy carbohydrate blocks and other semisolid items, such as energy bars, to fuel and settle their stomach. Experiment with these supplements. You may also want to consume liquid meals for a caloric boost during sections of the race where you power walk, as well as electrolyte tablets and drinks to prevent hyponatremia.

The foods and fluids provided on the racecourse can vary greatly. You may find fruit, pretzels, cookies, potato chips, M & Ms, peanut-butter-and-jelly sandwiches, salty broth, and/or baked potatoes at aid stations. Find out what will be available on the course and practice with these foods during training. Be sure to take along some tolerated salty food items and salt tablets to replace sodium losses during the race.

Start replacing fluid, carbohydrates, and sodium early so that you can finish the race. Know your sweat rate at the planned race intensity and in various race conditions. Once you become depleted, it can be difficult to dig yourself out of a nutritional hole. If your stomach feels bloated and is not emptying properly, you may be dehydrated. If your stomach does become overfull and you vomit, start consuming a sports drink slowly to rehydrate. It will empty from your stomach as quickly as water and provide needed carbohydrates and sodium.

Sodium losses vary greatly among individuals and in various weather conditions. Experiment in training with use of salt tablets to determine what works for you. Salty foods such as soup or broth may be available at aid stations for some electrolyte replenishment. Keep any salt tablets that you carry with you away from moisture so that they do not break down before you ingest them.

Wrapping them in plastic should work. Make sure that you ingest them with plenty of water. If you determine that you are losing weight during the race at check-ins, rehydrate with sodium-containing fluids that increase fluid retention. If you determine that you are gaining weight during the race, then lower your fluid intake and up your intake of sodium-containing products.

Drinking your calories is often your best option. Experiment with various drinks and flavors to prevent taste fatigue, and try to consume more than 250 calories per hour. Besides sports drinks, you may benefit from more concentrated sources such as high-carbohydrate supplements and meal replacements. These products are not as hydrating as sports drinks, but they provide needed carbohydrates. If you use these products, they will empty more comfortably from your stomach if you are well hydrated. Having access to a variety of foods during the race is a good idea because it gives you different options to choose from, which may make it easier for you to keep up with your calorie and fluid needs. It is fine if you decide not to use some of them—they will at least be there if you need them. They not only provide variety but may satisfy a craving or two along the way. Caffeine-containing soft drinks can provide an energy and mental boost later in the race. During long races, mental fatigue can occur, and a nice glucose boost from carbohydrates may be just what you need.

11

NUTRITION FOR
SWIMMING

INDIVIDUALS OF ALL AGES AND ABILITIES are involved in the sport of swimming at the recreational and competitive level. Swimmers train with local clubs, on high school teams, and in college under the National Collegiate Athletic Association (NCAA). The NCAA has a strong swimming program, with more than 7,000 men and 10,000 women participating in the sport (including diving) during the 2004 to 2005 season. U.S. Masters Swimming offers training and competition opportunities for athletes ranging from nineteen to eighty-plus years old and includes more than 45,000 members across the nation. Many masters teams train at local YMCA pools or at high school and university pools, but competitive swimming also includes open-water and long-distance swimming.

Competitive swimming requires a serious commitment to training at the high school, collegiate, and Olympic levels. These swimmers may complete anywhere from six to twelve sessions every week, each covering a training distance of 1,000 to 2,000 meters (for a sprinter in the taper phase) to 10 kilometers (for a distance swimmer in the base phase of training). Elite swimmers also incorporate land-based aerobic training, such as running and cycling, into their programs, as well as weight training. Swim training programs can vary greatly, however, depending on the swimmer's age, fitness level, competitive goals, and race events and distances. Elite swimmers tend to have pronounced upper-body muscle development. They are generally tall and usually have a low level of body fat, though it may not be as low as that of endurance athletes in land-based sports. Some body fat in the right distribution may, in fact, enhance buoyancy in the water.

Collegiate swim training is often very demanding, and in sharp contrast to the brevity of the competitive events for which these swimmers train, can require long periods of time in the pool. Collegiate swimmers can train up to 20 hours per week during the height of the season. They may schedule two sessions daily—one in the early morning or afternoon and another in the evening—to accommodate school and work schedules, although they may decrease their training load to 8 hours weekly out of season.

Masters and club swimmers are a diverse group, but even those who do not compete at meets are often serious about training. Masters swimmers may train at high intensities and anywhere from 1 to 2 hours daily. They may also participate in open-water events and in triathlons and various forms of land training. The amount of time that masters swimmers put into their weekly training varies greatly but often reaches levels that warrant an endurance training diet. Like athletes at the high school, college, and elite levels, masters swimmers will find that paying proper attention to nutrition will enhance their health, their fitness, and their performance in swimming.

TRAINING NUTRITION

Swim training intensities can include both aerobic and endurance-based training as well as anaerobic training sessions of interval work at different percentages of maximal heart rate. Clearly, swim workouts can rely heavily on muscle glycogen stores for fuel. Swimmers who regularly fail to replenish these stores after hard training sessions may find that they eventually become unable to complete sessions. Inadequate recovery can be compounded over the long haul. Even swimmers who frequently crosstrain, thus drawing on different muscle groups, may find that the benefits afforded by proper endurance nutrition are worth the effort it takes to pay attention to dietary matters.

Swimming competition itself often lasts only seconds or minutes, making competition highly anaerobic, though aerobic metabolism becomes more significant as the distance of the event increases. Olympic-level races last from 20 seconds to 15 minutes. Because of these relatively short race times at high intensities, swimming competition requires a unique set of nutritional strategies. Buildup of lactic acid, rather than depletion of fuel stores, is likely to be the limiting performance factor. Of course, an exception would be long-distance swimming, which draws more on the aerobic system and presents a real challenge to muscle fuel stores. Regardless of the competitive event, serious training requires adequate recovery nutrition.

RECOVERY NUTRITION
Energy

Calorie requirements for swimming increase as the volume and intensity of individual training sessions and of the program as a whole increase. Because of the wide range of training programs found among swimmers of all ages and competitive levels, calorie intake will vary from one athlete to the next. Refer to Chapter 4 for calorie recommendations. Moreover, an athlete's calorie requirements will vary from day to day depending on the intensity and distance of his or her swimming and crosstraining efforts. Match your calorie intake to your training for the day for optimal recovery, and pay close attention to eating well when you have several heavy training days in a row. An athlete who does not do so too often finds that fatigue and subpar performance can even halt training after just a few days of high-intensity effort.

Both male and female swimmers have special needs during their teenage years. Adolescent male swimmers, on the one hand, sometimes experience a period of heavy growth and muscular development that can result in significant short-term increases in energy needs. When combined with swim training, these growth spurts can use enough calories to outpace average intake, and during these times, it is best for optimal swimming performance if the athlete knows how to plan and carry out a healthy eating plan rather than just filling up on pizza and other fast foods. The danger for adolescent female swimmers, on the other hand, is falling prey to society's ideals of thinness, which can lead to inadequate calorie intake. Hormonal changes during these years can mean an increase in body fat for young women, and female swimmers may struggle to maintain low levels of body fat despite a high training load. But the energy needs of serious swimmers can exceed several thousand calories daily, as swimming may burn anywhere from 500 to 700 calories per hour. If excess body fat is truly a concern in regard to health and performance, following sensible weight-loss strategies may be warranted (see Chapter 6).

Carbohydrates

Adequate calorie intake is of course synonymous with consuming enough total carbohydrates for optimal recovery. Swim training typically lasts from 60 to 120 minutes per session. But it is not just long, steady-state sessions that can use up this important and limited fuel supply; shorter sessions of high-intensity interval or speed work can also deplete muscle glycogen stores. Match up your daily carbohydrate intake with your training as outlined in Chapter 4. After strenuous training sessions, consume adequate carbohydrates for recovery, aiming for 0.5 gram of carbohydrates per pound (about 1 g/kg) of body weight, or about 50 to 75 gram of carbohydrates, immediately after exercise to begin the synthesis of muscle glycogen before your next training session. You can combine these carbohydrates with small amounts of protein, if desired, but make sure carbohydrate intake is your first priority. Convenient items that can be brought to the pool for consumption include energy bars, high-carbohydrate supplements, bagels, crackers, juices, and fruit.

Fluid Requirements

Swimmers training in the steamy environment of a heated indoor pool or outdoors in the hot sun can have moderate sweat losses that may not be obvious to them because they are wet anyway.

Just how much a swimmer sweats in the water can vary depending on individual sweat rates and fitness levels. Nevertheless, sweat rates are also affected by water temperature, air temperature, and humidity, particularly in an outdoor pool.

Limited data currently indicate that sweat losses in the pool are relatively moderate when compared with other types of endurance training, even for athletes who spend a significant amount of time traveling up and down the pool. Though these sweat losses are not as heavy as those measured in cyclists or triathletes, they should still be replaced through fluid intake during training. As in any sport, one of the best techniques for monitoring your fluid loss is to weigh yourself before and after training (see the sidebar "Estimating Your Sweat Losses" in Chapter 5). For every pound of weight lost, drink 24 ounces of fluid during and after training. Keep in mind that sweat rates vary among individual athletes. Though average fluid losses among swimmers may be relatively moderate when compared with land athletes who train in the heat, some individuals may have higher sweat rates than others.

Fortunately, swim training presents a convenient opportunity to replace fluids whether the sweat loss is modest or significant. Leave your fluid bottle at the end of your lane for relatively long or intense swim sessions. Concentrate on taking gulps every 15 minutes or so or whenever the nature of the training session allows you to take a quick break without disrupting your interval work. Gauge whether your drinking habits are keeping up with your losses by weighing yourself before and after training. Sweat losses would be expected to be higher during anaerobic threshold sets than during steady swimming, but knowing your individual sweat rate in different types of sessions is the key.

When you monitor your before and after weight, check that you don't overhydrate. Because sweat losses are somewhat diminished when swimming, very motivated drinkers may exceed their fluid losses. For training sessions lasting more than 1 hour, and for shorter sessions that are high in intensity, consume a sports drink. These drinks provide carbohydrates to maintain adequate blood glucose levels and supply your muscles with fuel when body stores run low. Sports drinks can easily meet both your carbohydrate and fluid requirements if consumed in adequate amounts. They also increase the drive to drink and enhance fluid absorption. Hydrate leading up to practice, and consume 20 ounces of fluid for every pound (600 ml for every 2 kg) of weight loss during training.

NUTRITION ISSUES FOR SPECIFIC GROUPS

High School Swimmers

Many dedicated swimmers are in adolescence and experience dramatic physical changes in their bodies during this time. In order for them to reach their full growth potential, the energy demands of both growing and training must be met. This is especially true of adolescent boys, as mentioned earlier, who often require frequent meals and snacks in order to maintain both weight and growth. They should also include high-quality protein in their diet and may require up to 0.75 to 0.9 gram of protein per pound (1.6–2 g/kg) of body weight per day. These elevated protein requirements are easily provided in a well-balanced diet, particularly if energy needs are met. Protein supplements are not necessary for a high school swimmer's diet.

Swimmers who struggle to meet caloric requirements may simply find that their busy training and school schedules limit the amount of time they have to eat. Planning is essential for these high calorie-burning athletes. Close attention should be paid to recovery nutrition after early-morning training. Packing foods and fluids high in carbohydrates when getting ready for school is essential. If the schedule and classroom setting allow, a mid-morning snack will aid the recovery process. Lunch should not be left to some fatty choice in the school cafeteria; rather, it should be planned out and should consist of high-quality protein, adequate carbohydrates, and reasonable amounts of good fats. A pre-exercise snack is also useful for maintaining energy levels and steady blood glucose levels for afternoon training. Of course, a variety of foods is essential for a balanced diet, and young athletes should be sure to make good food choices to support muscle growth, recovery, and top performance.

Adolescent swimmers should consume water during breaks in training, or sports drinks for training lasting longer than 60 minutes. Sports drinks maintain hydration levels and provide fuel for athletes who have not eaten for several hours. High-intensity training sessions can also warrant the ingestion of sports drinks to provide glucose for fuel.

Consuming a high level of calories can ensure a diet adequate in vitamins and minerals, if planned wisely, but adolescents have higher calcium and iron requirements and need to plan accordingly. It is easy to fall short of these nutrients. Good intakes of calcium along with optimal training can help a young athlete achieve peak bone mass, reduce risk of stress fractures, and minimize the effects of bone loss later in life. Good sources of calcium should be emphasized in the diet (see Table 3.5). Iron intake is a particular concern for adolescent girls, who have increased iron losses with menstruation. Food sources high in iron should be emphasized in the diet (see Table 3.6). A multivitamin providing the RDA for iron may be beneficial, but higher doses should not be taken without a physician's supervision.

Overall, high school athletes should minimize their reliance on fast foods as much as possible to limit their intake of fatty foods and hydrogenated and saturated fats. Packing fruits to supplement school lunches is one good option. Low-fat milk and yogurt may also be available at most school cafeterias. Athletes can pack healthy low-fat lunches consisting of sandwiches, fruit, and other carbohydrate items such as pretzels and granola bars. Their parents should become involved in meal planning and assist them, especially when it comes to meals served at home. Their dinners should include quality protein sources and whole grains. An evening snack can provide additional nutritious calories.

Swimmers struggling with body-weight management issues, despite their high energy output during training, should not try to conform to an ideal promoted by the media and other elements of society. Young women especially need to realize that their body-fat levels are likely within a healthy range. They should appreciate that success in competition is related to a number of factors and not solely based on low body-fat levels. Following sensible strategies for controlling weight at a healthy level is best. It is especially important to avoid extreme diets, such as ones that eliminate almost all fat or restrict calories to an unreasonable level for keeping up with growth and training needs. In some cases, rigid dieting can lead to disordered eating or even full-blown eating disorders. Again, parents should be aware of the signs and symptoms of these disorders and provide and seek help if needed. (For more specific weight-loss guidelines for endurance athletes and more information about eating disorders, see Chapter 6.)

Collegiate Swimmers

Swimmers in college are limited by the NCAA to 20 hours of training during the regular season. Training often consists of two practice sessions daily. These athletes frequently weight-train, and running is often part of their training program.

Collegiate swimmers must meet high energy and carbohydrate requirements and carefully practice the principles of recovery nutrition, particularly when training twice daily. Inadequate carbohydrates between an early-morning and late-afternoon training session can compromise performance. Carbohydrates should be consumed immediately after training and should be followed by a high-carbohydrate meal or snack. They can also be consumed several hours prior to exercise to replenish liver glycogen stores and provide fuel for the second training session. Collegiate swimmers, like all athletes, should monitor their fluid losses during training by checking body weight before and after exercise, and they should drink water and sports drinks during high-intensity workouts or sessions that are relatively long in duration, as well as during strength training sessions, to replace their fluid and carbohydrate losses. The real challenge for collegiate athletes, however, is meeting their nutritional requirements when eating at the college dormitory or preparing meals in their own apartments.

Eating dorm food can present a new challenge to the college athlete accustomed to family-style home-cooked meals. Although an athlete may be able to keep foods in his or her dorm room and may have the opportunity to purchase foods near campus, the majority of his or her nutritional needs will have to be met at the dorm dining hall during breakfast, lunch, and dinner.

AGING AND THE MASTERS ATHLETE

Men and women are eligible to become masters swimmers regardless of ability, speed, age, or competitive swimming background. Masters swimming therefore encompasses swimmers ranging in age from nineteen to eighty and beyond. A wide variety of events are offered at swim meets, including freestyle events ranging from 50 to 1,500 meters as well as 50-, 100-, and 200-meter events for freestyle, backstroke, breaststroke, and butterfly. Relay events are also offered, as are open-water distance events longer than 1 mile and up to 10 kilometers.

In a survey conducted by United States Masters Swimming (USMS), over half the respondents indicated that they were "serious" swimmers. Most USMS members weight-train regularly and cycle and run to complement their swimming. Probably one of the most significant physiological changes that occurs with aging is a slight decrease in muscle mass after age thirty. Weight training can offset these muscle losses and provide the masters athlete with the benefits of maintaining strength and power. Muscle is metabolically active tissue. Weight training can strengthen weak body areas and improve one's strength-to-weight ratio. Masters athletes who are dedicated to resistance training should refer to the corresponding nutrition guidelines provided in Chapter 6.

Because of the large range of training commitments and schedules found among masters athletes in any endurance sport, calorie and carbohydrate requirements can vary. It is the intensity and volume of training that make the difference. Masters athletes should be aware that their nutritional requirements can change throughout the year as they make seasonal adjustments in training volume and focus. As athletes age, a decrease in calories may be necessary to maintain a healthy weight. However, the quality of the diet should not be compromised. Nutrient-dense foods become an even more important component of the diet when calorie requirements decrease.

Although aging is typically regarded as a function of chronological age, the number of years a person has been alive may be a very poor predictor of functional age. Masters athletes in their fifties and sixties often outperform sedentary persons in their twenties. But even well-conditioned and trained athletes will experience a decline in aerobic power after age thirty to thirty-five. VO_2max declines after age twenty-five, but at a slower rate in active individuals than in sedentary ones. Muscle strength plateaus at age thirty-five to forty and then declines, though muscle strength can be maintained and improved with a good resistance training program. Masters athletes adopt healthy lifestyles and appear to derive very tangible health benefits from

CONTINUES

AGING AND THE MASTERS ATHLETE   continued

these good habits and their training. These benefits may include more favorable blood lipid profiles and lower risk for developing hypertension, diabetes, and osteoporosis.

It is thought that for the most part, older athletes should follow the same recommendations for carbohydrate, protein, and fat intake as younger athletes with comparable training programs. Aging may increase the need for calcium in women to prevent osteoporosis, though men can also develop this debilitating condition. Vitamin D requirements increase after age fifty, as do vitamin B6 requirements. Continuing to choose nutrient-dense foods throughout a lifetime is useful for meeting the increases in vitamin and mineral needs that occur with aging. Masters athletes concerned about adequate vitamin and mineral intake can take a balanced low-dose multivitamin and mineral supplement. This supplement should also provide the daily value of vitamin B12 for individuals over age sixty, since gastric acid levels decrease with aging, reducing absorption of B12 by the body. Calcium supplementation may also be beneficial to meet higher calcium needs.

Calcium needs increase with age among both men and women. One study conducted by researchers at Tufts University that included both men and women over age sixty-five found that an average intake of 1,350 milligrams of calcium (500 of which came from a supplement), combined with a diet high in protein, produced higher bone mineral densities in the test subjects after three years. Lower calcium intakes—of 850 milligrams daily—did not work synergistically with the protein to improve bone density. Researchers are still trying to determine the underlying mechanisms and why the high protein intake was not accompanied by increased calcium excretion in the urine. The bottom line from this study is not for older individuals to eat excess protein but to meet their calcium requirements and maintain good protein intake within the recommended ranges for health and training.

Older athletes should also pay attention to fluid intake. Thirst sensation declines in older individuals, affecting their fluid regulation. At the same time, their fluid requirements actually increase, as more water is needed to remove waste products from their system. Generally, older athletes can tolerate exercise in the heat but should drink as much fluid as possible before and after the exercise session. They should aim for the high end of recommended fluid intake amounts during exercise, consuming 8 ounces every 15 minutes. Older athletes should also pay close attention to warning signs of dehydration and be aware of how any medications they are taking may affect heat regulation.

Dining hall hours may be limited, however, and it can be difficult to coordinate class, training, and meal times. Dining hall hours may not always be sufficient to accommodate a heavy schedule. The serious swimmer may not be able to meet his or her calorie requirements in just three meals daily—but falling short can lead to weight loss or suboptimal recovery from daily training. Athletes may also be overwhelmed by the variety of foods offered in a dorm cafeteria. If they are not familiar with sensible sports nutrition principles, they may not feel confident that their food choices match their training requirements. They may have no idea of how to estimate their carbohydrate needs, and even if they do, it may be difficult to know what ingredients are contained in various entrees offered. The food-preparation techniques used in the kitchen and the fat content of certain items may be a mystery, as the popular terminology for dorm protein offerings—"mystery meat"—implies.

It is also possible to overeat at a dining hall where portions and choices are unlimited. Moreover, many athletes may snack while studying and feel that they have fewer food restraints imposed upon them than they did at home. They can begin to feel somewhat out of control in regard to their food choices. Food may also be a large part of the social life at school, and it can be all too easy to consume excess calories when a typical evening includes going to a party, visiting the snack bar at the student union, or dropping in at the local pizza parlor or pastry-laden coffeehouse.

Nevertheless, with knowledge and planning, eating in the dorm cafeteria can support a healthy sports diet. Athletes should educate themselves about the carbohydrate content of various foods and balance these items with quality protein sources and healthy fats (see tables in Chapter 4). For example, a grilled chicken breast with rice, a steamed vegetable, and a salad topped with olive oil would make a good meal choice for a college athlete. Athletes should understand that they can include some fat in their diet. It is a matter of balancing their fat intake with the day's other food choices and the training plan for the day and the rest of the week.

When eating in a dorm, survey all the choices before deciding what to consume. Don't just pile up on everything; rather, try to balance the meal by incorporating items from several food groups. Remember that the menu in the cafeteria is provided on a cycle. Your favorite foods and other interesting items will come around again. Treats can be part of the diet as long as they are well-chosen items and in reasonable portions. It can be tempting to stay in the cafeteria and socialize with friends. However, this can lead to eating when you are not hungry. Let your food choices be well informed and based on rational decisions, and avoid the overeating that can happen when emotions or social situations govern eating habits.

For those athletes who cannot meet their nutritional requirements with the three daily meals offered, several options exist. Many cafeterias permit snacks such as sandwiches, fruit, or yogurt to be taken from the dining hall for consumption later. You can also keep a small fridge in your

MEN AND OSTEOPOROSIS

According to the National Osteoporosis Foundation (NOF), the number of men with osteoporosis and low bone mass reached a combined total of more than 14 million in 2002. This figure is expected to increase to more than 17 million in 2010 and to well over 20 million in 2020. The prevalence of osteoporosis alone is estimated to have affected more than 2 million men in 2002 and is projected to affect almost 3 million men in 2010 and well over 3 million men in 2020. Men of all races and ethnic groups are affected, though Caucasian men appear to be at the greatest risk.

According to the NOF, one-third of all hip fractures occur in men. Men also suffer from osteoporotic fractures of the spine, wrist, and other bones. Despite the fact that this disease significantly affects men, however, and the fact that osteoporosis risk among women has been well publicized in recent years, it remains underdiagnosed, underreported, and inadequately treated among male patients.

It has long been known that the proper type of exercise for stimulating production of osteoblasts, the cells that build bone, is weight-bearing activity and weight training. But some sports, such as swimming and cycling, do not offer these specific weight-bearing benefits. Swimmers and cyclists should crosstrain in other sports that do include weight-bearing activity and engage in a weight-training program. But nutrition also plays a role in preventing osteoporosis in men. Men's diets seem to become deficient in calcium around age twenty-five, with two-thirds of men not meeting the recommended intake of 1,000 milligrams (1,200 milligrams over age fifty) per day. Men should be sure to get adequate vitamin D as well, either through intake of 400 to 600 IU daily or through 10 minutes a day of sunlight exposure.

Low levels of the hormone testosterone are also a risk factor for osteoporosis in men, just as low estrogen levels are for women. Blood testosterone levels can fall during long-term exercise, and resting levels may be lower than normal in highly trained endurance athletes. Some researchers have theorized that the male reproductive system may in fact be blunted in response to endurance training. Testosterone levels do decline naturally with age.

More men do achieve greater peak bone mass levels than women and do not have the accelerated bone loss that women can experience at menopause. It is possible that some men will not achieve peak bone density for genetic reasons or due to smoking and/or excess alcohol intake. Certain medications, such as long-term glucocorticoid treatment, may also adversely affect bone mass. Some men develop osteoporosis for no identifiable reason. Whatever the reason, prevention is the best medicine; consult with your doctor.

dorm room and stock fruit, yogurt, milk, cereal, and granola bars. You may decide to purchase snacks on campus between classes as your schedule permits. Fruit smoothies make excellent recovery snacks and may be available at a juice bar. Purchase your favorite sports drink if possible to minimize fuel depletion, enhance your workouts, and ultimately improve your recovery. (See also the sidebar "Eating Well on Campus" in Chapter 12.)

COMPETITION NUTRITION

One of the ironies of competitive swimming is that hours and hours of preparation week after week and month after month culminate in races lasting just seconds or minutes. Although each race may be brief, however, swim meets may be held over several days' time—and international events can last even longer. Swimmers often compete in multiple heats and events over the course of the entire event. It is not unusual for a swimmer to compete in a heat in the morning and a final later that day or have several races scattered throughout one day. It may be necessary to travel to races, either by car, bus, or plane, and traveling not only can cause fatigue but also can take a toll on one's eating habits.

CARB LOADING

Before swimmers arrive for a competition, they likely have tapered their training for several days, increasing their muscle glycogen stores. If so, they have a better chance of being race-ready and well fueled. Although an athlete's calorie needs may decrease somewhat, or even greatly, depending on the extent of the taper, it is still necessary to eat enough carbohydrates to ensure plenty of available glycogen. A high percentage of the pre-race diet should therefore come from carbohydrates. Carbohydrate stores can be filled with 24 hours of proper eating on a high-carbohydrate diet combined with rest. Swimmers who follow a longer race taper should decrease their total calorie intake over that time period to prevent unwanted gains in body fat.

The pre-competition meal should replenish low liver glycogen stores in the morning and increase blood glucose levels. Swimmers may have to very carefully time their food and fluid intake throughout the competitive day in order to replenish stores between heats, semi-finals, and finals. Some well-tolerated choices are sports drinks, fruit juices, and gels when there is only a short period of time between races. For longer time intervals, swimmers can consume bagels, English muffins, energy bars, fruit, or sandwiches. Swimmers normally complete light warm-ups prior to competition and a swim-down after the event to improve recovery, so take all of this into consideration when planning your snacks and fluids for a competition day. Well-tolerated protein choices can augment this carbohydrate intake. Good choices include lean turkey, yogurt, dairy products and soy milk, and energy bars with a high protein content. If traveling to competition, bring some of your favorite and well-tolerated competition foods with you. In addition, drink fluids steadily—without overdrinking—but be aware that if the competition is being held in a warm and humid environment, you will need to increase your fluid intake accordingly. Your urine should be pale in color if hydration levels are adequate.

LONG-DISTANCE SWIMMING

The fuel demands of long-distance swimming are high, and swimmers specializing in this niche should consume adequate snacks and meals before and after all training sessions. They should also hydrate with a sports drink during their long training swims in order to provide fuel when muscle glycogen stores run low and develop a tolerance for these products, which will become even more essential when racing. Their carbohydrate intake should match their swim training volume, as outlined in Chapter 4.

EATING WELL ON THE ROAD

Swimmers and other athletes competing in their sport in high school and college may frequently be presented with the need to make healthy food choices on the road. It is important to consider how traveling affects your pre-competition nutrition program and plan accordingly. Special meals can be ordered on airlines with advance notice. When traveling—by road or plane—try to bring bottled water with you to make sure you maintain good hydration levels. Make healthy choices at airports whenever possible. Aim for turkey sandwiches or wraps for lower-fat choices and plenty of carbohydrates. Choose low-fat frozen yogurt, fruit juices, soft pretzels, low-fat milk, baked potatoes, and/or smoothies. Plan ahead, and pack some of your favorite nonperishable items, such as energy bars, granola bars, cereals, packets of instant breakfast mix, dried fruit, whole-grain crackers, powdered sports drinks, meal replacements, instant soups, fruit juices, and any other items that travel safely.

You can also investigate the food options at your destination before you leave. Call ahead to your hotel and find out about food establishments in the area. Internet searches can also provide valuable travel information.

Some healthy suggestions for various meal and snack choices when eating on the road are outlined in Table 11.1.

TABLE **11.1**	MEAL AND SNACK CHOICES WHILE TRAVELING

MEAL	FOOD CHOICES
Breakfast	Choose dry or cooked cereals, juices, fresh fruit, waffles, French toast, and/or pancakes. Keep margarine and butter to a minimum. Order skim milk and low-fat yogurt. Bagels and muffins with small amounts of peanut butter and jam are good choices as well. Omelets made with egg whites are fine, but go easy on the cheese. Ask for vegetable fillings instead.
Lunch	Try to frequent restaurants that have low-fat sandwiches made from poultry or lean meats. Low-fat tuna salads may be available. Go easy on the cheese, and ask for extra vegetable toppings whenever possible. Choose salads that include lean protein, baked potatoes, or chili. A regular-sized hamburger or cheeseburger is fine, but split a small order of French fries with a teammate.
Dinner	Choose lean meats, fish, or poultry that is broiled, grilled, baked, or blackened. Ask for potatoes, rice, pasta, or noodles to be prepared with less than the usual amount of fat. Consume breads and rolls, but go easy on the margarine or butter. Have fruit for dessert whenever possible. Order your salad with dressing on the side.
Snacks	Try fresh or dried fruit, granola bars, and energy bars. Buy milk chugs and low-fat yogurt whenever possible. Snack on low-fat crackers, instant soups, and pretzels. Drink water and other fluids.

Long-distance swimmers need to take extra care that they start any race, whether a 10K, which is now an Olympic distance, or a 25K—or even a 75K or an 88K, which are possible on the World Cup circuit—optimally fueled and hydrated. Typically these races take about 1 hour for every 5 kilometers, with women at a slightly slower pace than the men, which puts 10K finishes at over 2 hours and 25K finishes somewhere around 6 hours. Other race distances can take 7 to 10 hours to complete.

Because of the high fuel demands of distance swimming, competitors should carefully consume a high-carbohydrate diet during the race taper. High-carbohydrate supplements can make the carb-loading phase simpler, and swimmers should make sure they maximize this opportunity, as outlined in Chapter 5. Sports drinks, energy bars, and concentrated carbohydrate foods all are beneficial in preparing for these long events. Drink lots of fluids in the days leading up to the race, and carefully plan your pre-race meal. Carbohydrate-containing liquids and easily digested foods will fill your liver glycogen stores before the race and raise your levels of blood glucose.

Swimmers should be accustomed to taking and consuming "feeds" during a race. Events at the 5K and 10K levels have feeding stations, and athletes swimming these distances can be optimally fueled with a sports drink. Feeding cups typically provide 8 to 10 ounces (250–300 ml) of fluid such as a sports drink and can be consumed at each feeding station as needed, ideally every 15 minutes. An athlete's fluid requirements can be higher in hot weather than in cooler temperatures or cooler water conditions.

In events covering more than 10 kilometers, there should be a feed support boat. Swimmers should have a predetermined feed schedule, but they should be prepared to modify this schedule during the race as needed. Aim for 60 to 75 grams of carbohydrates per hour, and practice rolling on your back and drinking. Gels can be carried in your swimsuit and provided from the support boats. Have solid foods available to eat when you tire of drinking. Try cut-up energy bars or even a few bites of a banana. Aim to obtain feeds every 20 minutes.

Be aware of how air and water temperatures can affect your food and fluid needs during the race. Colder water temperatures make you burn fuel more quickly as your body attempts to keep itself warm. This may increase your need for carbohydrate sources such as gels and for a variety of solid items. Without proper fueling, strong hunger pains can set in. Hot-water feeds can also be warming during the swim. In warmer water, your fluid needs increase during competition. Try to keep your hydrating fluids cool in warm weather and be aware of your sweat rate in these conditions.

12

NUTRITION FOR
ROWING

ROWING IS AN INTENSE SPORT, with participants at the high school, collegiate, elite, and club levels, and places heavy physiological demands upon participants. Elite rowers at the top of their sport have developed both exceptional aerobic and anaerobic capacity as well as muscular strength and power. But although strength development is essential to rowing, endurance training is also a key component of race preparation. U.S. Rowing based in Princeton, New Jersey, provides development and support for the elite competitors who represent the United States in international competition, a junior national team, and the adaptive team that participates in the ParaOlympics. Many club rowers are highly dedicated and train in the early-morning hours in preparation for competition.

Rowing is divided into two main categories. In sweep rowing, each rower uses only one long oar, whereas in scull rowing, rowers use two shorter oars. Sweep rowing teams consist of two or four members, with or without a coxswain, or a team of eight rowers with a coxswain. Coxswains are responsible for steering the boat and calling out rowing commands to the crew. In sculling, a boat can include one or two rowers without a coxswain, a team of four with or without a coxswain, or a team of eight rowers and a coxswain.

Rowers mainly compete in open events that have no weight classification, but they may also compete in a lightweight division requiring compliance with specific weight regulations. In the men's lightweight division, the crew can average no more than 155 pounds (70 kg) each, and no individual rower can weigh more than 160 pounds (72.5 kg) (coxswains are not included). A single male sculler cannot weigh more than 160 pounds (72.5 kg). In the junior division (less than nineteen years of age), no individual rower can weigh more than 155 pounds (70 kg), and in the masters division no individual can weigh more than 160 pounds. In the women's lightweight category, no rower, including single scullers, can weigh more than 130 pounds (59 kg), and at the elite level the crew members must average no more than 125 pounds (57 kg) each. Coxswains have their own weight restrictions, with a minimum weight of 120 pounds (55 kg) for men's and junior men's, and 125 pounds (56.5 kg) for collegiate men. The minimum weight is 110 pounds (50 kg) for junior women's, women's, and mixed crew teams. In the United States, female coxswains can compete in male events, and male coxswains in female events.

The maximal aerobic capacities of rowers are some of the highest ever recorded. Top male heavyweight and female openweight rowers also tend to be taller and heavier, and have taller arm spans and sitting heights, than other endurance athletes. They have a high level of muscle mass, but because absolute mass is also important, they may not always have low body-fat levels. Since the load of the boat and coxswain is held constant, a larger and heavier crew in fact has an advantage over a smaller and lighter crew. Lightweight crews are noticeably smaller and lighter than other rowers and often have low body-fat levels in order to stay under the weight requirements. As in many sports that have weight divisions, rowers competing in the lightweight category are often sitting on the fence of their weight limit and struggle to fit under the cutoff. Rowers selected for the lightweight category should be individuals who are naturally lighter in weight and who have their lean physique built into them genetically; otherwise, it can be difficult and even harmful for them to maintain the proper weight and body composition.

TRAINING NUTRITION

Top rowers exhibit a unique mix of aerobic and anaerobic endurance, technique, and power. They require long hours of intense training even though competitive events may last only 5 to 8 minutes. Elite rowers train eight to ten months of the year, with sessions averaging 12 miles (20 km), and may train twice daily. High school teams train and compete in both the fall and spring seasons, and their training sessions can reach 2 hours in duration. Masters rowers may train for 2 hours in the morning or evening. Rowers can also undertake gym sessions that include weight training, and they may crosstrain with running and cycling. It is not unusual for collegiate swimmers to complete twelve training sessions weekly, and elite rowers may train even more.

In the fall, rowers build a good aerobic base, work on skills, and train for races of 4 to 6 kilometers. During the winter season, training usually moves indoors and shifts in focus. The goal becomes building an anaerobic base on indoor rowers and building power and strength through resistance training. Spring racing season focuses on maximizing both the aerobic and anaerobic systems and preparing for the races of 1 or 2 kilometers.

CALORIES AND CARBOHYDRATES

Rowers can have very high energy and carbohydrate requirements to match both the volume and intensity of their training throughout the season. Energy needs are further increased for heavyweight rowers, who weight-train to add muscle mass. Collegiate male rowers may struggle to keep their energy levels and body weight up. They need to make sure they eat adequately to recover from one training session to the next, particularly during two-a-day practices. Collegiate male rowers often require more than 6,000 calories daily, and female rowers may need at least 3,000 calories daily.

A rower's energy and carbohydrate requirements can vary in different training phases of the season as training intensity and volume change, but proper meal and snack timing is essential at any time of the training year. You may need frequent meals and snacks in order to take in adequate carbohydrates before, after, and between training sessions, while working within food and fluid tolerances close to training. (See Chapter 4 for carbohydrate requirements based on daily training levels.)

Rowers often train in the early hours, and for some, it may be possible to stomach only a light snack before training, reserving a full breakfast for later. Because of low morning liver glycogen stores, rowers should nevertheless attempt to consume at least 50 grams of easily tolerated carbohydrates before an early-morning practice. Fluids could provide the majority of these carbohydrates, if necessary. Some early-morning choices that provide at least 75 grams of carbohydrates are:

- 2 slices of toast with 2 tbsp. (40 ml) jam and 8 oz. (240 ml) juice
- 3 oz. (90 g) bagel with 2 tbsp. (40 ml) of jam and 12 oz. (360 ml) sports drink
- 12 oz. (360 ml) yogurt smoothie made with milk and fruit
- 1 energy bar and 1 large banana with 8 oz. (240 ml) juice

For afternoon or evening training, rowers must consume enough carbohydrates during the day to begin their session with adequate fuel stores. To top off your muscle glycogen stores and increase your blood glucose levels as well as your liver glycogen stores, consume a snack within 2 hours of training. Aim for 50 to 75 grams of carbohydrates during this same time frame. Some good afternoon carbohydrate choices are:

- 8 oz. (240 ml) yogurt mixed with fruit and raisins
- Peanut-butter-and-jelly sandwich with an apple
- 10 crackers with hummus, carrots, and 8 oz. (240 ml) juice
- 8 oz. (240 ml) pasta salad with a piece of fruit
- ½ cup (120 ml) muesli or granola mixed with 6 oz. (180 ml) yogurt and raisins

Rowers who train twice daily should adopt a grazing pattern that continues throughout the day. Grazing can begin with a light to moderate breakfast before training, which can be followed by a moderate-sized recovery breakfast containing whole grains, fruit, and protein. Lunch can follow shortly thereafter, and an afternoon pre-training snack can ensue a bit later on. An hour after training, or even sooner, is a good time for dinner. This meal should include a mix of healthy carbohydrate sources and some protein. Because of the high amount of calories they burn in one day, rowers can also eat a high-carbohydrate evening snack. If dinner is delayed by a couple of hours, it is a good idea to have a carbohydrate and protein recovery snack within 30 minutes of the evening training session. The well-balanced dinner can then follow 2 hours later. Recovery drinks and energy bars can be very useful in helping rowers to meet their carbohydrate and energy requirements. Carbohydrate intake should be rounded out with the required amounts of protein and fat, as outlined in Chapter 4.

FLUID AND MINERAL REQUIREMENTS

Long training sessions on the water can result in significant fluid losses from sweating, particularly when training twice daily. Because drinking during practice is not always handy or convenient, make sure to start all training sessions well hydrated. For early-morning sessions, rowers can hydrate with carbohydrate-containing fluids such as sports drinks, high-carbohydrate drinks, juice, milk, and water.

Drink fluids right up to the start of the training session. Bring bottles of fluid on the boat during practice. During training sessions, sports drinks are the best choice for sessions lasting more than 75 minutes because of the carbohydrates and sodium they provide. Try to quickly consume some fluids every 15 to 20 minutes or between training sets. While taking your hand off the oars and reaching for a bottle may not always be feasible or safe, drink fluids whenever you have a chance. Better yet, wear a back-mounted hydration system to keep from having to take your hands off the oars.

Rowers must be persistent in their rehydration efforts to match their sweat losses during training, especially since their sweat losses are so high. They should check their weight before and after training to determine the extent of their sweat losses that have not been replaced (for technique, see the sidebar "Estimating Your Sweat Losses" in Chapter 5). Every pound (or 0.5 kg) of weight lost represents a fluid loss of 16 ounces (480 ml). Rowers should consume 150 percent of their fluid losses to compensate for both urine and sweat losses. Therefore, for each pound (0.5 kg) of weight lost, consume 24 ounces (720 ml) of fluid. Sodium should be part of the recovery mix to enhance rehydration. Lightweight rowers should be aware that any weight loss that occurs during training reflects fluid loss rather than changes in body fat.

Female rowers have greater iron requirements than sedentary women because of their heavy training load and should be sure to consume adequate iron in their diet. Regular monitoring of iron stores by a physician is recommended. Male rowers may also be at risk for iron deficiency during the periods of rapid growth that can occur in the high school and college years. Both male and female high school and collegiate rowers should take extra care to meet their calcium requirements by consuming 3 to 4 servings of high-calcium foods daily. Calcium food sources such as milk and yogurt are usually available at dining halls and school cafeterias. Calcium-forti-fied products can also be included in the rower's diet to ensure that optimal bone mass levels are reached. Inadequate calcium intake can be compensated for by use of a daily calcium supplement. Many multivitamin and mineral supplements contain the Daily Value of iron, but consult with a physician before taking higher iron doses.

WEIGHT AND BODY FAT

Lightweight Rowers

Rowers who compete in the lightweight category should be realistic about their weight goals, body type and genetics, and ability to healthily reach and maintain the lightweight requirements. Those who are too small to compete in the heavyweight division may attempt to "make weight" to com-pete in the lightweight division. This can be tricky. Rowers wanting to compete in the lightweight division should receive expert advice on how to determine their optimal competition weight and how likely it is that they can achieve this weight without compromising their health.

Both male and female lightweight rowers who do attempt to follow a strict diet to stay within the limits can become obsessed with food and develop patterns of disordered eating. Their diet practices can cause them to be underfueled for hard training sessions and can lead to subpar per-formance, poor nutritional recovery, chronic fatigue, and symptoms of overtraining. Strict dietary practices can even alter one's metabolic efficiency. When that happens, weight loss becomes more difficult as the adaptive mechanisms programmed into our bodies fight to retain weight and body fat. One assessment of elite Australian lightweight rowers determined that those who had lower body fat and greater total muscle mass were more successful. But strict dieting can compromise both muscle mass and strength.

Scientific data indicate that rowing is a sport in which eating issues related to weight are fairly prevalent. One survey found that lightweight rowers exhibited more unhealthy eating practices than heavyweight rowers, and that females displayed more of these practices than males. An-other study, which monitored the body composition of lightweight rowers throughout the season, found that seasonal weight fluctuations were related to changes in fat, but that dietary and weight restrictions could limit beneficial increases in muscle mass.

Rowers who have excess body-fat levels but could realistically compete in the lightweight category should begin their body-fat loss efforts early in the season. They should develop their body-fat and weight-loss goals in a context of good training nutrition, and focus on gradual changes instead of rapid weight loss. It is essential that they fuel adequately for their training sessions and take in more calories as their training intensifies during the season.

Heavyweight and Openweight Rowers

The situation for heavyweight and openweight rowers is vastly different from the lightweight rower's situation. Rowers in the heavyweight division can actually benefit from increased mass. Nevertheless, there is a limit to the amount of excess fat they should carry. Although increases in muscle mass certainly can improve performance, levels of body fat that are too high need to be addressed. Heavyweight and openweight rowers who do need to decrease their body-fat levels should focus on sensible weight-loss practices (see Chapter 6). For rowers who also wish to build muscle mass, following the nutritional guidelines outlined in this chapter are the best bet. Many heavyweight rowers find that excess body fat takes care of itself if they simply follow sensible nutritional guidelines during heavy training periods. Focused calorie restriction is usually not required, since the calorie needs of rowers are so high.

Female rowers who are fairly new to the sport should have their body composition monitored periodically as the season progresses. Increases on the scale usually reflect increases in muscle mass and strength, not increased body fat, and are due to the intense weight-training component of their program.

COMPETITION NUTRITION

In contrast to training sessions in rowing, which are often long and may fall into a wide range of intensities, rowing competitions are super-intense and short. Standard 2K (2,000 m) races can last over 7 minutes for single racers and around 5 minutes for teams of eight. Masters races are 1 kilometer (1,000 m) in distance, and high school athletes compete in races that are 1.5 kilometers (1,500 m) long. These sprints usually take place in the spring and summer. Longer races may also take place in the fall and early winter and range from 4.5 to 6 kilometers in distance. Race distances are often dictated by course availability, and some high school–level races can even last up to 30 minutes.

Fall regattas often last only one day, but competitions, or regattas, in the springtime can last several days and sometimes up to a week. Competitors first compete in heats, then in semi-finals and finals. Rowers can race once daily in the larger competitions, and they can race hard for

EATING WELL ON CAMPUS

College food services usually offer a wide selection of foods for students living in dorms or group home settings such as sororities and fraternities. Campus food courts also provide selections in a variety of locations near classrooms, and of course there is the ever-present vending machine. The college athlete's task is to seek out items that support athletic training, recovery, and good health.

Eating on campus presents several challenges. One is the "all-you-can-eat" setting, with unlimited returns to the table and a wide variety of hot and cold foods that may or may not be prepared with moderate to high amounts of fat. You need to become a savvy consumer in these settings and make wise choices just as you would at any restaurant or fast-food establishment.

Although dorm dining hall hours of operation are usually fairly generous, students do need to review their class and practice schedules and plan when and where they will be eating each day of the week. Late nights of studying may necessitate evening snacking, so keep a stash of healthy choices in your room as well. Remember, you are not on a 9-to-5 schedule. You need to be flexible with your meal and snack times while giving yourself the consistent mealtime structure required for a healthy diet.

Although it may be tempting to sleep in, make sure that you always start your day with breakfast. Dorm-style breakfast offerings include many choices with wholesome carbohydrates and protein. Consider the standard cold and hot cereals, and gravitate toward whole-grain, low-sugar choices. Skim milk and yogurt add more carbohydrates and high-quality protein to the mix. Be sure to include fruit and whole-grain breads as desired. Peanut butter adds some protein, as do eggs— any style. If you do sleep late, try to at least catch the tail end of breakfast time. You can also keep some simple breakfast items in your room, such as cereal, milk, fruit, and yogurt, so that skipping breakfast is not necessary even if you do sleep in.

Breakfast choices on campus often go beyond the simple items typically available at home. Food fare that was once limited to weekend brunches, such as omelets, waffles, pancakes, sausage, and bacon, may be available every day. These items can be part of your breakfast choices, but keep portions of high-fat items to reasonable levels.

Most athletes get hungry every 3 to 4 hours, and sometimes even at shorter intervals if a long training session takes place. Although you should sit down to eat lunch and dinner regularly, it

CONTINUES

EATING WELL ON CAMPUS   continued

is also important to plan some snacks in your sports diet. Quick items like yogurt and fruit can be purchased on campus, as can granola bars and sandwiches. Carry snacks with you as needed, and stake out various campus locations close to your classrooms for healthy choices.

Try not to arrive for your meals famished. You want to have time to look over the hot and cold choices that are available and make healthy selections, rather than rushing to buy the first thing that looks good. If you are overly hungry, you might eat too fast and eat more than you intended. Some food services and group homes post their menus for the week ahead of time, which can be helpful for meal planning. Make your choices based on what looks good and what best fits your nutritional needs. Keep an eye out for whole grains, fruits, and vegetables. Standard items offered usually include a salad bar, a sandwich bar, soups, baked potato bar, several hot entrées, and a decent variety of desserts.

The salad bar can certainly supplement a healthy meal, but choose wisely if it is your main course. Plenty of fresh vegetables such as carrots, mushrooms, cucumbers, and peppers are great, as are leafy greens such as lettuce and spinach. If the salad is to be a main focus of the meal, be sure to include proteins such as cottage cheese, eggs, tuna, cheese, chickpeas, kidney beans, tofu, and turkey. Prepared salads such as pasta salad, potato salad, and marinated vegetable salads also add carbohydrates, but they may contribute some fat as well, so do control your portions with these items. Watch out for foods loaded with mayonnaise if you are trying not to overdo your fat intake.

If you like sandwiches at lunchtime, gravitate toward whole-grain breads, but also vary your choices with pita bread and sandwich wraps. Turkey, tuna, peanut butter, and ham all supply good protein. Round out your sandwich with a bowl of soup, some fruit, vegetables, and yogurt or a glass of milk. Higher-calorie items would include a large bagel or submarine sandwich, French fries, and milkshakes. Baked potato bars, like sandwich bars, can provide a nice balance of protein and carbohydrates. Spuds can be topped with vegetables, cheese, yogurt, chili, turkey, or various sauces.

Hot entrées are available at both lunch and dinner in college dining halls and can run the gamut from healthy stir-fries to high-fat fried foods, though a wider variety of healthy entrées seem to be offered at dorm food services in recent years than in the past. Ask questions about how

CONTINUES

EATING WELL ON CAMPUS | continued

the foods have been prepared, and request specific portion sizes. You can also ask for sauces to be served on the side so that you can control your own portion sizes of these items, which are often high in fat. Veggie and turkey burgers make good low-fat choices, as do pasta plates with red sauces, grilled or broiled fish, and other grilled meats. Regularly offered sides often include steamed rice, baked potatoes, skim milk and yogurt, fresh fruit, and soups.

Desserts are often in abundant supply at the dorm food service. A self-serve frozen yogurt machine and side toppings make a popular choice. Ice cream, cakes, and pies may also be available on a regular basis, but they are probably the highest in calories. More reasonable options include fruit bars, yogurt bars, and popsicles as well as sorbet and baked or fresh fruit. But set limits on your consumption of desserts. One a day or several per week may be fine, depending on your energy needs.

several consecutive days. They can even race twice daily if they compete in a repechage, in which boats that lost a previous heat compete against one another in an attempt to still qualify for the semi-finals, and they sometimes have less than 12 hours of recovery time before a race the next morning. Lightweight competitors are required to weigh in on the morning of each race, which can complicate pre-race meal and hydration strategies.

Rowers must arrive on race morning well fueled, well hydrated, and with a comfortable stomach. If a competition is going to last several days, recovery between events is essential. Even with light training the day before a race, rowers can eat adequately to replenish their muscle glycogen stores and rehydrate. They should keep their protein and fat intake at moderate levels, however, and combine this strategy with reduced training volume in preparation for a race.

Follow the guidelines outlined in Chapter 5 for planning your pre-race meal and your carbohydrate intake as the race approaches. Allow for 2.5 to 3 hours of digestion time prior to your hard race effort. Racing in the rowing position with a stomach that is too full can be uncomfortable. It is best to experiment with timing and tolerances in training, and then reproduce what works best for you on race day. Liquid meals may be better tolerated for early-morning race starts or to top off an early pre-race breakfast before a late-morning or early-afternoon race start. Plan out meal timing carefully for your race start, particularly if you are to race more than once in a day. Some pre-race foods to consider are breakfast cereals with soy or dairy milk, toast with jam, juice, fruit, crackers, rice, and pasta.

Pay close attention to hydration as well. You can become dehydrated from warm-ups, racing, and being out in the heat during the day and watching the competition. Hydrate leading to the race start, but allow adequate time for your stomach and bladder to empty. Carry a bottle of water or sports drink to maintain your fluid levels over the course of a day.

Plan ahead and organize your foods, fluid, and sports nutrition supplements for a day of competition or for multiple-day events. If you are traveling for a day of competition, plan to pack a cooler of supplies. In some cases, you may have to arrive very early in the morning with your team and support crew only to wait until afternoon to race. Consider packing sandwiches, fresh or dried fruit, low-fat muffins, yogurt, energy bars, cereals, soy and dairy milk, and liquid meal supplements. Pack your favorite sports drink as well, along with water.

Pay close attention to recovery nutrition when racing over multiple days. Replenish with carbohydrates and fluids immediately after the race, and have your next snack or meal within 2 hours. If you compete over several days, outline your meals ahead of time. Where will you eat, and what will be on the menu? Call ahead to find out about restaurants, delis, and grocery stores available in the area of the competition, or check the Internet for information.

LIGHTWEIGHT ROWING

Unfortunately, many lightweight rowers practice unhealthy eating behaviors to "make weight" for competition. If rowers were guided into competing in the lightweight category only when this was their optimal competitive weight division, perhaps this would not happen. Lightweight rowers should be able to stay within their weight limitations without having to compromise their health. Current guidelines from the International Federation of Rowing Associations (Fédération Internationale des Sociétés d'Aviron, FISA) specify that an athlete be no more than 2.25 pounds (5 kg) above weight for 5 to 6 months before competition and no more than 1.4 pounds (3 kg) above weight for 2 to 3 months before competition. These rules are intended to keep lightweight rowers at a stable weight during the training season and prevent crash dieting before competition, but unhealthy behaviors around making weight persist in the sport.

One Australian study evaluated the weight-management practices of lightweight rowers before a regatta. The researchers found that the majority of the racers used both long-term and short-term weight-loss strategies to make weight. Most of the respondents were within FISA body-weight guidelines. Nevertheless, they used weight-loss strategies such as increased training sessions and dietary and fluid restrictions. These practices can deplete body-fuel reserves and fluid stores prior to competition and are not in keeping with optimal pre-competition nutrition guidelines. Researchers also evaluated the nutritional recovery practices of rowers in the time between their weigh-ins and the start of competition. In general, fluid and sodium intakes after

MEAL PLAN OUTLINE

Arower with an early-afternoon start time could consume a large breakfast to top off both muscle and liver glycogen stores, allowing plenty of time for digestion. A meal plan based on a 1:30 p.m. race time might be as follows:

Breakfast, 9:00 a.m.

2 eggs

2 slices toast

2 tbsp. (40 ml) jam

¾ oz. (20 ml) cereal

8 oz. (240 ml) skim milks

12 oz. (360 ml) juice

1 small banana

12 almonds

Snack, 11:30 a.m.

1 large energy bar

12 oz. (360 ml) high-carbohydrate drink

It is important to hydrate with a sports drink in the hours leading up to the race. After the race, the priority is to refuel by consuming plenty of carbohydrates to prepare for the next day's race. If this rower has an earlier start time the next day, such as at 9:00 a.m., there is less than a 24-hour recovery time.

Post-race lunch

Turkey sandwich (4 oz. turkey, 2 slices bread)

1½ oz. (45 g) pretzels

1 medium orange

8 oz. (240 ml) skim milk

Snack

6 oz. (180 ml) yogurt

1 medium-sized piece of fruit

Dinner

4 oz. (120 g) fish

2 c. (480 ml) cooked rice

1 c. vegetable

3–4 tsp. (20–25 ml) cooking oil

8 oz. (240 ml) juice

DO NUTRITIONAL NEEDS OF MALES AND FEMALES DIFFER?

Despite the well-established physiological differences between female and male athletes, female athletes are routinely given sports nutrition advice based on scientific data derived from male test subjects in research studies. Fortunately, the number of studies focusing on the specific nutritional needs of female athletes has increased over the past decade. Much of this research has looked at endurance exercise, and female athletes participating in these sports can benefit from a few key findings. The emerging research, including several studies from McMaster University and the University of Guelph, both in Ontario, Canada, provides gender-specific guidance for women relating to carbohydrate loading, nutritional intake during training, and recovery strategies.

Training before a race can optimize body glycogen fuel stores for female athletes just as it can for their male counterparts. In order to glycogen load effectively, women need to consume an adequate number of grams of carbohydrates per pound of body weight. Female endurance athletes should taper and carbohydrate load before extended competition even though they have been found to derive less benefit from the process than their male counterparts following the same glycogen-loading protocol.

Researchers at McMaster University have also studied gender differences in carbohydrate consumption during exercise, with useful results. Female athletes may not respond as robustly as men to carbohydrate loading, but they can consume sports drinks during exercise to compensate for storing less glycogen. Test subjects cycled at 60 percent VO_2max for 90 minutes while consuming an 8 percent carbohydrate beverage (1 gram carbohydrate per kilogram of body weight). When female athletes performing endurance exercise were provided with sports drinks during exercise, they oxidized, or burned, more of the sports drink than males. Overall, however, women still burn more fat than carbohydrate, during exercise when compared with men. Carbohydrate consumption during higher training intensities would also be expected to benefit female athletes.

Other research from McMaster University has shown that consuming carbohydrates immediately after training improves muscle glycogen resynthesis and recovery in women just as efficiently as in men. Males and females appear to store glycogen at similar rates when carbohydrates are given immediately after endurance exercise, and they benefit from this strategy equally. Future research is needed to determine how this nutritional recovery strategy affects training programs specific to endurance athletes.

CONTINUES

DO NUTRITIONAL NEEDS OF MALES AND FEMALES DIFFER?   continued

Another recent study pointed to the need for more data to fine-tune the knowledge of the unique daily nutritional requirements of female athletes and the effect of diet manipulations on performance, particularly for carbohydrate intake. Researchers had well-trained female triathletes and cyclists follow three separate protocols and consume either a low-carbohydrate diet of 1.4 grams per pound (3 g/kg) of body weight, a moderate-carbohydrate diet of 2.25 grams per pound (5 g/kg) of body weight, and a high-carbohydrate diet of 3.5 grams per pound (8 g/kg) of body weight for six days. Subjects then cycled to exhaustion. Interestingly, on the high-carb diet subjects had difficulty consuming the prescribed amount of carbohydrates. When completing a time trial after cycling at 70 percent VO_2max, no significant performance differences were found among the three diets. More performance testing of various carbohydrate dietary levels in female athletes is needed. Earlier studies have demonstrated a difference in fuel metabolism between men and women, but more research is needed in this area before nutritionists can draw any real conclusions about what it all means in practical terms. In any case, nutritional recommendations may become more sex-specific in the future as awareness of metabolic differences in men and women increases.

Another recent finding is that women have a greater increase in core temperature during exercise, given similar heat exposure, when compared with men. The onset of sweating may occur at higher body temperatures, and sweat rates may be lower. However, there are likely more differences in sweat rates among individual women athletes than between men and women. Female athletes should still consume enough fluid during and after exercise to match their fluid losses, while staying within their gastrointestinal tolerances. Another study indicated that replacing body fluids after exercise is not affected by the phase of the menstrual cycle.

Although the protein needs of female athletes are higher than those of the general population, there appear to be no significant differences between men and women athletes in this regard. Protein intake should be based on body weight and specific training programs, and it can vary with the amount of calories and carbohydrates consumed. Of course, adequate calorie intake allows for more optimal utilization of the protein consumed.

There has been growing concern among some researchers that as a greater number of female athletes attempt to reach lower body-fat levels, their health could be compromised. Women have to work harder than men to achieve the same level of leanness. When a female athlete's intake of calories is inadequate, her body may be more prone to making adjustments to defend or maintain

CONTINUES

her current weight than a male athlete's body would, given the same dietary and training factors. Recent data indicate that inadequate calorie intake is the main trigger for hormonal imbalances, absence of menstruation, and compromised bone health.

Although more specific nutritional training recommendations for women need to be tested and formulated, women athletes should still practice focused strategies to ensure optimal performance. Based on the current research, female athletes can be confident that they will benefit from consistently practicing optimal recovery nutrition following hard training, glycogen loading in combination with adequate calorie intake, and consuming enough carbohydrates during training and competition to keep up their glucose levels.

the weigh-ins were not sufficient to fully restore hydration levels, a factor that could significantly affect performance. Restrictive dietary practices to make weight could result in depleted muscle glycogen stores. Although this may not have a huge impact on a race lasting only a few minutes, racing with low muscle glycogen levels could have a negative effect on performance in multiple races or impact a rower's health over time. For their own good, lightweight rowers need to determine weight strategies for competition day that do not compromise their health or performance. Sensible nutrition is always the best policy.

THE LIFE OF A COXSWAIN

Although coxswains are simply along for the ride during competition, they do have their own training regimens designed to keep them at the lowest weight possible allowed for competition. Presiding over a boat of competitive athletes who must maintain a unified stroke is an important task. Because of the low body-weight profile of the position, many coxswains come from other sport backgrounds, such as gymnastics, cross-country running, or wrestling. Their own training programs are designed to keep them fit and lean. They spend hours in the boat with very few calories burned, but they must also make time for their own fitness program. It is best to choose a coxswain who truly fits the job requirements: Someone who is genetically endowed with a small frame and lean physique is less likely to become entangled in an unhealthy cycle of calorie restriction than someone who must work hard to keep the pounds off. Coxswains who do need to lose weight should set realistic goals. Their body-fat loss should be achieved through a healthy nutrition and exercise plan, not by undereating or overexercising. Coxswains should also avoid using dehydration and other techniques for manipulating fluid balance in order to make weight.

13

NUTRITION FOR
ADVENTURE RACING

ADVENTURE RACING HAS BEEN PART OF the New Zealand landscape for several decades, but as a modern sport receiving international attention it was launched onto the scene in 1989 with the now-defunct Raid Gauloises, which after its inception in New Zealand traveled around the world to locations such as Costa Rica, Madagascar, and Ecuador as well as Tibet and Nepal. Teams of five, with at least one female per team, competed by trekking, mountain biking, paddling, using rope skills, and navigating by map and compass in a multiday event. Many North Americans are familiar with the Eco-Challenge, which was held in the United States, Canada, and other parts of the world from 1995 to 2002. Other highly challenging multiday races remain on the adventure-racing scene, including the Primal Quest Expedition Race, but mid-length, shorter, and entry-level adventure racing has also become popular, opening the sport to a greater field of competitors. The United States Adventure Racing Association (USARA) now primarily sanctions hundreds of sprint, weekend, and 24-hour adventure races across the country year-round. Adventure racing places an emphasis on both teamwork and individual achievement, and completing a race in itself is often considered a victory.

Because of the variety of race distances and types of challenges in adventure racing, there are several categories in which teams and individuals can compete. The longer races now often allow or even require a support crew of one or two people to transport the team's gear to transition areas along the racecourse. In "unsupported" races, in contrast, race personnel transport the gear. Typically adventure races have no official rest times, and the competitors must make their own decisions about when to stop, rest, or even catch short periods of sleep. The shorter races normally have a single transition area for all competitors, so that support team assistance is not required. Many races are designed to have a coed team, though this factor can vary among race categories.

Adventure racing offers new and fun challenges to cyclists, runners, hikers, and water sports enthusiasts. Races may include a variety of sports, such as mountain biking, trekking, mountaineering, race navigation or orienteering, and rafting, canoeing, or kayaking. Longer races may even include horseback riding, whitewater swimming, and caving. Some races have special tests that focus on team-building and problem-solving skills. Racers know ahead of time what disciplines their race will include, but not the duration and succession of these disciplines, which, of course, are part of the adventure of adventure racing.

Adventure racing can be categorized according to the amount of time required to complete the race. The main categories are expedition-style races, one-day races, and sprint races.

Expedition-style races. In the early days of adventure racing, competitors would take from 2 to 10 days or longer to complete a course covering 250 to 500 miles or more. A handful of these races are still held around the world, though in recent years not as many in the United States. These races are extremely challenging and besides the typical multisport events can include paddling events and extensive mountaineering and rope work. With the trend toward shorter races, shorter expedition races became more common. The term "expedition race" is now used to refer to any adventure race taking more than 24 hours to complete.

One-day races. One-day events, which may last anywhere from 8 to 24 hours, have become a popular race option. Sleep deprivation is a factor for the longer racing times, and races lasting 8 to 12 hours usually require some navigation and orienteering.

Sprint races. Completion times for these shorter races are under 8 hours. This category can also include urban races lasting from 2 to 4 hours. Navigation is not required.

No matter how long a particular race is, or what athletic disciplines it requires competitors to master, good fueling strategies are essential to bringing each team and racer to the finish. These strategies should cover not only the type and amount of fuel but also the timing of fuel consumption. The longer the race, the more complicated the nutrition plan will be—and the more difficult it will be to master the logistics of staying well fed and hydrated. Good nutrition is essential during both training and competition. During training, it provides for daily recovery and gives racers practice in working out fueling strategies.

TRAINING NUTRITION

Training programs for adventure racing vary because they must be determined by the makeup and distance of the adventure race in which an athlete will be competing. All adventure racing requires a good endurance and strength base and the necessary skills for various sporting disciplines. Most adventure racers train for 10 to 12 hours or more weekly, depending on the goal they have in mind—that is, whether it is finishing or winning.

Adventure racers training for endurance generally build an endurance base at 60 to 70 percent of maximum heart rate and train for more than an hour at this intensity. Generally these workouts include cycling and/or running. Their endurance training also consists of long, hard workouts of back-to-back sports, such as hiking followed by canoeing, topped off with a bike or run. These sessions work out all areas of the body and help simulate an adventure race. To further simulate race conditions, athletes should practice carrying a pack in training and bring foods and fluids with them as they work out. Adventure race training may include any or all of the following workouts:

TREKKING: Training for trekking consists of long slow trail runs, fast hikes, and running and trekking sessions of 2 to 3 hours using a pack. Runs and hill work are incorporated into these trekking sessions. In the winter, snowshoeing and cross-country skiing are great activities for maintaining an aerobic base. Indoor training on a treadmill or NordicTrack can also help a trekker maintain fitness.

MOUNTAIN BIKING: Weekly sessions may consist of road training for 2 to 3 hours and longer rides lasting up to 5 or 6 hours. Off-road skills may also be required on the mountain bike.

PADDLING: Training for this section of the race also calls for endurance, as racing may require several hours of paddling. Training sessions should last 2 to 3 hours.

STRENGTH TRAINING: Adventure racers may schedule two or three sessions with the weights weekly to build strength. These sessions should cover the whole body.

INTERVAL TRAINING: Interval workouts can be useful in running, hiking, or cycling.

Endurance training is the main priority when preparing for an adventure race and requires a focus on the proper training nutrition strategies. Because your training can vary with your next scheduled race and the makeup of your race, your training nutrition plan may need to be adjusted throughout the season. Some of the nutritional fundamentals that you can follow for any training program are described below.

Post-exercise recovery nutrition. Endurance training requires that you begin the recovery process shortly after exercise. After training sessions lasting longer than 90 minutes, focus on consuming 0.5 gram of carbohydrates for every pound (1 g/kg) of body weight, and add 10 to 20 grams of protein into the mix. Consume 24 ounces of fluid for every pound of weight lost during exercise. Include sodium in your post-exercise intake, particularly after training in the heat and humidity.

Daily recovery nutrition. Recovery nutrition continues for the next 24 hours or until the next training session. Refer to Chapter 4 to ensure that your carbohydrate intake matches that day's training and recovery requirements. Round out your meals with adequate amounts of protein and fat. If you plan to train twice in one day, make sure that several meals and snacks are consumed every 2 to 3 hours between training sessions.

Hydrate and fuel during training. Train yourself to drink during exercise so that it will be easy for you to use various hydration strategies during the race. Your focus is on consuming optimal amounts of fluids, carbohydrates, and electrolytes.

Here are some other tips for staying hydrated and well fueled in adventure racing:

- Practice consuming 4 to 8 ounces of fluid every 15 to 20 minutes. Experiment to determine your favorite brands of sports drinks so that you can consume a variety of flavors while racing. Aim for 30 to 60 grams of carbohydrates per hour, and up to 75 to 100 grams per hour for ultraendurance sessions.
- Experiment with a variety of carbohydrate sources such as gels and bars. You will need these foods during longer training sessions and competitions and may benefit from them even during short races.
- During adventure racing, you may want to consume a variety of foods to relieve any taste boredom, particularly in the longer races. Experiment with pretzels, granola bars, sugary candy, dried fruit, gorp, Pop Tarts, paninis, beef jerky, and anything that appeals to you and is well tolerated. Heavier foods can be consumed on days when your training efforts will be relatively low in intensity.
- You may be allowed to bring along foods such as instant soup and powdered mashed potatoes when you compete. Experiment with different items during training to discover what works for you.
- Train with high-sodium products if you anticipate racing in hot and humid conditions, and particularly if you are a salty sweater. Experiment with sports drinks that are relatively high in sodium, as well as sodium tablets, if needed.

Practice nutrition guidelines for resistance training. Since strength training is an important part of preparation for adventure racing, it is important that you practice the nutrition principles outlined in Chapter 6. If your goal is to build muscle mass, you may be able to take in 350 to 400 extra calories daily above your current training requirements. In addition, time your protein intake properly before and after training. During training you can also consume a sports drink to provide carbohydrates to your muscles and enhance the quality of your exercise sessions. Practice good recovery nutrition techniques after intense strength training sessions, particularly when they occur back to back with an endurance training session.

Practice eating while exercising when training for any length race and with equipment and strategies specific to your race profile and length. This is especially crucial for expedition racing, where racers must eat well and stay well hydrated day after day to be successful. Learning to eat comfortably at low exercise intensities and at transition areas is essential. Practice eating as much as possible during training. Purposely run, hike, or bike at a slow, steady pace after eating to give your system a chance to digest this fuel. This will train your system to make the most of refueling opportunities and allow you to determine your tolerances and learn new strategies for staying fed and hydrated during racing. If you practice, you will know what portions and foods to consume at varying intensities. Generally, gels and liquid products work best during high-intensity efforts, while solid foods are a welcome change at relatively low intensities. Many adventure racers, particularly those competing in the longer distances, can train their stomachs to tolerate a higher level of fullness during exercise than other endurance athletes usually can manage.

Refer to the sport-specific nutrition fueling and hydration guidelines provided in previous chapters. For each discipline in your training program, there are specific techniques that are best for fueling and hydrating. Practice these techniques and become accustomed to using various types of support equipment, such as a back-mounted hydration system, a hydration belt, and a pack. Seal electrolyte tablets in plastic to keep them dry, and pack solid food items efficiently for easy access. Some of the logistical challenges of staying hydrated during adventure racing can be solved with practice. Here are some methods to try:

- Keep a bladder hydration system in your backpack for readily available fluid. Have the bite valve accessible.
- Learn to carry and drink fluid when running. Rigging a system where a straw for drinking is available right at your mouth can be helpful.
- Have a drinking system that works with the personal flotation device (PFD) that you wear when paddling. One team actually sewed their drinking system onto the top of their PFDs so that they could easily hydrate when on the water.

COMPETITION NUTRITION

When racing, always start out with a fueling and hydration plan that matches the duration, intensity, and profile of your race. The longer the race, the more detailed and complex your nutrition plan needs to be.

Race foods and fluids can be divided into several categories: sports nutrition supplements, processed foods, real foods, and cooked (or meal) foods for the transition area. How far you move through all the race food categories depends upon the race distance. For the shorter races, the sports nutrition supplements available on the market should be adequate. A list of these foods and fluids is provided in the sidebar "Sports Nutrition Supplements."

RACE FOODS AND FLUIDS

Sports Nutrition Supplements
Sports drinks
Gels
Energy bars
High-energy carbohydrate drinks
Liquid meal replacements
Electrolyte tablets

Processed Foods
Pop Tarts
Gummy Bears
Sour Patch Kids
Potato chips
Snickers candy bar
Pretzels
Starbursts
Fruit Roll-Ups
M & Ms
Twinkies
Chocolate

Real Foods
Sandwiches (peanut butter, honey, jam)
Dried fruit
Nuts and seeds
Trail mix
Jerky
String cheese

Transition-area foods
Pasta or ravioli
Rice
Oatmeal
Soup
Sandwiches
Bagels
Yogurt
Soy milk
Chocolate milk

SPRINT RACE

Pre-race. When preparing for a race lasting from 4 to 8 hours, make it a priority to rest for 24 to 48 hours before the starting time and consume the carbohydrate amounts recommended for carb-loading as outlined in Chapter 5. Hydrate steadily, and consume plenty of sodium from foods and fluids in the days leading up to the race. For very early start times, plan for simple solid and liquid foods to consume to refill your liver glycogen stores before the race.

During the race. Although relatively short adventure-racing competitions may be called "sprints," they can still require up to a full 8 hours of race time. Races of this length include much steady-state activity along with periods requiring the competitors to move into higher gear. Nutrition plans for sprints should be based on the level of exercise intensity that is expected and your toler-ance level for various food items. Sprint racers should be familiar with their sweat rate in specific race and weather conditions, and sports drinks should be their fluid and fuel staple. By race time, they should have developed drinking techniques and strategies for each race discipline. For races lasting 2 to 4 hours, gels can also contribute some important carbohydrate fuel. In the longer

BREAKING THROUGH THE ICE: COLD-WEATHER HYDRATION STRATEGIES

When training outside during the off-season, you are often reminded of the cold, hard fact that water solidifies at temperatures below 32° Fahrenheit (0° Celsius), making optimal hydration a challenge. Endurance sport athletes who train in cold weather can practice a few warming strategies to keep the fluids flowing.

Sports drinks can be heated before training and placed inside a thermos or a bottle covered with an insulating warmer. Experiment with drinks and flavors that appeal to you when heated. Warm sports drinks should be easier to down on a cold winter day than cold ones and can help to maintain your core body temperature.

Tube-fed winter hydration systems are also now available for training in the cold. There are some relatively new models that are designed for the cold—but in the coldest temperatures you cannot fight the freeze indefinitely. Hydration systems are handy, as they do not require that you reach for your bottle with cold fingers and thick gloves. In order to prevent the drink tube from freezing, you can now buy products with an insulated hose and bite valves covered with insulating caps. In full-on winter weather, make sure that you fill the fluid reservoir with warm or hot fluid. You should also blow back into the drink tube after you have taken a hydrating gulp to prevent fluid from sitting and freezing in the drink tube. And keep the fluid reservoir and hose as close to your body as possible so that your body heat can keep the system warm.

sprint races—that is, those lasting over 4 hours—you can also use more solid items, like Gummy Bears, Fruit Roll-Ups, and energy bars. Any solid items should be consumed with ample amounts of water. Find the mix of semisolid and solid items that works best for you by experimenting during training. Caffeine-containing gels and cola can also provide a needed brain and endurance boost for racers hitting the 8-hour mark.

After the race. Some weight loss from fluid depletion is expected during even a sprint race, but competitors should rehydrate steadily with sodium-containing fluids to minimize this as much as possible. Recovery nutrition emphasizing carbohydrates (with some protein) is recommended. Food sources containing sodium should also be included.

ONE-DAY RACE

Pre-race. Carb loading for 48 hours before the race is recommended for any race lasting from 8 to 24 hours. The day before a race, high-carbohydrate supplements can be used to keep fiber intake low. Finish your carb-loading menu early in the evening on the night before the race so that you wake up hungry for the pre-race meal. Hydrate optimally in the days leading up to the race, and consume plenty of sodium-containing foods and fluids.

During the race. For races lasting from 12 to 24 hours, a competitor may bring along more of the processed and real foods, while always paying close attention to hydration needs. Sports drinks should continue to be a staple, but you should carefully consume more solid items on a steady schedule. Aim for 0.5 to 0.6 gram of carbohydrates per pound (1.1–1.3 g/kg) of body weight per hour. For races lasting longer than 10 hours or so, it is expected that the competitors will need some real food. Sandwiches, fruit, and trail mix can be stored in your gear at the transition areas. Think about what you may crave during a race, and pack a variety of items so that you have appealing choices throughout the event. Liquid meals can also work very well for the longer races. Of course, this should all be practiced in training to determine personal tolerances. Don't try new foods out on race day. Some racers may also need salt and electrolyte tablets, and be sure to use a high-sodium sports drink if you are a salty sweater or prone to muscle cramping.

After the race. Your recovery will take several days, but start with some recovery nutrition strategies. Muscle damage from a full 24 hours of racing can delay muscle glycogen repletion, so refuel steadily. Rehydrate, and include sodium-containing foods and fluids in the recovery mix.

EXPEDITION RACE

Pre-race. Obviously, expedition races present the greatest challenge in regard to fueling, hydration, and the logistics of transporting and preparing food items. If you are traveling overseas to your adventure race, you may want to be careful about consuming local foods in exotic locations. Contracting a bacterial infection is a poor way to start the race. Bring some of your own items, and practice good travel hygiene.

You should also consider carbohydrate loading before your multiday event. Rest for several days beforehand (you may be traveling anyway), and consume a high percentage of carbohydrates in your diet. This will supercompensate your muscles with much-needed glycogen. Maintain optimal hydration levels and plenty of sodium in your diet.

During the race. Although carbohydrates should predominate, you also will need to consume a mix of protein and fat during the race. During the more intense races, you will burn several thousand calories daily. Aim to consume 300 to 400 calories per hour to replace these losses. Every racer has his or her own personal tolerances, but aim for the maximum that your body can handle. Even with your best efforts, you still may end up with a calorie deficit over the course of the race.

As in most ultraendurance competitions, in your expedition race you will need to maintain a high carbohydrate intake to keep your blood glucose levels up and supply your muscles with fuel.

Your body should provide enough stored fat for your endurance efforts. Aim for at least 0.6 g carbohydrates per pound (1.3 g/kg) of body weight per hour during the race. You can also consume small amounts of proteins as tolerated when refueling during these long races.

Carrying your food and fluid with you is a key component of adventure racing. Foods that are light in weight, calorically dense, low in volume, appealing, and nonperishable and that will not melt are likely to work best. Carry your favorite energy bars or gels, meal replacements, and some real foods. Good food choices include trail mix, candy such as Gummy Bears, Fruit Roll-Ups, dried fruit, and beef and turkey jerky. Some racers may even carry heavier items, such as a sandwich or burrito, which can be consumed early on in the race to lighten your load. You can even rehydrate items such as mashed potatoes, powdered milk, and stuffing that have been sealed in small plastic bags. Organize your foods for several days of racing. Each day's menu can be placed in a large plastic bag and then labeled properly. This system makes it easy to locate the appropriate bag at the transition area.

Bringing bottled water is essential. You should also carry water-purification tablets to treat water found along the course. Powdered sports drinks can be reconstituted. Plan to carry fluids in a bladder hydration system. You may also want to experiment with waist belts or water-bottle holsters that attach to your backpack. Determine how much water you will need to carry with you during the race, depending on the placing of transition areas and availability of other sources of water along the course, if possible (make sure that you carry some local currency!). Aim to drink enough to offset sweat losses based on your own sweat rate (see the sidebar "Estimating Your Sweat Losses" in Chapter 5). You may require several quarts or liters of fluids daily. Plenty of salty foods should also be carried, as well as salt packets and salt tablets. Remember to drink on a schedule. A carbohydrate- containing sports drink not only fuels your brain but also provides much-needed sodium. Adequate sodium intake is essential to prevent the development of hyponatremia, which can occur over the course of a long race even when you are steadily hydrating. Keep in mind that dehydration can also increase your risk for developing hyperthermia or hypothermia. To prevent dehydration, drink before you are thirsty. Other signs of dehydration are headache, loss of appetite, infrequent urination, rapid heart rate, shortness of breath, and fatigue.

Eat on a schedule as well. Know what your total food consumption should be for each day of the race, based on the sport and the intensity level. Try to plan the best times to eat based on the activity and terrain. Save your liquid carbohydrates for high-intensity endeavors and eat the solid foods when the intensity slows up a bit. Protein foods that may be appealing during the run include jerky, string cheese, peanuts, peanut butter, and canned tuna. Keep food readily accessible in pockets and waistbands so that the effort of obtaining food is not too great. Practice consuming small, consistent amounts throughout the race. Plan to eat every 30 to 60 minutes, and set a watch

NUTRITION AND YOUR IMMUNE SYSTEM

Periods of heavy training are sometimes associated with depressed immune function, and compromised immune function can be further aggravated by inadequate nutrition. Combining training with school and/or work can overtax your resources, stress your body, and compromise your ability to fight infection. A strong immune system should result in fewer colds and other viruses, and when you do get sick, should enable you to make a quicker recovery.

Specific foods can strengthen your immune system and help to prevent unwanted halts to your training program due to illness. Vitamin C has a widespread reputation as an immune system booster, but it is not a magic pill for preventing the common cold. It should, however, be part of your daily diet in adequate amounts. Though a daily multivitamin and mineral supplement may contain the Daily Value (DV) of vitamin C, don't underestimate the importance of ample food sources of this nutrient. Athletes can consume more than 3 servings of fresh fruit and up to 2 cups of cooked vegetables daily for ample amounts of dietary vitamin C. Megadoses of vitamin C in supplement form have not been shown to protect the immune system—250 milligrams is adequate to saturate body stores.

Fruits and vegetables contain hundreds of phytochemicals that provide many preventative health benefits and are also excellent sources of carotenoids that boost the activity of the white blood cells called *lymphocytes*. Beta-carotene can also be converted to vitamin A, an important nutrient for the immune system. Other nutrients important for a strong immune system are zinc, iron, and vitamins B6 and B12. A good daily multivitamin and mineral supplement providing 100 percent of the DVs ensures adequate nutrient intake. Megadosing with vitamins and minerals can compromise the immune system, and excessive intakes of iron, zinc, and vitamin E are not advised. A balanced diet that includes a large variety of foods provides many nutrients that work together to keep your immune system healthy, and a moderate-dose supplement ensures that you are obtaining all the nutrients that you need.

Consuming adequate calories is not only beneficial for an athlete's recovery and energy levels but also important for maintaining a healthy immune system. Falling short of your calorie requirements can compromise your immune system, as can poorly planned and low-calorie diets, especially those low in protein. Diets too low in calories can result in inadequate intake of vitamins and minerals, which also decreases immunity. Training with optimal stores of glycogen obtained from a diet adequate in calories and carbohydrates not only provides fuel for your workouts but also

CONTINUES

NUTRITION AND YOUR IMMUNE SYSTEM   continued

boosts your immune system. Levels of certain stress hormones normally rise during exercise, but athletes who train in the carbohydrate-depleted state experience a greater increase in these hormones than those who are well fueled. Consuming carbohydrates during exercise also seems to diminish some of the immunosuppressive effects of intense training. Overall, good carbohydrate replacement supports your immune system.

to remind yourself and your teammates to eat. Remember, you are only as fast as your slowest teammate. Before the race, you should be used to working together and planning your food and fluid intake according to the same principles for optimal performance.

For longer races that allow a support crew, the transition area provides a great opportunity to fill up with calories. This is your chance to replenish your sagging energy stores. Your crew can provide you with a substantial meal while you prepare for the next event. Burritos, stews, grilled cheese sandwiches, rice, meat, and pasta are all good choices for these meals. Liquid meal replacements that provide more than 300 calories can also be helpful at this time. Rely on dehydrated meals, if necessary. Unsupported races require that you plan your transition meals carefully and have items ready for consumption in your pack.

After the race. You likely will need to rest for a few weeks after such a long race. Practice the same recovery nutrition principles by steadily consuming carbohydrates, protein, fluid, and sodium. Your damaged muscle fibers will need at least several days of recovery time. Enjoy the wide variety of foods and fluids available to you after the limited menu of adventure racing.

Appendixes

A

GLYCEMIC INDEX OF
FOODS

FOOD	SERVING SIZE	GRAMS OF CARBOHYDRATES PER SERVING	GLYCEMIC LOAD PER PORTION	INDEX FOR 50 GRAMS
High-Glycemic Foods (GI > 70)				
Glucose	(test portion)	50	–	100
Potatoes, instant, mashed	5 oz. (150 g)	22.8	22.1	97
Baguette	1 oz. (30 g)	15.9	15.1	95
Potato, baked	6.5 oz. (195 g)	29	27.3	94
Rice, instant	5 oz. (150 g)	42	36.5	87
Cornflakes	1 oz. (30 g)	25	21.5	86
Pretzels	2 oz. (60 g)	39	32.2	83
Rice Krispies	1 oz. (30 g)	29	24	82
Waffles	2 oz. (60 g)	24.7	19.2	76
Doughnut	1.6 oz. (48 g)	19	14.3	76
Total cereal	1 oz. (30 g)	25	19	76
Waffle	2 oz. (60 g)	25	19.3	76
Soda crackers	0.8 oz. (24 g)	17.8	13.1	74
Cheerios	1 oz. (30 g)	25	18.5	74
Watermelon	8 oz. (240 g)	12	8.6	72
Bagel, white	2.25 oz. (68 g)	35.5	25.5	72
Millet	5 oz. (150 g)	34.8	24.7	71
Bread, white	2 oz. (60 g)	26.8	18.8	70
Pancakes, from mix	2.7 oz. (81 g)	32.5	21.8	67

CONTINUES

GLYCEMIC INDEX OF FOODS	continued

FOOD	SERVING SIZE	GRAMS OF CARBOHYDRATE PER SERVING	GLYCEMIC LOAD PER PORTION	INDEX FOR 50 GRAMS
Moderate-Glycemic Foods (GI 55–70)				
Croissant	1.9 oz. (57 g)	14.7	22	67
Shredded Wheat	1 oz. (30 g)	21.7	14.6	67
Cream of Wheat	1 oz. (30 g)	20	13.2	66
Pineapple	4 oz. (120 g)	9.6	6.3	66
Oat kernel bread	2 oz. (60 g)	25.6	16.6	65
Raisins	2 oz. (60 g)	42.7	27.3	64
Rye crispbread	1 oz. (30 g)	16	10.1	63
Muffin	1.9 oz. (57 g)	27.7	17.2	62
Corn, sweet	2.6 oz. (78z g)	16	9.5	62
Ice cream	1.6 oz. (48 g)	9.9	6.1	62
Couscous	5 oz. (150 g)	14.3	8.7	61
Bran muffin	1.9 oz. (57 g)	20.9	12.5	60
Spaghetti, white	6 oz. (180 g)	44.3	25.6	58
Pita bread	1 oz. (30 g)	16	9.2	57
Orange juice	9 oz. (270 ml)	21	12	57
Muesli	2 oz. (60 g)	32	17.9	56
Oat bran, raw	2 oz. (60 g)	30	16.5	55
Popcorn	2 oz. (60 g)	19	10.5	55
Pumpernickel bread	1 oz. (30 g)	13.4	7.4	55
Low-Glycemic Foods (GI < 55)				
Pound cake	1.75 oz. (53 g)	25	13.4	54
Buckwheat	5 oz. (150 g)	28.8	14.6	51
Bread, whole-grain	2 oz. (60 g)	23	12	51
Banana, ripe	4 oz. (120 g)	23.9	12.1	50
All-Bran	2 oz. (60 g)	36.8	18.4	50
Rice, brown	5 oz. (150 g)	47.7	23.9	49
Porridge oatmeal	8 oz. (240 ml)	20.3	9.9	48
Sweet potato	5 oz. (150 g)	26	12.5	48
Bulgur	5 oz. (150 g)	26	11.9	46
Lactose	(test portion)	50	–	43

CONTINUES

GLYCEMIC INDEX OF FOODS   continued

FOOD	SERVING SIZE	GRAMS OF CARBOHYDRATE PER SERVING	GLYCEMIC LOAD PER PORTION	INDEX FOR 50 GRAMS
Chickpeas	5 oz. (150 g)	21	8.6	42
Grapefruit juice	8 oz. (240 ml)	15.7	7.5	41
Pear, Bartlett	4 oz. (120 g)	11.3	4.6	40
Apple juice	8 oz. (240 g)	26	10.4	40
Apple	4 oz. (120 g)	14.6	5.9	33
Apricots, dried	2 oz. (60 g)	25	8	32
Fettucine	4 oz. (120 g)	30	9.6	32
Yogurt, fruited	6.5 oz. (195 g)	33	10.9	32
Milk, skim	8 oz. (240 g)	13	4.1	32
Spaghetti, whole-meal	4 oz. (120 g)	30	9.6	28
Peach	8 oz. (240 g)	15	4.2	28
Lentils	5 oz. (150 g)	14.9	4.1	28
Kidney beans	5 oz. (150 g)	24	5.5	23
Fructose	(test portion)	50	–	20

B

COMPARISON OF
VITAMINS AND MINERALS

VITAMINS	DRIs	MAJOR SOURCES	MAJOR FUNCTIONS
Water-Soluble			
Thiamin (vitamin B1)	**Males** 14–70 yrs: 1.2 mg **Females** 14–70 yrs: 1.1 mg	Wheat germ, whole-grain breads and cereals, organ meats, lean meats, legumes	Energy production from carbohydrates, essential for healthy nervous system
Riboflavin (vitamin B2)	**Males** 14–70 yrs: 1.3 mg **Females** 14–18 yrs: 1.0 mg 18–70 yrs: 1.1 mg	Milk and dairy products, green leafy vegetables, lean meats, beans	Energy production from carbohydrates and fats, essential for healthy skin
Niacin (nicotinamide, nicotinic acid)	**Males** 14–70 yrs: 16 mg **Females** 14–70 yrs: 14 mg	Lean meats, fish, poultry, whole grains, peanuts	Energy production from carbohydrates, synthesis of fat, blocks release of FFA
Vitamin B6 (pyridoxine)	**Males** 14–50 yrs: 1.3 mg 51–>70 yrs: 1.7 mg **Females** 14–18 yrs: 1.2 mg 19–50 yrs: 1.3 mg 51–>70 yrs: 1.5 mg	Liver, lean meats, fish, poultry, legumes, bran cereal	Plays role in protein metabolism, necessary for formation of hemoglobin and red blood cells and synthesis of essential fatty acids; required for glycogen breakdown
Vitamin B12 (cobalamin)	**Males** 14–>70 yrs: 2.4 mcg **Females** 14–>70 yrs: 2.4 mcg	Lean meats, poultry, dairy products, eggs	Plays role in formation of red blood cells and metabolism of nervous tissue; involved in folate metabolism, formation of DNA

CONTINUES

COMPARISON OF VITAMINS AND MINERALS   continued

VITAMINS	DRIs	MAJOR SOURCES	MAJOR FUNCTIONS
Folic acid (folate)	**Males** 14–>70 yrs: 400 mcg **Females** 14–>70 yrs: 400 mcg	Green leafy vegetables, legumes	Plays role in red blood cell and DNA formation
Biotin	**Males** 14–18 yrs: 25 mcg 19–>70 yrs: 30 mcg **Females** 14–18 yrs: 25 mcg 19–>70 yrs: 30 mcg	Meats, legumes, milk, egg yolks, whole grains	Plays role in metabolism of carbohydrates, protein, fat
Pantothenic acid	**Males** 14–>70 yrs: 5 mg **Females** 14–>70 yrs: 5 mg	Liver, lean meats, eggs, salmon, all animal and plant foods	Plays role in metabolism of carbohydrates, protein, fat
Vitamin C	**Males** 14–18 yrs: 75 mg 19–>70 yrs: 90 mg **Females** 14–18 yrs: 65 mg 19–>70 yrs: 75 mg	Citrus fruits, green leafy vegetables, broccoli, peppers, strawberries, potatoes	Essential for connective tissue development, plays role in iron absorption; antioxidant; plays role in wound healing

Fat-Soluble RDAs

VITAMINS	DRIs	MAJOR SOURCES	MAJOR FUNCTIONS
Vitamin A (retinol, provitamin carotenoids)	**Males** 14–>70 yrs: 900 mcg **Females** 14–>70 yrs: 700 mcg	Liver, milk, cheese, fortified margarine, carotenoids in plant foods (orange, red, deep green in color)	Maintains healthy tissue in skin and mucous membranes, essential for night vision; plays role in bone development
Vitamin D (cholecalciferol)	**Males** 14–50 yrs: 5 mcg 51–70 yrs: 10 mcg >70 yrs: 15 mcg **Females** 14–50 yrs: 5 mcg 51–70 yrs: 10 mcg >70 yrs: 15 mcg	Vitamin D–fortified milk and margarine, fish oil, metabolized by sunlight on skin	Increases intestinal absorption of calcium, promotes bone and tooth formation, plays role in preventing colon cancer and autoimmune diseases, such as type 1 diabetes and rheumatoid arthritis
Vitamin E (tocopherol)	**Males** 14–>70 yrs: 15 mg **Females** 14–>70 yrs: 15 mg	Vegetable oils, margarine, green leafy vegetables, wheat germ, whole-grain products	Plays role in formation of red blood cells; antioxidant
Vitamin K (phylloquinone)	**Males** 14–18 yrs: 75 mcg 19–>70 yrs: 120 mcg **Females** 14–18 yrs: 75 mcg 19–>70 yrs: 90 mcg	Liver, soybean oil, spinach, cauliflower, green leafy vegetables	Essential for normal blood clotting

CONTINUES

COMPARISON OF VITAMINS AND MINERALS   continued

VITAMINS	DRIs	MAJOR SOURCES	MAJOR FUNCTIONS
Major Minerals			
Calcium	**Males** 14–18 yrs: 1,300 mg 19–50 yrs: 1,000 mg 51–>70 yrs: 1,200 mg **Females** 14–18 yrs: 1,300 mg 19–50 yrs: 1,000 mg 51–>70 yrs: 1,200 mg	Milk, cheese, yogurt, dried peas and beans, dark green leafy vegetables	Plays role in bone formation, enzyme activation, nerve impulse transmission, muscle contraction
Phosphorus	**Males** 14–18 yrs: 1,250 mg 19–>70 yrs: 700 mg **Females** 14–18 yrs: 1,250 mg 19–>70 yrs: 700 mg	Protein foods such as meat, poultry, fish, eggs, milk, cheese, dried peas and beans, whole grains	Plays role in bone formation, cell membrane structure, B-vitamin activation, component of ATP-CP and other important organic compounds
Magnesium	**Males** 14–18 yrs: 410 mg 19–>70 yrs: 420 mg **Females** 14–18 yrs: 360 mg 19–30 yrs: 310 mg 31–>70 yrs: 320 mg	Milk, yogurt, dried beans, nuts, whole grains, tofu, green vegetables, chocolate	Plays role in protein synthesis, glucose metabolism, muscle contraction
Trace Minerals			
Iron	**Males** 14–18 yrs: 11 mg 19–>70 yrs: 8 mg **Females** 14–18 yrs: 15 mg 19–50 yrs: 18 mg 51–>70 yrs: 8 mg	Organ meats, lean meats, poultry, shellfish, dried peas and beans, whole-grain products, green leafy vegetables	Plays role in hemoglobin formation, oxygen transport
Zinc	**Males** 14–>70 yrs: 11 mg **Females** 14–18 yrs: 9 mg 19–>70 yrs: 8 mg	Organ meats, meat, fish, poultry, shellfish, nuts, whole-grain products	Involved in energy metabolism, immune function
Copper	**Males** 14–18 yrs: 890 mcg 19–>70 yrs: 900 mcg **Females** 14–18 yrs: 890 mcg 19–>70 yrs: 900 mcg	Organ meats, meat, fish, poultry, shellfish, nuts, bran cereal	Plays role in use of iron and hemoglobin by body, involved in connective tissue formation and oxidation

CONTINUES

COMPARISON OF VITAMINS AND MINERALS   continued

VITAMINS	DRIs	MAJOR SOURCES	MAJOR FUNCTIONS

Fluoride	*ADEQUATE INTAKE*
	Males
	  14–18 yrs: 3 mg
	  19–>70 yrs: 4 mg
	Females
	  14–>70 yrs: 3 mg
		Milk, egg yolks, drinking water, seafood	Plays role in tooth and bone formation

Selenium	**Males**
	  14–>70 yrs: 55 mcg
	Females
	  14–>70 yrs: 55 mcg
		Meat, fish, poultry, organ meats, seafood, whole grains and nuts from selenium-rich soil	Forms part of antioxidant enzyme

Chromium	**Males**
	  14–50 yrs: 35 mcg
	  51–>70 yrs: 30 mcg
	Females
	  14–18 yrs: 24 mcg
	  19–50 yrs: 25 mcg
	  51–>70 yrs: 20 mcg
		Organ meats, meats, oysters, cheese, whole-grain products, beer	Enhances insulin function as glucose tolerance factor

Iodine	**Males**
	  14–>70 yrs: 150 mcg
	Females
	  14–>70 yrs: 150 mcg
		Iodized table salt, seafood, water	Forms part of thyroxine, which plays a role in reactions involving cellular energy

Manganese	*ADEQUATE INTAKE*
	Males
	  14–18 yrs: 2.2 mg
	  19–>70 yrs: 2.3 mg
	Females
	  14–18 yrs: 1.6 mg
	  19–>70 yrs: 1.8 mg
		Beet greens, whole grains, nuts, legumes	Plays role in essential enzyme systems

Molybdenum	**Males**
	  14–18 yrs: 43 mcg
	  19–>70 yrs: 45 mcg
	Females
	  14–18 yrs: 43 mcg
	  19–>70 yrs: 45 mcg
		Legumes, cereal grains, dark green leafy vegetables	Plays role in essential enzymes involved in carbohydrate and fat metabolism

C

COMPARISON OF
SPORTS NUTRITION PRODUCTS

PRODUCT	TYPE OF CARBOHYDRATE	CARBOHYDRATE CONCENTRATION (%)	CALORIES	CARBO-HYDRATES (g)	SODIUM (mg)
Commercial Sports Drinks (8 oz. or 240 ml serving)					
Accelrade	Sucrose, fructose, maltodextrin (also contains 4 gm protein per serving)	7.75	93	17	127
All Sport	Fructose, sucrose	8	70	19	55
Amino Vital	Fructose (also contains 740 mg of amino acids)	3.3	35	8	10
Body Fuel	Maltodextrin, fructose	7	70	17	70
Cytomax	Fructose, maltodextrin, polylactate, glucose	8	83	19	70
E Fuel	Maltodextrin, fructose	7	70	18	130
EFS	Complex carbohydrates, sucrose, dextrose (also contains 1.5 g of amino acids)	7.5	72	18	188
Endura	Glucose polymers, fructose	6	60	15	92

CONTINUES

COMPARISON OF SPORTS NUTRITION PRODUCTS continued

PRODUCT	TYPE OF CARBOHYDRATE	CARBOHYDRATE CONCENTRATION (%)	CALORIES	CARBO-HYDRATES (g)	SODIUM (mg)
Endurathon	Maltodextrin, trehalose, ribose, fructose, glucose, sucrose (also contains 4 g of protein)	6.7	90	16	200
Exceed	Glucose polymer, fructose	7	70	17	50
Gatorade	Sucrose, glucose	6	50	14	110
Gatorade Endurance Drink	Sucrose, glucose	6	60	15	200
Gookinaid	Glucose, fructose	5	43	10	69
GU20	Maltodextrin, fructose	5.5	52	13	120
HEED	Maltodextrin	5	48	12	31
Hydra Fuel	Glucose polymer, fructose, glucose	7	66	16	25
Hydro-BOOM	Maltodextrin, sucrose, glucose, fructose	7	70	17	160
Met-Rx ORS	Rice syrup solids, glucose	8	70	19	125
Perform	Glucose, fructose, maltodextrin	7	60	16	110
Performance	Maltodextrin, fructose	10	100	25	115
Power Ade	Fructose, sucrose	6	55	14	50
PowerBar Endurance Sports Drink	Maltodextrin, dextrose, fructose	7	70	17	160
PR Solution	Maltodextrin, fructose	12.5	120	30	50
Red Bull	Sucrose, glucose	12	112	28	215
Replenisher	Maltodextrin	1.25	10	3	37.5
Revenge	Maltodextrin, amylopectin starch	9	90	23	100

CONTINUES

COMPARISON OF SPORTS NUTRITION PRODUCTS   continued

PRODUCT	SERVING SIZE	CALORIES	CARBO-HYDRATES (g)	PROTEIN (g)	FAT (g)
Recovery Drinks					
Boost	8 oz. (240 ml)	240	33	15	6
EndoroxR4 (vanilla)	2 scoops (74 g) for 12 oz. (360 ml)	260	50	13	1
Endura Optimizer	2 scoops (78 g)	280	58	12	1
Ensure	8 oz. (240 ml) can	250	40	9	6
Gatorade Energy Drink	12 oz. (360 ml)	310	78	0	0
Gatorade Nutrition Shake	11 oz. (325 ml) can	360	55	20	8
Met-Rx (vanilla)	1 packet (72 g)	250	20	37	2.5
Metabolol Endurance Formula	1 packet (52 g)	200	24	14	5
Metabolol II	1 packet (66 g)	260	40	18	3
Physique	½ cup (57 g)	210	38	14	0.5
Race Recovery	1 packet (87 g)	300	53	20	0
UltraFuel	16 oz. or 2 scoops (480 ml)	400	100	0	0
Ultragen	12 oz. (360 ml)	320	60	20	0

PRODUCT	SERVING SIZE	CALORIES	CARBO-HYDRATES (g)	SODIUM (mg)
Carbohydrate Gels				
Accel Gel	1.4 oz (41 g) packet	90	20 (plus 5 g protein)	95
Carb BOOM	1.4 oz (41 g) packet	110	27	50
Clif Block	3 pieces (30 g)	100	25	70
Clif Shot	1.1 oz (32 g) packet	100	25	50
E-Gel	1.9 oz (55 g) packet	150	37	230
Gu	1.1 oz (32 g) packet	100	30	20
Honey Stinger	1.3 oz (37 g) packet	120	29	50
Power Gel	1.1 oz (41 g) packet	110	33	50
Pro-BOOM	3.0 oz (88 g) packet	150	26	180

CONTINUES

COMPARISON OF SPORTS NUTRITION PRODUCTS continued

GLYCEMIC INDEX OF SELECTED SPORTS NUTRITION PRODUCTS AND CARBOHYDRATE SOURCE

Product/Source	Glycemic Index
Gatorade	89
XLR8	68
Powerade	65
Cytomax	62
Allsport	53
Fructose	22–24
Galactose	22–24
Sucrose	65
Honey	69–73
Glucose	100
Maltodextrin	105

D

CREATING THE OPTIMAL
TRAINING DIET

MEAL PLANNING DOES NOT NEED to be a frustrating experience for dedicated endurance athletes—and you don't have to employ your own personal chef or learn to make gourmet meals. But like your training program, meal planning does require forethought, organization, and flexibility. With practice, your meal-planning skills will become second nature. Some of the fundamentals of meal planning follow.

PLANNING YOUR DAILY MEALS

Have a well-organized and well-equipped kitchen. Make sure that you have all the convenience items that you need, including a microwave, a steamer, a toaster oven, a set of microwave-proof cookware, and a slow cooker. Other handy items include a large stovetop skillet or wok, a rice cooker, a lasagna dish, and sharp knives. Always store items in the same places: Knowing where everything is located will make putting together quick and easy meals that much easier.

Plan out your week's meal ideas beforehand. Think ahead to what meals you will need to cook, pack, or eat out based on that week's schedule. Determine how many dinners you will cook that week at home, and leave room for healthy takeout, eating out, and leftovers. Think about where you will be for lunch. Do you need to pack a full lunch, or some extras, like pretzels and fruit? Determine whether your training schedule requires you to have energy bars or carbohydrate drinks on hand. Perhaps you prefer quick recovery nutrition items to tide you over until your next full meal. Make a shopping list as you plan; if you only can shop once for the whole week, plan to consume the fresh vegetables and fruit early on and save the frozen or canned items for later.

Develop a meal schedule. For example, you could always have chicken on Monday nights, fish on Thursdays, and stir-fries on Fridays. Try to vary the types of vegetables and side dishes that you consume. Sometimes it is easier to obtain variety when you can prepare dinner for an entire family; when cooking for just one or two people, try to obtain variety on a weekly basis, switching the grains, fruits, and vegetables you consume.

Keep nonperishable stock food items amply supplied. Having a well-stocked cupboard of items such as rice, pasta, whole grains, instant couscous, and other dry items and canned goods can help you in a pinch when fresh food supplies run low or during heavy training weeks. Some quick meals made from these ingredients are black bean burritos (freeze the tortillas); pasta and tomato sauce; stir-fries made from frozen chicken, instant rice, and frozen vegetable mixes; and canned chili with bread or crackers.

Go grocery shopping every week for fresh items. Have a designated grocery-shopping day and time and make it part of your weekly schedule. Don't put off shopping until it is convenient to go—it may never be convenient! And in the long run, going shopping once a week is much less time-consuming than having to make several quick trips to the store as the week progresses to grab just a few needed items each time. Try to find one supermarket that can supply all the items you need. Go during off-peak times to avoid crowds, and don't mull over items that are not on your shopping list. If you can't make it to the supermarket some weeks, try an increasingly popular alternative and find a grocery store or online grocery system that accepts phone, fax, or Internet delivery orders.

Keep a running list of items that need to be replenished. Have a pad and pen handy in the kitchen. When you notice that items are running low or are used up, add them to your list. Trying to re-member everything you need while shopping at the grocery store may not be the best strategy for a busy athlete.

Batch cook meals, make extra portions, and freeze single servings. This strategy can be a great time saver. You can set aside a lighter training day to cook items such as soup, chili, and lasagna. When cooking regular meals, making an extra one or two portions for the next day can save dinner preparation time or provide you with a nice midday meal. Freeze single-item portions in plastic containers or oven-ready aluminum foil pans for later use on heavy training days.

Pack meals, snacks, and food supplements for the next training day the night before. If your next day's schedule is full, consider packing your foods and snacks the night before. Having some portioned items and fresh foods in the fridge will make this task as simple as possible. Plan snacks that can be eaten on the run.

Acquire a repertoire of quick and easy-to-prepare meals. Anyone can become a proficient cook, and it does not have to be a time-consuming project. Be on the lookout for quick and simple recipes. Ask friends for some of their quick meal ideas. Focus on recipes like stir-fries, risottos, burritos, and pastas.

SIMPLE SUGGESTIONS FOR STOCKING YOUR PANTRY

For the Freezer
Chicken tenders
Cooked shrimp
Lean ground beef
Lean pork filets
Cubed meat for stir-fries
Soy and garden burgers
Textured vegetable proteins
Egg substitute

Variety of breads
Waffles
English muffins
Muffins
Tortillas
Pre-cooked pasta and rice

Frozen vegetables
Stir-fry mixes

Sorbet
Frozen fruit

For the Refrigerator
Fresh fruit
Fresh vegetables (including pre-washed salad greens, mini-carrots)

Juices

Milk (dairy, soy, rice)
Yogurt
Eggs
Reduced-fat cheese

Butter or margarine

Lean deli meats
Fresh pasta

Sauces and condiments (including salsa, marinades)

For the Cupboard
Dried pasta
Rice
Couscous
Quinoa
Pilaf
Tabouleh
Canned beans and chickpeas

Canned tuna
Peanut butter and other nut butters
Instant stuffing mixes
Canned soup
Instant soup and grain cups
Seasoning mixes

Cold cereal assortment
Oatmeal and farina

Low-fat crackers
Dried fruit
Granola bars
Nuts and sunflower seeds
Pretzels
Fig Newtons

Take advantage of food shortcuts. Purchase chicken tender strips, beef stir-fry strips, frozen pre-cooked shrimp, and rotisserie chickens. Also try frozen vegetable stir-fry mixes, pre-cut fruits, pre-seasoned and cut tofu, ready-to-heat soups, instant couscous mixes, fresh pastas (you can freeze them), and canned beans, chickpeas, and other legumes.

BREAKFAST, LUNCH, AND SNACKS

Breakfast is one of the most important meals of the day. It revs up your body's metabolism and refills liver glycogen stores that have become depleted overnight. It may even be an important recovery meal after a solid early-morning training session. If you, like so many other Americans, tend to skip breakfast, eat a medium-sized lunch, and feast at dinner, you may be not only compromising your recovery but also cheating your body of important nutrients. Skipping breakfast is also a terrible weight-management strategy because it can set you up for increased hunger and overeating later in the day.

Breakfast should keep you feeling satisfied for 3 hours or so until you are hungry again. Inserting a mid-morning snack into your eating plan can enable you to stretch out the span of time between breakfast and lunch. If your energy needs are high, try to have a substantial breakfast. Eat calorically dense cereals such as granola or muesli. A large glass of juice can add a substantial amount of calories and carbohydrates—which is good if you need the carbs to supply energy for your morning workout. Adding some protein to your breakfast can help keep you comfortably full until the next meal.

Depending on your schedule, you may need to consume breakfast on the fly. Bringing breakfast with you as you leave for work or school is better than skipping it altogether. Quick choices can include fruit smoothies made with yogurt and granola, yogurt, bananas, dried fruit, bagels, and muffins.

Your lunch should provide you with quality carbohydrates balanced with a healthy proportion of proteins and fats. Eat lunch when hunger first sets in, as this is a sign that your body needs fuel. Packing a lunch takes a little more time and planning than purchasing one at a restaurant or fast-food establishment, but it is well worth the effort because you can ensure that you have lean proteins and the right type and amount of fats. Some people enjoy eating leftovers from the previous night's dinner, but sandwiches are always a good place to start if last night's leftovers seem too repetitive. Some good protein options are lean beef, hummus, turkey, chicken, tuna, and low-fat cottage cheese. Liven up that turkey sandwich with add-ons such as avocado, lettuce leaves, cucumber, tomato, sprouts, and low-fat cheese. High-carbohydrate items that you can include with your lunch are fruits, pretzels, raw vegetables, yogurt, low-fat chips, low-fat crackers, and vegetable and bean soups.

When your energy needs are high, snacks give you a nice calorie boost. They can also provide you with fuel before training sessions and keep hunger at bay until you can sit down for a full meal. Many elite athletes swear by snacking. Plan some serious snacking in your diet. If there is a particular time of day when you experience an energy lull, snacking may make all the difference. The sidebar "Breakfast and Snack Ideas" lists some tasty breakfast and snack ideas.

BREAKFAST AND SNACK IDEAS

Breakfast

Cooked oatmeal with raisins, cinnamon, and low-fat milk

Open-face English muffin halves broiled with cheese, and fruit on the side

Omelet made with egg substitute and vegetables, with toast, juice, and milk

Yogurt with fresh fruit and a low-fat muffin

Whole-grain cereal with milk and fruit

Fruit smoothie made with yogurt, fresh or frozen fruit, and granola

Whole-grain bread with peanut butter, banana, and honey

Any leftovers that sound appealing

Snacks

Peanut-butter-and-jelly sandwich

Hard and soft pretzels

Baked potato with low-fat cheese

Crackers with peanut butter

Muffin or bagel with jam and low-fat cream cheese

Yogurt with fruit

Bowl of soup with crackers

Pasta or bean salad

Fresh fruit, low-fat cheese, and nuts

Cottage cheese and fruit

Instant breakfast mix and fruit

Hummus and crackers or pita bread

Fruit smoothie

Milk and fruit

LABEL-READING TIPS

Food labels can help you determine the nutritional breakdown of foods. The ingredients list is a good place to start. Because the ingredients are listed by weight, the ingredient that makes up the largest percentage of a food by weight will be the first item listed; the one that makes up the next largest percentage by weight will be the second listed, and so on. So, for example, if you are trying to incorporate more whole-wheat flours and other whole grains into your diet, this part of the label will help you decide among brands of bread, pastas, and the like. Look for whole-wheat flour to be the first ingredient.

Before going any further, look for the part of the label that lists the serving size, and compare it with the amount that you actually eat. The portions you consume may be double those on the package, and you should adjust the nutrition information accordingly. To evaluate whether a food will significantly impact your carbohydrate intake, check for the total grams of carbohydrates per serving. You can then determine how far that particular food will go toward providing the carbohydrates you need to help you meet your training requirements for the day.

Total fat grams as well as calories from fat are also listed. To determine the percentage of calories from fat, divide the fat calories per serving by the total calories per serving and multiply by 100. Keep high-fat foods in perspective. Your fat intake needs to be considered in the context of an entire day. Your total day's intake should include some foods that contain healthy fats—as long as you don't go overboard with fatty foods or eat the wrong type of fats. Some foods, such as dried pasta, are very low in fat, while others, such as margarine, provide a relatively high amount of fat. As long as the percentage of fat for the day averages out to 20 to 25 percent of your total intake, you are in the ballpark. (See Chapter 2 for more information on healthy versus unhealthy fats.)

The Daily Value (DV) for various vitamins and minerals provided on the nutrition label are based on a 2,000-calorie intake. The percent can tell you if a food is high or low in a nutrient such as calcium, fiber, iron, or vitamin C. A food is considered to be a good source of a nutrient if it provides 20 percent of the DV. Besides increasing your intake of foods high in specific nutrients, you can use the DV to avoid excess fat, saturated fat, and cholesterol.

DIETARY RULES FOR RESTAURANTS

Like many North Americans, chances are that you eat out several times weekly. Lunch is the meal most frequently eaten away from home, followed by dinner and then breakfast. Currently, more than 45 percent of the money spent on food in the United States goes toward restaurant meals and other foods consumed away from home. You may eat out at restaurants, in a cafeteria, at your desk, and even in your car.

Regardless of where you eat your meal out, the basic strategies are the same. Watch out for hidden and added fats, and keep a close eye on the portions. Despite your high energy requirements for endurance training, not all restaurant meals fit nicely into your nutrition plan. They may be too high in fat to become a frequent indulgence and may not provide the healthy ingredients that you require. It is important to learn what healthy food choices are available at your favorite restaurants. Ask questions about how foods are prepared, and don't hesitate to request modifications. Often you can creatively outsmart the menu and enjoy your meal knowing that it will be good for you.

FAST FOOD

Fast food—especially supersized meals and grease-laden French fries—can provide excessive amounts of fat. But it is possible to make choices that fit into a sports diet at some fast-food establishments. Have a small hamburger that provides only 2 or 3 ounces of meat rather than the large one. Order baked potatoes over French fries whenever possible. Broiled chicken sandwiches are decent choices, whereas chicken pieces are generally fried. The same goes for fish sandwiches, as they come dripping with plenty of unwanted oil. Order skim milk or juice whenever possible instead of sugary sodas. Salads and vegetables may be on the menu, but watch out for the dressings. Limit the sauces and toppings whenever possible, too.

Many fast-food establishments now provide good sandwich choices. You can choose lean roast beef, ham, turkey, or chicken and limit oils, mayonnaise, and cheese. Go for baked chips and pretzels when offered. Chicken fajitas or tacos sometimes also make good lower-fat choices. Frozen yogurt and low-fat milkshakes are better for you than deep-fried pastries or cookies.

Another fast-food choice that can fit into your sports nutrition plan is a vegetarian thin-crust pizza. Some establishments also have a soup and baked potato bar. Bean burritos and soft tacos may also be available, or possibly chili, bagels, English muffins, waffles, pancakes, and cereals.

ETHNIC CUISINE

If you eat out frequently, you have probably enjoyed many types of ethnic cuisines. These cultural edibles can fit into a healthy training diet if you know what choices to make and can avoid consuming hidden fats. The sampling of ethnic cuisine below is only a few of the many cultural options available in most large and medium-sized cities. You can use a commonsense approach for any ethnic cuisine, whether Indian, Thai, Vietnamese, African, Russian, or Middle Eastern, looking for lean protein options and low-fat alternatives.

Italian Cuisine

Italian food is a popular favorite—especially since it includes pizza—and can be consumed at a variety of settings—upscale, family style, or fast-food. With an emphasis on grains and vegetables, Italian eating can be quite healthy. Some relatively light, low-fat choices include starches such as spaghetti, risotto, and polenta; vegetables such as zucchini and even tomato-based sauces; and lean meats such as chicken, veal, shrimp, and grilled fish. Herbs, vinegar, garlic, and crushed red peppers may be available at the table to spice up your food. Fill up on minestrone, and top your pasta with marinara or red clam sauce. Order your salad dressing on the side, and have an Italian ice for dessert. You can also make special requests—for example, you can ask your waiter to remove the olive oil from the table or have the chef remove the skin from your chicken.

There are also plenty of heavier choices at Italian restaurants. Starches such as garlic bread and focaccia are usually loaded with fat, as are fried vegetables and meats like salami, prosciutto, and sausage. Watch out for high-fat cheeses and dishes prepared with cream, butter, and even olive oil, which may be relatively healthy as far as oils go but still contains plenty of fat calories. Go easy on the antipasto plate and the olive oil served with bread. Alfredo sauce, Italian sausage, lasagna, and parmigiana dishes are all high in fat because of the ingredients and methods of preparation.

Mexican Cuisine

Like Italian food, Mexican cuisine contains both light and heavy choices. Many staples of Mexican cuisine can be considered low-fat, including items such as whole beans, refried beans prepared without oil, tortillas, rice cooked without oil, grilled vegetables, and salsa. Grilled proteins, such as shrimp, fish, and chicken, are also good choices, as are whole black beans. You can also fill up on gazpacho, marinated vegetables, and burritos (but go easy on the cheese).

Some heavier choices at Mexican restaurants would be tortilla chips, chimichangas, and taco shells. Avocados (guacamole), olives, sour cream, and cheese are also high in fat. Also watch out for chorizo, cheese, sour cream, and oil used in cooking, which may contribute a significant amount of fat, especially saturated fat, to a meal. Avoid items on the menu with descriptions that say "smothered in cheese."

Chinese Cuisine

Chinese cuisine, providing a variety of regional cooking styles, is a frequent favorite at mall eateries and small neighborhood restaurants. Although there are light choices in Chinese cooking, there are also many high-fat pitfalls. To keep your meal on the light side, look for stir-fried vegetables. Almost every Chinese restaurant will have a variety to choose from, such as peapods, bamboo shoots, water chestnuts, cabbage, baby corn, and broccoli.

Lean proteins found in Chinese dishes include shrimp, chicken, tofu, and lean cuts of beef and pork, usually mixed with vegetables in some sort of stir-fry combination. Chinese dishes may also contain low-fat fruits, such as pineapple and orange sections. Condiments such as mustard, soy sauce, ginger, sweet sauce, and garlic will not increase the fat content of your meals.

Chinese cuisine also contains plenty of high-fat choices, however. Everyone is familiar with the fatty breaded and fried sweet-and-sour dishes. Fried rice has twice the calories of steamed rice, with all the additional calories coming from oil. Fried noodles and egg rolls can also up your fat intake. Try to stay away from fried seafood, pork, spare ribs, and duck with skin. Stir-fried dishes that contain nuts and peanuts will also be much higher in fat, as will any choices in which oil is used heavily. Request that your dish be prepared with as little oil as possible, and try to split entrees, as portions are often large.

MEAL PLANNING TIPS FOR VEGETARIANS

- Include a protein-rich food at all meals and snacks.
- Add milk, fortified soy or rice milk, or yogurt to every meal or snack.
- Use nuts, butters, hummus, and low-fat cheeses (soy and regular) for toppings on breads, bagels, and crackers.
- Add nuts and seeds to a fruit and yogurt snack.
- Make tofu and tempeh stir-fries.
- Experiment with quick and easy bean recipes to make burritos, casseroles, and salads.
- Make thick soups and stews with beans and lentils.
- Experiment with all the meat-replacer soy products on the market, such as tofu dogs and burgers.
- Make casseroles, lasagna, and stuffed shell recipes with tofu.
- Most health-food stores and the health-food sections of many supermarkets provide a wide selection of vegetarian food choices and convenience items.
- The number of textured vegetable protein products has increased significantly in the past several years. You can now buy products that resemble and taste like hotdogs, burgers, or breakfast sausage. Many of these products make quick and easy lunch ideas.
- Tofu can be substituted for chicken in most recipes. Seasoned tofu is available, and you can also season the recipe to spice up tofu's milder taste.
- You can substitute vegetable broth when recipes call for beef or chicken stock. Vegetable broth is available in many supermarkets and most health-food stores.
- Canned lentils, chickpeas, and beans are a quick and nutritious vegetarian option. When time allows, soak the dried lentil and bean versions. Bean and lentil recipes can be batch cooked and frozen for later use.
- If you need assistance, find a vegetarian cookbook that provides meal ideas suited to athletes.
- Include protein-rich foods at every meal. Because vegetarian options are not as concentrated in protein as animal sources, you need to include adequate portions at most meals and snacks.
- Purchase calcium-fortified soy and rice milks if you drink these products instead of dairy milk.
- Purchase iron-fortified cereals and consume them with products high in vitamin C, such as orange juice.

SALAD BARS

Visits to the salad bar are often well intended but can result in surprisingly high-fat meals. Beside those healthy raw vegetable items like spinach, tomatoes, broccoli, and green peppers are plenty of items mixed with fat or sitting in oil. Some of the less healthy choices are pasta salad, potato salad, marinated vegetables, cheeses, and bean salads made with oil. Go easy on portions of these items. Of course, try to keep salad dressing portions reasonable as well.

Salad bars have plenty of carbohydrates and fiber and can help you keep your protein portions low and reasonable. Obviously, fresh greens and plain raw vegetables are your best bet. Starches on the salad bar may include chickpeas, kidney beans, green peas, crackers, and pita bread. Lean protein salad-bar choices include plain tuna, cottage cheese, hard-boiled egg, ham cubes, and feta cheese. Try to avoid most cheeses and pepperoni. Keep marinated vegetable portions small, and especially watch out for salads made with mayonnaise, such as tuna or chicken salad, seafood salad, macaroni salad, and potato salad. Peanuts, sesame seeds, and sunflower seeds provide good fats and can be used in small amounts.

E

SAMPLE
MENUS

NUTRITIONAL REQUIREMENTS NEED TO BE TAILORED to the unique needs of individual athletes, and they will change even for individual athletes at various phases in their training program. A periodized nutrition plan requires adjustments in total intake of carbohydrates, proteins, and fats through each training cycle as well as for various types of training sessions within a training cycle (see Chapter 4).

The sample menus provided below are therefore not meant to be followed precisely—individual athletes must design their own menus that are appropriate for their own nutrient and energy needs; however, they can serve as a guide to how food intake might be balanced for various levels of training. If you know your calorie intake and nutrient needs, you may find that you can choose menus from the list that are a fairly good match for your current training cycle and use them to help you get started in improving your sports nutrition diet, then learn how to make adjustments for your own tastes and exact requirements. Experiment with various food items and portion sizes to find out what works best for you.

Because of the timing of training most common among endurance athletes—and the frequency of training, with some athletes training twice daily—most of these menus provide one or two snacks a day. In some of the menus, one of these is a light snack that can be consumed before very early morning training, a time when a full breakfast may not be tolerated. The timing of food and fluid intake can, and should, be adjusted to accommodate individual tolerances and training schedules. Consult Chapter 5 for more information on making adjustments in meal and snack timing before and after training. Also, many endurance athletes may need additional amounts of water and other fluids for adequate daily hydration. Monitor your weight before and after different types of training sessions so that you will be familiar with your sweat rate, and then be sure to drink enough fluids to replace these losses adequately (see the sidebar "Estimating Your Sweat Rate" in Chapter 5).

Sports nutrition supplements such as sports drinks and gels can also be added to these sample menus. You may choose to use sports nutrition products in place of some of the snacks because of their convenience. If so, keep in mind that these products would typically replace a grain or fruit serving in the menus.

Of course, you may want to enlist the services of a sports dietitian or nutritionist, who would be able to provide you with your own personalized meal plans as you prepare for an event or competition.

BASE CYCLE MEAL PLANS

2,200 CALORIES **340 G CARBOHYDRATES (60%)** **99 G PROTEIN (18%)** **56 G FAT (22%)**	**2,400 CALORIES** **346 G CARBOHYDRATES (58%)** **99 G PROTEIN (17%)** **68 G FAT (25%)**	**2,700 CALORIES** **380 G CARBOHYDRATES (55%)** **130 G PROTEIN (19%)** **75 G FAT (25%)**

Breakfast
Orange juice, 1 c. (240 ml)
French toast, 2 slices
Syrup, ½ c. (120 ml)
Strawberries, 1 c. (240 ml)

Lunch
Low-fat cheese, 2 oz. (60 g)
Bread, 2 slices
Tomato, 1 medium
Yogurt with fruit, 1 c. (240 ml)
Pear, 1 medium

Snack
Crackers, 8 small
Hummus, ½ c. (120 ml)
Skim milk, 8 oz. (240 ml)

Dinner
Rice, cooked, 1½ c. (360 ml)
Shrimp, cooked, 6 oz. (180 g)
Red pepper, 1 whole
Broccoli, cooked, 1 c. (240 ml)
Sesame seed oil, 1 tbsp. (15 ml)

Snack
Frozen yogurt, 1 c. (240 ml)
Fruit slices, ½ c. (120 ml)

Breakfast
English muffin
Cream cheese, 2 tbsp. (30 ml)
Jam, 2 tbsp. (30 ml)
Grapefruit juice, 12 oz. (360 ml)
Egg, 1 medium

Lunch
Pinto beans, ½ c. (120 ml)
Rice, cooked, 1 c. (240 ml)
Tortilla, 1 medium
Salsa, 4 tbsp. (60 ml)
Cheese, 1 oz. (30 g)
Avocado, ¼ whole

Snack
Granola bar
Peaches, 2 medium
Almonds, 1 tbsp. (15 ml)

Dinner
Pasta, cooked, 2 c. (480 ml)
Lean beef, 3 oz. (90 g)
Marinara sauce, 1 c. (240 ml)
Green salad, 2 c. (480 ml)
Salad dressing, 2 tbsp. (30 ml)

Snack
Frozen yogurt, 1 c. (240 ml)
Blueberries, ½ c. (120 ml)

Breakfast
Oatmeal, cooked, 1½ c. (360 ml)
Skim milk, 8 oz. (240 ml)
Wheat germ, 4 tbsp. (60 ml)
Bread, 2 slices
Jam, 2 tbsp. (30 ml)
Orange juice, 8 oz. (240 ml)

Lunch
Chicken, 4 oz. (120 g)
Bread, whole-grain, 2 slices
Mayonnaise, light, 2 tbsp. (30 ml)
Rice and bean salad, ½ c. (120 ml)
Grapes, 1 c. (240 ml)

Snack
Energy bar
Banana, 1 medium
Yogurt with fruit, 8 oz. (240 ml)

Dinner
Tofu, 6 oz. (180 g)
Asian noodles, cooked, 2 c. (480 ml)
Vegetables, 2 c. (480 ml)
Sesame seed oil, 2 tbsp. (30 ml)

CONTINUES

BASE CYCLE MEAL PLANS | continued

3,000 CALORIES 450 G CARBOHYDRATES (60%) 115 G PROTEIN (15%) 83 G FAT (25%)	3,400 CALORIES 510 G CARBOHYDRATES (60%) 130 G PROTEIN (15%) 95 G FAT (25%)	3,800 CALORIES 570 G CARBOHYDRATES (60%) 140 G PROTEIN (15%) 105 G FAT (25%)

3,000 CALORIES

Snack
Toast, 1 slice
Jam, 1 tbsp. (15 ml)
Juice, 8 oz. (240 ml)

Breakfast
Oatmeal, cooked, 1 c. (240 ml)
Skim milk, 8 oz. (240 ml)
Raisins, 2 tbsp. (30 ml)
Banana, 1 large
Juice, 8 oz. (240 ml)

Snack
Granola bar, 1 medium

Lunch
Chicken salad, 3 oz. (100 g)
Bread, whole-grain, 2 slices
Avocado, 3 slices
Potato salad, low-fat, 1 c. (240 ml)
Grapes, 15

Snack
Cottage cheese, ½ cup
Pretzels, 1½ oz. (45 g)
Apple, 1 medium

Dinner
Pork, cooked, 5 oz. (150 g)
Stir-fry vegetable mix, 1 cup
Canola oil, 1 tbsp. (15 ml)
Brown rice, cooked, 1½ c. (360 ml)

Snack
Yogurt, 6 oz.
Peach, 1 medium

3,400 CALORIES

Snack
Energy bar
Juice, 8 oz. (240 ml)
Banana, 1 medium

Breakfast
Granola, 1 cup (240 ml)
Soy milk, 8 oz. (240 ml)
Nuts, 12
Berries, 1 c. (240 ml)
Juice, 8 oz. (240 ml)

Snack
Bagel, 3 oz. (90 g)
Jam, 2 tbsp. (30 ml)
Orange, 1 medium

Lunch
Roast beef, 4 oz. (120 g)
Cheese, low-fat, 1 oz. (30 g)
Roll, 2 oz. (60 g)
Pasta salad, ½ cup (120 ml)
Pear, 1 medium

Snack
Yogurt with fruit, 6 oz. (180 ml)
Nuts, 24

Dinner
Burrito:
Beans, 1 c. (240 ml)
Rice, cooked, ⅔ c. (160 ml)
Chicken, 4 oz. (120 g)
Tortilla, 1 large, 2 oz. (60 g)
Salsa, ½ c. (120 ml)
Vegetable mix, 1 c. (240 ml)

Snack
Ice cream, low-fat, 1 c. (240 ml)
Fruit, ½ cup (120 ml)

3,800 CALORIES

Snack
Toast, 2 slices
Jam, 2 tbsp. (30 ml)
Peanut butter, 1 tbsp. (15 ml)
Juice, 8 oz. (240 ml)

Breakfast
Muesli, 1 c. (240 ml)
Skim milk, 8 oz. (240 ml)
Raisins, 3 tbsp. (45 ml)
Juice, 8 oz. (240 ml)

Snack
Yogurt with fruit, 6 oz.
Nuts, 24
Banana, 1 medium

Lunch
Tuna salad, 4 oz. (120 g)
Bread, whole-grain, 2 slices (60 g)
Pretzels, 2 oz. (60 g)
Vegetable mix, 1 c. (240 ml)
Plums, 2 small

Snack
Crackers, 2 oz. (60 g)
Cream cheese, 1 tbsp. (15 ml)
Dried apricots, 12

Dinner
Fish, 5 oz. (150 g)
Sweet potato, 1 large
Salad mix, 2 c.
Salad dressing, 3 tbsp. (45 ml)
Vegetables, cooked, 1 c. (240 ml)
Bread, 2 slices

Snack
Frozen yogurt, 8 oz.
Berries, 1 c.

BUILD CYCLE MEAL PLANS

2,200 CALORIES 370 G CARBOHYDRATES (67%) 100 G PROTEIN (18%) 33 G FAT (15%)	2,500 CALORIES 410 G CARBOHYDRATES (66%) 120 G PROTEIN (19%) 42 G FAT (15%)	2,800 CALORIES 455 G CARBOHYDRATES (65%) 125 G PROTEIN (18%) 53 G FAT (17%)

Breakfast
Toast, 2 slices
Jam, 2 tbsp. (30 ml)
Juice, 8 oz. (240 ml)
Egg, 1 medium
Banana, 1 medium

Snack
Crackers, 1 oz. (30 g)
Hummus, 2 tbsp. (30 ml)
Apple, 1 medium

Lunch
Ham, 3 oz. (100 g)
Bread, 2 slices
Kidney bean salad, 1 c. (240 ml)
Grapes, 30

Snack
Granola bar
Pear, 1 small
Nuts, 12

Dinner
Stir-fry:
Shrimp, 5 oz. (150 g)
Vegetable mix, 1 c. (240 ml)
Brown rice, cooked, 1½ c. (360 ml)
Sesame seed oil, 1 tbsp. (15 ml)

Breakfast
Bagel, 4 oz. (120 g)
Jam, 2 tbsp. (30 ml)
Peanut butter, 1 tbsp. (15 ml)
Juice, 8 oz. (240 ml)

Snack
Yogurt, 8 oz. (240 ml)
Granola, ½ cup (120 ml)
Raisins, 1 tbsp. (15 ml)

Lunch
Burrito:
Beans, ½ c. (120 ml)
Tortilla, 1 large
Chicken, 3 oz. (90 g)
Salsa, ½ c. (120 ml)
Rice, cooked, ⅔ c. (180 ml)
Peppers, ½ c. (120 ml)

Snack
Pretzels, 2 oz. (60 g)
String cheese, 1 oz. (30 g)
Plums, 2 medium

Dinner
Fish, 6 oz. (180 g)
Baked potato, 1 medium
Bread, 2 slices
Vegetable, 1 c. (240 ml)

Breakfast
Cereal, 1½ oz. (45 g)
Soy milk, 8 oz. (240 ml)
Juice, 8 oz. (240 ml)
Berries, 1 c. (240 ml)

Snack
Bagel, 4 oz. (120 g)
Honey, 2 tbsp. (30 ml)
Peanut butter, 1 tbsp. (30 ml)
Juice, 8 oz. (240 ml)

Lunch
Turkey, 3 oz. (90 g)
Bread, 2 slices
Lentil salad, ½ c. (120 ml)
Vegetable mix, 1 c. (240 ml)
Juice, 8 oz. (240 ml)

Snack
Yogurt, 8 oz. (240 ml)
Raisins, 3 tbsp. (45 ml)
Nuts, 12

Dinner
Pasta, cooked, 2½ cups (600 ml)
Marinara sauce, 1 c. (240 ml)
Salad, 2 c.
Salad dressing, 4 tbsp. (60 ml)
Chicken breast, 3 oz. (90 g)

CONTINUES

BUILD CYCLE MEAL PLANS continued

3,000 CALORIES	3,700 CALORIES	4,500 CALORIES
430 G CARBOHYDRATES (58%)	**630 G CARBOHYDRATES (68%)**	**775 G CARBOHYDRATES (67%)**
176 G PROTEIN (23%)	**130 G PROTEIN (14%)**	**140 G PROTEIN (12%)**
63 G FAT (19%)	**75 G FAT (18%)**	**105 G FAT (21%)**

Breakfast
Bagel, 4 oz. (120 g)
Peanut butter, 2 tbsp. (30 ml)
Citrus juice, 12 oz. (360 ml)
Banana, 1 medium
Yogurt, plain, 1 c. (240 ml)

Lunch
Tuna, 4 oz. (120 g)
Mayonnaise, 1 tbsp. (15 ml)
Pita bread, 1 round
Pretzels, 1½ oz. (45 g)
Raw vegetable salad, 1 c. (240 ml)

Snack
Soy or dairy milk, 12 oz. (360 ml)
Peach slices, 1 c. (240 ml)
Granola, low-fat, ¼ c. (60 ml)

Dinner
Halibut, 8 oz. (240 g)
Buckwheat, cooked, 1½ c.
 (360 ml)
Asparagus, 1 c. (240 ml)
Canola oil, 2 tsp. (10 ml)

Snack
Sorbet, 1 c. (240 ml)
Fig cookies, 3 small

Breakfast
Grits, cooked, 1 c. (240 ml)
Raisins, 2 tbsp. (30 ml)
Yogurt, nonfat, plain, 1 c. (240 ml)
Dried cherries, 10
Cashews, 1 tbsp. (15 ml)

Lunch
Hummus, ½ c. (120 ml)
Pita bread, 2 rounds
Celery, pepper, carrots, 2 c.
 (480 ml)
Apple juice, 12 oz. (360 ml)

Snack
Bagel, 2 oz. (60 g)
Nut butter, 2 tbsp. (30 ml)
Apple, 1 large

Dinner
Pork tenderloin, 8 oz. (240 g)
Rice, cooked, 1½ c. (360 ml)
Corn, ½ c. (120 ml)
Mushrooms, 1/4 c. (60 ml)
Bread, 2 slices
Olive oil, 4 tsp. (20 ml)

Snack
Sherbet, 1 c. (240 ml)
Raspberries, 1 c. (240 ml)

Breakfast
Pancakes, 4 small
Maple syrup, ¾ c. (180 ml)
Banana, 1 medium
Raisins, 2 tbsp. (30 ml)
Nuts, 1 tbsp. (15 ml)
Soy milk, 12 oz. (360 ml)

Sports drink, 40 oz. (1,200 ml)

Lunch
Burrito:
Chicken, 5 oz. (150 g)
Rice, cooked, 2 c. (480 ml)
Pinto beans, cooked, 1 c. (240 ml)
Avocado, ¼ whole
Salsa, ½ c. (120 ml)

Dinner
Linguine, cooked, 3 c. (720 ml)
Mixed vegetables, 1 c. (240 ml)
Bread, 2 slices
Olive oil, 2 tbsp. (30 ml)
Salad, 2 c. (480 ml)
Salad dressing, 2 tbsp. (30 ml)

Snack
Frozen yogurt, 2 c. (480 ml)
Cookies, 2
Strawberries, 1 c. (240 ml)

TRANSITION CYCLE MEAL PLANS

2,200 CALORIES, **290 G CARBOHYDRATES (51%)** **143 G PROTEIN (25%)** **60 G FAT (24%)**	**2,500 CALORIES** **415 G CARBOHYDRATES (64%)** **110 G PROTEIN (17%)** **53 G FAT (19%)**	**2,600 CALORIES** **335 G CARBOHYDRATES (51%)** **139 G PROTEIN (21%)** **83 G FAT (28%)**

Breakfast
Cooked grain cereal, 1 c. (240 ml)
Banana, 1 medium
Cottage cheese, ½ c. or egg,
  1 medium
Nuts, 1 tbsp. (15 ml)

Snack
Recovery smoothie:
12 oz. soy or dairy milk (360 ml)
Frozen fruit, 1 c. (240 ml)

Lunch
Low-fat tuna salad, 3 oz. (90 g)
Bread, 2 slices
Lentil or pasta salad, ½ c. (120 ml)

Dinner
Salmon, 6 oz. (180 g)
Buckwheat or rice, cooked, 1 c.
  (240 ml)
Asparagus, 1 c. (240 ml)
Salad, 2 c. (480 ml)
Olive oil, 2 tsp. (10 ml)
Salad dressing, 2 tbsp. (30 ml)

Snack
Sorbet or frozen yogurt, ½ c.
  (120 ml)
Peach, 1 medium

Breakfast
Oatmeal, cooked, 1 c. (240 ml)
Apple, 1 medium
Juice, 8 oz. (240 ml)

Snack
Yogurt, 6 oz. (180 ml)
Strawberries, 1 c. (240 ml)

Lunch
Chicken, 3 oz. (100 g)
Bread, whole-grain, 2 slices
Pretzels, ¾ oz. (22 g)
Pear, 1 large

Snack
Bagel, 3 oz. (90 g)
Peanut butter, 1 tsp. (5 ml)

Dinner
Beef strips, 3 oz. (90 g)
Noodles, cooked, 2 c. (480 ml)
Bread, 1 slice
Olive oil, 2 tsp. (10 ml)
Mixed vegetables, 1 c. (240 ml)

Breakfast
Muesli, ¾ c. (180 ml)
Apple, 1 medium
Raisins, 2 tbsp. (30 ml)
Soy or dairy milk, 1 c. (240 ml)
Almonds, 2 tsp. (10 ml)

Snack
Granola bar
Peach, 1 medium

Lunch
Chicken tacos:
Chicken, 3 oz. (90 g)
Kidney or pinto beans, cooked,
  ½ c. (120 ml)
Rice, cooked, 1 c. (240 ml)
Tortillas, corn, 2
Oil, 2 tsp. (10 ml)

Snack
Papaya, 1 medium
Crackers, 2 oz. (60 g)
Cream cheese, 2 tbsp. (30 ml)

Dinner
Risotto:
Beef, 4 oz. (120 g)
Broccoli, 1 c. (240 ml)
Rice, 1½ c. cooked (360 ml)
Bread, 2 slices
Oil, 2 tsp. (10 ml)

CONTINUES

TRANSITION CYCLE MEAL PLANS   continued

2,800 CALORIES	3,800 CALORIES	4,300 CALORIES
405 G CARBOHYDRATES (58%)	550 G CARBOHYDRATES (58%)	610 G CARBOHYDRATES (56%)
125 G PROTEIN (18%)	160 G PROTEIN (17%)	168 G PROTEIN (15%)
90 G FAT (24%)	105 G FAT (25%)	137 G FAT (29%)

Breakfast
Waffles, 4 squares
Syrup, ½ c. (120 ml)
Berries, 1 c. (240 ml)
Hard-boiled egg, 1
Soy or dairy milk, 12 oz. (360 ml)

Lunch
Roast turkey, 3 oz. (90 g)
Avocado or hummus, 2 tbsp.
 (30 ml)
Toasted pita, 1 round
Plums, 3 medium
Soy or dairy milk, 8 oz. (240 ml)
Yogurt, nonfat, 6 oz. (180 g)

Snack
Pear, 1 large
Crackers, 12

Dinner
Pasta, 3 c. (720 ml) cooked
Marinara sauce, 1½ c. (360 ml)
Lean beef, 3 oz. (90 g)
Bread, 2 slices
Salad, 2 c. (480 ml)
Olive oil, 1 tbsp. (15 ml)
Salad dressing, 2 tbsp. (30 ml)

Breakfast
Raisin bran, 1½ c. (360 ml)
Milk, 8 oz. (240 ml)
Grapefruit, 1 medium
Bagel, 3 oz. (90 g)
Cheese, low-fat, 2 oz. (60 g)

Snack
Recovery smoothie:
Skim milk, 16 oz. (480 ml)
Juice, 4 oz. (120 ml)
Granola, ½ c. (120 ml)
Banana, 1 medium

Lunch
Peanut butter, 1 tbsp. (15 ml)
Jam, 2 tbsp. (30 ml)
Bread, 2 slices
Pear, 1 medium

Snack
Orange, 1 medium
Yogurt with fruit, 8 oz. (240 ml)
Granola bar, 1 medium
Nuts, 24

Dinner
Grilled chicken, 6 oz. (180 g)
Sweet potatoes, 10 oz. (300 g)
Peas, cooked, 1 c. (240 ml)
Bread, 2 slices
Olive oil, 5 tsp. (50 ml)
Fruit salad, 1 c. (240 ml)

Snack
Sorbet, 1 c. (240 ml)
Strawberries, 1 c. (240 ml)

Breakfast
Bran flakes, 1 c. (240 ml)
Milk, 1 c. (240 ml)
English muffins, 2
Cheese, low-fat, 2 oz. (60 g)
Smoothie:
Soy or dairy milk, 12 oz. (360 ml)
Banana, 1 medium
Wheat germ, 1 tbsp. (15 ml)
Sports drink, 40 oz. (1,200 ml)

Lunch
Beef and bean burritos:
Beef, 8 oz. (240 g)
Rice, cooked, ½ c. (120 ml)
Beans, 1 c. (240 ml)
Tortillas, 2 large
Salsa, 1 c. (240 ml)
Canola oil, 4 tsp. (35 ml)

Snack
Gingersnaps, 6
Juice, 8 oz. (240 ml)

Dinner
Tofu stir-fry:
Tofu, 4 oz. (120 g)
Brown rice, 1½ c. cooked (360 ml)
Sweet peppers and broccoli,
 cooked, 1 c. (240 ml)
Sesame seed oil, 1 tbsp. (15 ml)

Snack
Granola bar
Ice cream, 1 c. (240 ml)
Chocolate syrup, 2 tbsp. (30 ml)
Nuts, 2 tsp. (10 ml)

VEGETARIAN MENUS

2,200 CALORIES 348 G CARBOHYDRATES (62%) 95 G PROTEIN (17%) 53 G FAT (21%)	2,400 CALORIES 390 G CARBOHYDRATES (63%) 105 G PROTEIN (17%) 56 G FAT (20%)	3,000 CALORIES 475 G CARBOHYDRATES (67%) 102 G PROTEIN (14%) 60 G FAT (19%)

Breakfast
Farina, cooked, 1 c. (240 ml)
Skim milk, 8 oz. (240 ml)
Nuts, 1 tbsp. (15 ml)
Apple, 1 medium
Orange juice, 12 oz. (360 ml)

Lunch
Soy burger, 1 patty
Bun, 1 whole
Cheese, low-fat, 1 oz. (30 g)
Lentil or bean salad, ½ c.
 (120 ml)
Vegetables, raw, 1 c. (240 ml)
Avocado, ¼ whole

Dinner
Kidney beans, 1 c. (240 ml)
Rice, cooked, 1 c. (240 ml)
Tortilla, 1 medium
Green salad, 1 c. (240 ml)
Salad dressing, 2 tbsp. (30 ml)

Snack
Granola bar
Peach, 1 medium
Yogurt with fruit, 8 oz. (240 ml)

Breakfast
Muesli, ¾ c. (180 ml)
Soy or dairy yogurt, 8 oz. (240 ml)
Blueberries, 1 c. (240 ml)

Lunch
Garbanzo beans, ⅓ c. (80 ml)
Salad greens/vegetables, 3 c.
 (720 ml)
Pita, 1 large
Cheese, low-fat, 2 oz. (60 g)
Grapefruit juice, 8 oz. (240 ml)

Snack
Energy bar, 1 medium
Apple, 1 medium

Dinner
Tempeh, ¾ c. (180 ml)
Rice, cooked, 1½ c. (360 ml)
Broccoli, cooked, 1 c. (240 ml)
Sesame seed oil, 1 tbsp. (15 ml)

Snack
Orange, 1 medium
Almond, 2 tsp. (10 ml)

Breakfast
Waffles, 2 small
Maple syrup, 4 oz. (120 ml)
Raspberries, 1 c. (240 ml)
Skim milk, 1 c. (240 ml)

Lunch
Hummus, ½ c. (120 ml)
Rice, cooked, ½ c. (120 ml)
Lentil salad, ½ c. (120 ml)
Pita bread, 1 round
Carrots and celery, 2 c.
 (480 ml)

Snack
Bagel, 4 oz. (120 g)
Cheese, low-fat, 2 oz. (60 g)
Apple, 1 medium

Dinner
Tofu, 4 oz. (120 g)
Soba noodles, cooked, 2 c.
 (480 ml)
Greens, cooked, 1 c. (240 ml)
Sesame seed oil, 1 tbsp. (15 ml)

Snack
Pear, 1 large

CONTINUES

VEGETARIAN MENUS | continued

2,900 CALORIES **470 G CARBOHYDRATES (62%)** **113 G PROTEIN (15%)** **78 G FAT (23%)**	**3,400 CALORIES** **550 G CARBOHYDRATES (65%)** **120 G PROTEIN (14%)** **77 G FAT (21%)**	**3,700 CALORIES** **610 G CARBOHYDRATES (66%)** **134 G PROTEIN (14%)** **83 G FAT (20%)**

Breakfast
Pancakes, 4 small
Syrup, 6 tbsp. (90 g)
Raisins, 2 tbsp. (30 ml)
Apple juice, 8 oz. (240 ml)
Eggs, 2 medium

Snack
Soy or dairy yogurt with fruit, 8 oz. (240 ml)
Almonds, 2 tbsp. (30 ml)

Lunch
Bean soup, 1½ c. (360 ml)
Rye crackers, 4
Vegetable salad, 1 c. (240 ml)
Soy milk, 12 oz. (360 ml)

Dinner
Potato, 1 large
Kidney beans, 1 c. (240 ml)
Cheese, low-fat, 1 oz. (30 g)
Green salad, 2 c. (480 ml)
Salad dressing, 3 tbsp. (45 g)

Snack
Frozen yogurt, 1 c. (240 ml)
Banana, 1 medium

Breakfast
Oatmeal, cooked, 1½ c. (360 ml)
Skim milk, 1 c. (240 ml)
Wheat germ, 2 tbsp. (30 ml)
Orange juice, 12 oz. (360 ml)
Yogurt, 1 c. (240 ml)
Apple, 1 large
Sports drink, 40 oz. (1200 ml)

Lunch
Thin-crust pizza, cheese, 3 slices
Green salad, 2 c. (480 ml)
Salad dressing, 2 tbsp. (30 ml)
Soy milk, 8 oz. (240 ml)

Snack
Pretzels, 2 oz. (60 g)
Hummus, ½ c. (120 ml)
Raw vegetables, 1 c. (240 ml)

Dinner
Spaghetti, cooked, 3 c. (720 ml)
Marinara sauce, 2 c. (480 ml)
Parmesan cheese, 3 tbsp. (45 ml)
Italian bread, 2 slices
Olive oil, 1 tbsp. (15 ml)

Snack
Sorbet, 1½ c. (360 ml)
Fig bars, 2

Breakfast
Bran flakes, 1½ c. (360 ml)
Wheat germ, 2 tbsp. (30 ml)
Soy or dairy milk, 8 oz. (240 ml)
Peach, 1 medium
Nuts, 12

Recovery Drink
Juice, 12 oz. (360 ml)
Yogurt, 1 c. (240 ml)
Banana, 1 medium

Lunch
Nut butter, 2 tbsp. (30 ml)
Bread, 2 slices
Bean soup, 1 c. (240 ml)
Raw vegetables, 1 c. (240 ml)

Dinner
Tofu, 8 oz. (240 g)
Peas, 1 c. (240 ml)
Noodles, cooked, 2 c. (480 ml)
Rolls, 2
Vegetable oil, 2 tbsp. (30 ml)
Green salad, 2 c. (480 ml)
Salad dressing, 2 tbsp. (30 ml)
Sports drink, 40 oz. (1,200 ml)

Snack
Yogurt, 8 oz (240 ml)
Mango, 1 large
Crackers, 12

Selected Bibliography

Armstrong, L.E. 2000. *Performing in Extreme Environments*. Champaign, IL: Human Kinetics.

Armstrong, L.E. 2002. Caffeine, body fluid–electrolyte balance, and exercise performance. *International Journal of Sport Nutrition and Exercise Metabolism* 12(2): 189–206.

Armstrong, L.E. 2005. Fluid, electrolyte, and renal indices of hydration during 11 days of controlled caffeine consumption. *International Journal of Sport Nutrition and Exercise Metabolism* 15(3): 252–265.

Ball, T., et al. 1995. Periodic carbohydrate replacement during 50 minutes of high intensity cycling improves subsequent sprint performance. *International Journal of Sport Nutrition* 5(2): 151–158.

Beals, K. 2004. *Disordered Eating Among Athletes*. Champaign, IL: Human Kinetics.

Beals, K., and M. Manore. 1994. The prevalence and consequences of subclinical eating disorders in female athletes. *International Journal of Sports Nutrition* 4(2): 175–195.

Below, P., et al. 1995. Fluid and carbohydrate ingestion independently improve performance during 1 hour intense exercise. *Medicine and Science in Sports and Exercise* 27: 200–210.

Benson, J., et al. 1996. Nutritional aspects of amenorrhea in the female athlete triad. *International Journal of Sport Nutrition* 6(2): 134–145.

Berning, J. 1996. The role of medium chain triglycerides in exercise. *International Journal of Sport Nutrition* 6(2): 121–133.

Blom, T., et al. 1987. The effects of different post-exercise sugar diets on the rate of muscle glycogen resynthesis. *Medicine and Science in Sports and Exercise* 19: 491–496.

Brand-Miller, Jennie, et al. 2003. *The New Glucose Revolution Complete Guide to Glycemic Index Values*. New York: Marlowe and Company.

Brooks, G., et al. 1991. Increased dependence on blood glucose after acclimatization to 4,300 meters. *Journal of Applied Physiology* 70(2): 919–927.

Brown, G., et al. 2000. Effect of anabolic precursors on serum testosterone concentrations and adaptations to resistance training in young men. *International Journal of Sport Nutrition and Exercise Metabolism* 10(3): 340–359.

Bruce, C.R. et al. 2000. Enhancement of 2000-m rowing performance after caffeine ingestion. *Medicine and Science in Sports and Exercise* 32(11): 1958–1963.

Burke, L.M., and JA. Hawley. 2002. Effects of short-term fat adaptation on metabolism and performance for prolonged exercise. *Medicine and Science in Sport & Exercise* 34(9): 1492–1498.

Burke, L.M., et al. 1993. Muscle glycogen storage after prolonged exercise: Effect of the glycemic index of carbohydrate feedings. *Journal of Applied Physiology* 75(2): 1019–1023.

Burke, L.M., et al. 1996. Muscle glycogen storage after prolonged exercise: Effect of the frequency of carbohydrate feedings. *American Journal of Clinical Nutrition* 64: 115–119.

Burke, L.M., et al. 2000. Effect of fat adaptation and carbohydrate restoration on metabolism and performance during prolonged cycling. *Journal of Applied Physiology* 89(6): 2413–2421.

Burke, L.M., et al. 2002. Adaptations to short-term high-fat diet persist during exercise despite high carbohydrate availability. *Medicine and Science in Sports and Exercise* 34(1): 83–91.

Burke, L.M., et al. 2004. Carbohydrate and fat for training and recovery. *Journal of Sport Sciences* 22(8): 15–30.

Burke, L.M. et al. 2005. Effect of carbohydrate intake on half-marathon performance of well-trained runners. *International Journal of Sport Nutrition and Exercise Metabolism* 15(6): 573–589.

Butterfield, G., et al. 1992. Increased energy intake minimizes weight loss in men at high altitude. *Journal of Applied Physiology* 72(5): 1741–1748.

Campbell, W., et al. 1997. Effects of chromium picolinate and resistance training on body composition in older men. *Medicine and Science in Sports and Exercise* 29(5): S277.

Carey, A., et al. 2001. Effects of fat adaptation and carbohydrate restoration on prolonged endurance exercise. *Journal of Applied Physiology* 91(1): 115–122.

Catlin, D., et al. 2000. Trace contamination of over-the-counter androstenedione and positive urine test results for a nandrolone metabolite. *Journal of the American Medical Association* 284(20): 2618–2621.

Chryssanthopoulos, C., et al. 2002. The effect of a high carbohydrate meal on endurance running capacity. *International Journal of Sport Nutrition and Exercise Metabolism* 12(2): 157–171.

Clancy, S., et al. 1994. Effects of chromium picolinate supplementation on body composition, strength and urinary chromium loss in football players. International Journal of Sport Nutrition 4: 142–153.

Clarkson, P. 1991. Nutritional ergogenic aids: Chromium, exercise, and muscle mass. *International Journal of Sport Nutrition* 1: 289–293.

Clarkson, P. 1992. Nutritional ergogenic aids: Carnitine. *International Journal of Sport Nutrition* 2: 185–190.

Conley, M., and M. Stone. 1996. Carbohydrate ingestion/supplementation for resistance exercise and training. *Sports Medicine* 21(1): 7–17.

Cox, G.R., et al. 2002. Effect of different exercise protocols of caffeine intake on metabolism and endurance performance. *Journal of Applied Physiology* 93(3): 900–909.

Coyle, E. 2004. Fluid and fuel intake during exercise. *Journal of Sports Sciences* 22(8): 39–55.

Coyle, E., et al. 2001. Low-fat diet alters intramuscular substrates and reduces lipolysis and fat oxidation during exercise. *American Journal of Endocrinology and Metabolism* 280(3): E391–E398.

Crowe, M.J., et al. 2003. The effects of B-hydroxy-B-methylbutarate (HMB) and HMB/creatine supplementation on indices of health in highly trained athletes. *International Journal of Nutrition and Exercise Metabolism* 13(2): 184–197.

Davis, J. 1996. Carbohydrates, branched chain amino acids and endurance: The Central Fatigue Hypothesis. *Gatorade Sports Science Exchange* 9(2).

Decombaz, J., et al. 1993. Effect of L-carnitine on submaximal exercise metabolism after depletion of muscle glycogen. *Medicine and Science in Sports and Exercise* 25: 733–740.

Dunford, Marie. 2006. *Sports Nutrition: A Practice Manual for Professionals.* Chicago: American Dietetic Association.

Fallowfield, J., et al. 1995. The influence of ingesting a carbohydrate-electrolyte beverage during 4 hours of recovery on subsequent endurance capacity. *International Journal of Sport Nutrition* 5: 285–299.

Febbraio, M.A., et al. 1996. Carbohydrate feedings before prolonged exercise: Effect of glycemic index on muscle glycogenolysis and exercise performance. *Journal of Applied Physiology* 81(3): 1115–1120.

Fiala, K.A. 2004. Rehydration with a caffeinated beverage during the nonexercise periods of 3 consecutive days of 2-a-day practices. *International Journal of Nutrition and Exercise Metabolism* 14(4): 419–429.

Foster-Powell, K., and J. Brand-Miller. 1995. International tables of glycemic index. *American Journal of Clinical Nutrition* 62 (supplement): 871–893.

Gleeson, M., et al. 2004. Exercise, nutrition, and immune function. *Journal of Sports Sciences* 22(8): 115–125.

Graham, T., and L. Spriet. 1996. Caffeine and exercise performance. *Gatorade Sports Science Exchange* 9(1).

Grandjean, A.C., et al. 2000. The effect of caffeinated, non-caffeinated, caloric and non-caloric beverages on hydration. *Journal of the American College of Nutrition* 19(5): 591–600.

Green, H., et al. 1992. Altitude acclimatization and energy metabolic adaptation in skeletal muscle during exercise. *Journal of Applied Physiology* 73 (6): 2701–2708.

Haff, GG, et al. 2000. Carbohydrate supplementation attenuates muscle glycogen loss during acute bouts of resistance exercise. *International Journal of Sport Nutrition and Exercise Metabolism* 10(3): 326–339.

Havemann, L., et al. 2006. Fat adaptation followed by carbohydrate-loading compromises high-intensity sprint performance. *Journal of Applied Physiology* 100(1): 194–202.

Hellsetn-Westing, Y., et al. 1993. The effect of high-intensity training on purine metabolism in man. *Acta Physiologica Scandinavica* 149: 405–412.

Ivy, J.L., et al. 1988. Muscle glycogen storage after different amounts of carbohydrate ingestion. *Journal of Applied Physiology* 64(5): 2018–2023.

Ivy, J.L., et al. 1988. Muscle glycogen synthesis after exercise: Effect of time of carbohydrate ingestion. *Journal of Applied Physiology* 64(4): 1480–1485.

James, A.P., et al. 1999. Muscle glycogen supercompensation: Absence of gender-related differences. *European Journal of Applied Physiology* 85(6): 533-538.

Jentjens, R.L.P., et al. 2004. High oxidation rates from combined carbohydrates ingested during exercise. Medicine and Science in Sports and Exercise 36(9): 1551–1558.

Jentjens, R.L.P., et al. 2004. Oxidation of combined ingestion of glucose and fructose during exercise. Journal of Applied Physiology 96(4): 1277–1284.

Jeukendrup, A., et al. 1997. Carbohydrate-electrolyte feedings improve 1 hour time trial cycling performance. International Journal of Sports Medicine 18(2): 125–129.

Kang, J., et al. 1995. Effect of carbohydrate ingestion subsequent to carbohydrate supercompensation on endurance performance. *International Journal of Sport Nutrition* 5: 329–343.

Kenney, W.L. 2004. Dietary water and sodium requirements for active adults. *Gatorade Sports Science Institute: Sports Science Exchange* 17(1): 1–6.

Kimber, N.E., et al. 2002. Energy balance during an Ironman triathlon in male and female triathletes. *International Journal of Sport Nutrition and Exercise Metabolism* 12: 47–62.

King, D., et al. 1999. Effect of oral androstenedione on serum testosterone and adaptation to resistance training in young men. *Journal of the American Medical Association* 281(21): 2020–2028.

Kirwan, J.P., et al. 1988. Carbohydrate balance in competitive runners during successive days of intense training. *Journal of Applied Physiology* 65(6): 2601–2606.

Kovacs, E.M.R., et al. 2002. Effect of high and low fluid intake on post-exercise rehydration. *International Journal of Sport Nutrition and Exercise Metabolism* 12: 14–23.

Kreider, R., et al. 1998. Creatine supplement: Analysis of ergogenic value, medical safety, and concerns. *Journal of Exercise Physiology online* 1(1): 1–11.

Lambert, E., et al. 2001. High-fat diet versus habitual diet prior to carbohydrate loading: Effects on exercise metabolism and cycling performance. *International Journal of Sport Nutrition and Exercise Metabolism* 11: 209–225.

Lemon, P., et al. 1992. Protein requirements and muscle mass/strength changes during intensive training in novice bodybuilders. *Journal of Applied Physiology* 73(2): 767–775.

Lemon, P., et al. 1995. Do athletes need more dietary protein and amino acids? *International Journal of Sport Nutrition* 5: S39–61.

Loucks, A.B., and J.R. Thuma. 2003. Luteinizin hormone pulsatility is disrupted at a threshold of energy availability in regularly menstruating women. *Journal Clinical Endocrinology and Metabolism* 88(1): 297–311.

Macdermid, P.W., and S.R. Stannard. 2006. A whey supplemented high protein diet versus a high carbohydrate diet: Effects on endurance cycling performance. *International Journal of Sport Nutrition and Exercise Metabolism* 16(1): 65–77.

Madsen, K., et al. 1996. Effects of glucose, glucose plus branched-chain amino acids, or placebo on bike performance over 100 km. *Journal of Applied Physiology* 81(6): 2644–2650.

Manore, M.M. 2002. Dietary recommendations and athletic menstrual dysfunction. *Sports Medicine* 32(14): 887–901.

Mason, W., et al. 1993. Carbohydrate ingestion during exercise: Liquid versus solid feedings. *Medicine and Science in Sport and Exercise* 25: 966–969.

McConnell, G., et al. 1996. Effect of timing of carbohydrate ingestion during exercise performance. *Medicine and Science in Sport and Exercise* 28: 1300–1304.

Millard-Stafford, M., et al. 1992. Carbohydrate-electrolyte replacement improves distance running performance in the heat. *Medicine and Science in Sports and Exercise* 24: 940–943.

Millard-Stafford, M., et al. 2005. Recovery from run training: Efficacy of a carbohydrate-protein beverage? *International Journal of Sport Nutrition and Exercise Metabolism* 15(6): 610–624.

Miller, S.L., et al. 2003. Independent and combined effects of amino acids and glucose after resistance training. *Medicine and Science in Sports and Exercise* 35(3): 449–455.

Nicholas, C.W., et al. 1997. Carbohydrate intake and recovery of intermittent running capacity. *International Journal of Sport Nutrition* 7(4): 251–260.

Nissen, S., et al. 1996. Effect of leucine metabolite B-hydroxy-B-methylbutarate on muscle metabolism during resistance training exercise. *Journal of Applied Physiology* 81(5): 2095–2104.

Parkin, J., et al. 1997. Muscle glycogen storage following prolonged exercise: Effect of timing of ingestion of high glycemic index food. *Medicine and Science in Sports and Exercise* 29(2): 220–224.

Pascoe, D., and L. Gladden. 1996. Muscle glycogen resynthesis after short term, high intensity exercise, and resistance exercise. *Sports Medicine* 21(2): 98–118.

Paul, D.R., et al. 2001. Carbohydrate-loading during the follicular phase of the menstrual cycle: Effect on muscle glycogen and exercise performance. *International Journal of Sport Nutrition and Exercise Metabolism* 11(4): 430–441.

Peters, E., et al. 1993. Vitamin C supplementation reduces the incidence of postrace symptoms of upper-respiratory-tract infection in ultramarathon runners. *American Journal of Clinical Nutrition* 57(2): 170–174.

Pizza, F., et al. 1995. A carbohydrate loading regimen improves high intensity, short duration exercise performance. *International Journal of Sport Nutrition* 5: 110–116.

Reed, M.J., et al. 1989. Muscle glycogen storage postexercise: Effect of mode of carbohydrate administration. *Journal of Applied Physiology* 66(2): 720–726.

Roy, B., and M. Tarnopolsky, et al. 1998. Influence of differing macronutrient intakes on muscle glycogen resynthesis after resistance exercise. *Journal of Applied Physiology* 84(3): 890–896.

Roy, R., et al. 1997. Effect of glucose supplement timing on protein metabolism after resistance training. *Journal of Applied Physiology* 82(6): 1882–1888.

Sawka, M.N., et al. 2005. Human Water Needs. *Nutrition Reviews* 63(6): S30–S39.

Sherman, W.M., et al. 1989. Effects of 4 hour preexercise carbohydrate feedings on cycling performance. *Medicine and Science in Sports and Exercise* 21(5): 598–604.

Sherman, W.M., et al. 1991. Carbohydrate feedings 1 hour before exercise improves cycling performance. *American Journal of Clinical Nutrition* 54(5): 866–870.

Shirreffs, S., et al. 1996. Post-exercise rehydration in man: Effect of volume consumed and drink sodium content. *Medicine and Science in Sports and Exercise* 28(10): 1260–1271.

Simonsen, J.C., et al. 1991. Dietary carbohydrate, muscle glycogen, and power output during rowing training. *Journal of Applied Physiology* 70(4): 1500–1505.

Slater, G. et al. 2001. B-hydroxy-B-methylbutarate (HMB) supplementation does not affect changes in strength and body composition during resistance training in trained men. *International Journal of Sport Nutrition and Exercise Metabolism* 11(3): 384–396.

Slater, G.J., et al. 2006. Preparation of former heavyweight oarsmen to compete as lightweight rowers over 16 weeks: Three case studies. *International Journal of Sport Nutrition and Exercise Metabolism* 16(1): 108–121.

Smith, J.S., et al. 2002. The effect of pre-exercise glucose ingestion on performance during prolonged swimming. *International Journal of Sport Nutrition and Exercise Metabolism* 12(2): 136–144.

Stanko, R., et al. 1990. Enhanced leg exercise endurance with a high-carbohydrate diet and dihydroxyacetone and pyruvate. *Journal of Applied Physiology* 68(5): 1651–1656.

Stanko, R. et al. 1990. Enhancement of arm exercise endurance capacity with dihydroxyacetone and pyruvate. *Journal of Applied Physiology* 68(1): 119–124.

Tarnolpolsky, Mark, ed. 1999. *Gender Differences in Metabolism*. Boca Raton, FL: CRC Press.

Tarnopolsky, M.A., et al. 2001. Gender differences in carbohydrate loading are related to energy intake. *Journal of Applied Physiology* 91(1): 225–230.

Tarnopolsky, M.A. 1997. Postexercise protein-carbohydrate and carbohydrate supplements increase muscle glycogen in men and women. *Journal of Applied Physiology* 83(6): 1877.

Thompson, D., et al. 2001. Prolonged vitamin C supplementation and recovery from demanding exercise. *International Journal of Sport Nutrition and Exercise Metabolism* 11: 466–481.

Thompson, J., et al. 1996. Effects of diet and diet-plus-exercise programs on resting metabolic rate: A meta-analysis. *International Journal of Sport Nutrition* 6: 41–61.

Tipton, K.D., R.R. Wolfe, 2004. Protein and amino acids for athletes. *Journal of Sports Science* 22(1): 65–79.

Volek, J., and W. Kramer. 1996. Creatine supplementation: Its effect on human and muscular performance and body composition. *National Strength and Conditioning Association, Journal of Strength and Conditioning Research* 10(3): 200–210.

Walker, L., et al. 1997. Effect of chromium picolinate on body composition and muscular performance in collegiate wrestlers. *Medicine and Science in Sports and Exercise* 29(5): S278.

Wojcik, J.R., et al. 2001. Comparison of carbohydrate and milk-based beverages on muscle damage and glycogen following exercise. *International Journal of Sport Nutrition and Exercise Metabolism* 11(4): 406–419.

Yaspelkis, B., et al. 1993. Carbohydrate supplementation spares muscle glycogen during variable-intensity exercise. *Journal of Applied Physiology* 75(4): 1477–1485.

Index

Page numbers in *italics* denote tables.

About the Author

Monique Ryan, MS, RD, LDN, is a nationally recognized nutritionist who has been practicing since 1984. She is founder of Personal Nutrition Designs, a nutrition consulting company based in the Chicago area. Started in 1992, Personal Nutrition Designs provides nutrition programs for diverse groups of people with an emphasis on long-term follow-up and support programming. Monique has developed thousands of nutrition plans for clients in the areas of sports nutrition, weight management, women's health, eating disorder recovery, various medical and health concerns, and disease prevention and wellness. She provides her clients with practical, cutting-edge nutrition information based on current scientific research.

In addition to her work with top age-group endurance sport competitors, Monique was a member of the Performance Enhancement Team for USA Triathlon, USA Cycling (Women's Road Team), and Synchro Swimming USA up to the 2004 Athens Olympic Games. She works with the Timex Multisport Team, consults with the Chicago Fire Soccer Team, and was the nutritionist for the Saturn Cycling Team for the 1994 to 2000 racing seasons. She has also consulted with many professional endurance triathletes, the Volvo-Cannondale Mountain Bike, Rollerblade Racing, and the Trek-Volkswagen and Gary Fisher Mountain Bike Teams. Monique has lectured extensively on sports nutrition to coaches, trainers, and amateur athletes who train at all levels. For several months in 2000, Monique was at the Australian Institute of Sport in Canberra, Australia, one of the world's top training and physiology and sport nutrition research centers. She has presented across the U.S., Canada, Brazil, and Australia. Monique is quoted frequently in sports nutrition articles, and her comments have appeared in the *Chicago Tribune, New York Times, Chicago Sun-Times, Runner's World, Fitness, Men's Journal, Men's Health, Outside,* and *Oxygen,* among other publications.

Monique is a prolific nutrition writer and is author of *Performance Nutrition for Winter Sports* and *Performance Nutrition for Team Sports.* She is the author of over 175 published articles. She has written regularly for *VeloNews* since 1991, for *Inside Triathlon* since 1994, and is a regular contributor to *Outside.* She has also contributed to *Her Sports, Triathlete,* and *Women's Sports & Fitness.* She has appeared on CLTV, FOX TV, and the WGN, ABC, and CBS news. She has a Bachelor of Science degree in Nutrition and Dietetics and a Master of Science degree in Nutrition, and she is an Amercian College of Sports Medicine Health Fitness Instructor. Monique participates in the sports of cycling, running, and snowshoeing.